Marijuana Horticulture Fundamentals

A Comprehensive Guide to Cannabis Cultivation and Hashish Production

Greg:
Thank you for publishing a great magazine.

Kenneth Morrow

By K of Trichome Technologies

GREEN CANDY PRESS

Marijuana Horticultural Fundamentals
A Comprehensive Guide to Cannabis Cultivation and Hashish Production
by K of Trichome Technologies

Green Candy Press
San Francisco, CA
www.greencandypress.com

Cover Photo: Original Amnesia Autoflowering by Dinafem Seeds, dinafem.org
Photography: Andre Grossman, AsturJaya, Better, Bubbleman, Cannanetics, David Strange, Dinafem Seeds, Dr. Dog and Blackra1n, Dru West, Ed Borg, Franc, Freebie, General Hydro, Hanna Bliss, Jasmin, Jeff Goldberg, K, Kangativa, Krane, Lochfoot, Mandala Seeds, MedicinalAlchemy.com, Mel Frank, MG Imaging, MoD, Pepper Design, Samson Daniels, Swiss Hortycolture, Todd McCormick, Trichome Technologies, Weado.

Trichome Tech poster illustrations by Chris Shaw www.chrisshawstudio.com

Printed in China by Oceanic Graphic International
Massively distributed by P.G.W.

This book contains information about illegal substances, specifically the plant Cannabis Sativa and its derivative products. Green Candy Press would like to emphasize that cannabis is a controlled substance in North America and throughout much of the world. As such, the use and cultivation of cannabis can carry heavy penalties that may threaten an individual's liberty and livelihood.

The aim of the Publisher is to educate and entertain. Whatever the Publisher's view on the validity of current legislation, we do not in any way condone the use of prohibited substances.

ISBN 978-1-937866-34-1

Morrow, Kenneth, author.
    Marijuana horticulture fundamentals : a comprehensive
guide to cannabis cultivation and hashish production /
by Kenneth Morrow.
    pages cm
    Includes index.
    ISBN 978-1-937866-34-1

1. Cannabis. 2. Marijuana.   I. Title.

SB295.C35M67 2016   633.7'9
                    QBI15-600196

Contents

CONTENTS

CONTENTS

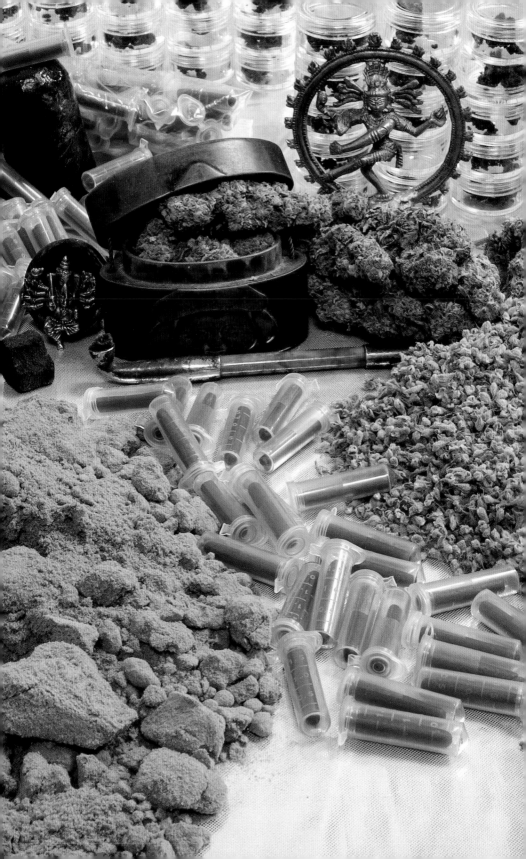

Foreword

Zorro

It was Denis Peron who once told me, "There is no such thing as the recreational use of marijuana. It's all medicinal." He was right!

It is one of the most profound statements I've heard in my thirty-eight years as a cannabis smoker. Whether you use it to alleviate stress or boredom, to relax after a hard day's work, or to alleviate the symptoms of multiple sclerosis, you are using it as a medicine. Recreational drugs are those such as LSD, MDMA, and the like: drugs that are taken to party with. Not that I would know much about them, as I left that crazy lifestyle behind in my teens. I am fifty-two years old now, and like to think of myself as being somewhat wiser than I was in those days.

Throughout the years, I've heard a lot of garbage governmental propaganda about the dangers of marijuana. Way back, when I was in grade school, perhaps eight or nine years old, I was made to sit in an auditorium with my fellow classmates and was force-fed the film *Reefer Madness* as part of my educational curriculum! It only got worse from there.

Although I live in what I lovingly refer to as Sleepy Hollows, England, I have traveled the world seeking out and tasting the best hash in the world. I've been through the tribal areas of Pakistan, to Manali and Manala, to the mountains of Nepal, to the Rif Mountains of Morocco, to

◀ Isolated bracts on the right; kif on the left; jelly hash in the blue tubes; water hash in the clear containers; and a 100-year-old pipe.

Photo: Samson Daniels

West and South Africa. I've tasted the best from everywhere. I was even made an official Sadhu at a gathering of Sadhus on Shiva's birthday at the great Hindu temple of Pashupatinath, just outside of Kathmandu, Nepal. And I do it all for a living. That's my job! And how cool a job is that? All of my adventure travel, hash-smoking articles were published in England's *Red Eye Magazine*.

It was through these articles that I first met K from Trichome Technologies. He had stumbled on a copy of one of the mags and managed to get my number through the international cannabis grapevine. Kind of like an old boy's network. K and I became really good friends over the next twelve years and I managed to convince him to write some grow articles for *Red Eye*. As we knew each other so well, I personally worked hand in hand with Kenny on editing and laying out a whole series of the best grow articles that *Red Eye* ever printed.

I have met all of the greats in the cannabis world, including Sam the Skunk Man, Rob Connell Clarke, Jorge Cervantes, Mel Frank, and Soma, to name a few. K, with his expert knowledge of the cannabis plant, stands out among them all. How else would he have earned the "Best Grow Operation in the Twenty-Five Year History of *High Times*," otherwise?

I learned everything I know about growing from K, and I'm now pretty damn good at it, if I do say so myself. Unfortunately, I haven't mastered the art of not getting busted on a regular basis! "Codswallop to them all, if they can't take a joke," that's what I say.

I've been with K through every stage of the writing of this book, and I know that his heart and soul have gone into every page. If it teaches the reader anything near what I have learned from this true master of cannabis growing, then this book will change your life.

I opened this foreword with a profound quote, and I'll be damned if I'm not going to close with one too. I'd like to quote Steve Gaskin, an aging old hippie like myself, who founded a working commune called "The Farm" in Tennessee along with three hundred and twenty other San Francisco hippies in 1971. The Farm still flourishes today and is one of the most successful communes in the U.S. of A. Steve, while speaking at the *High Times* Cannabis Cup, said, referring to pot smoking, "If you find yourself confronted by people who don't understand your lifestyle, don't ram your lifestyle down their throats and flaunt your joints in their face, you'll win nothing through confrontation. If you really do want to win the war, just get them to like you for who you are."

—Zorro, *Red Eye Magazine*, UK

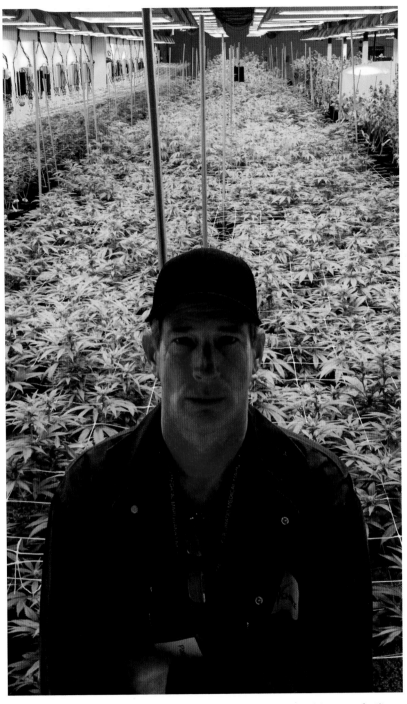

The author at work. K of Trichome Technologies in a cannabis grow facility.

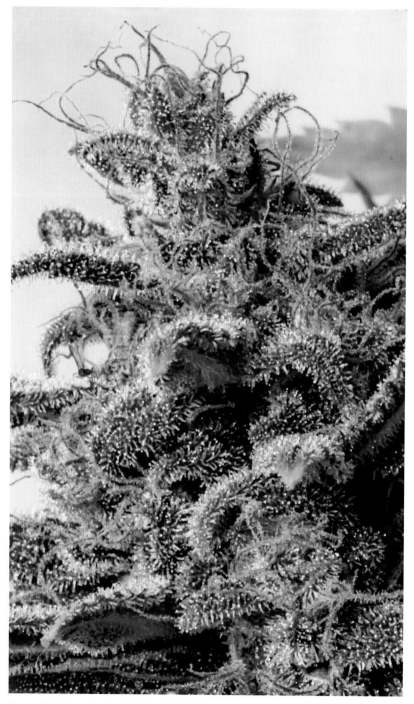

Photo: Mel Frank

Cannabis flower laden with trichomes.

Mel Frank

K, from Trichome Technologies, has long been known in the subculture of Northern California for his thorough professionalism and constant innovation in growing techniques. His determined research toward better understanding all aspects of marijuana growing, including increasing potency and yields, and breeding award-winning cultivars, has earned him high praise, admiration, and well-earned respect from his peers. With his very low public profile, he received little notice for devising a truly practical hashish-making technique for both the home and commercial gardener, first explained in *High Times*, April 2000. His refined approach became the basic procedure for both American and European hashish-makers.

Here, in his first book, K brings his experience and knowledge to the benefit of the greater marijuana-growing public. Hopefully, his guidance will long serve all of us into the time when our era of Reefer Madness is rightfully relegated to the designated dumpster for legislative lunacy, and marijuana and hemp consumption and growing will once again be legal as it was through our first 161 years as a free nation.

— Mel Frank, *Marijuana Grower's Guide Deluxe* and
Marijuana Grower's Insider's Guide

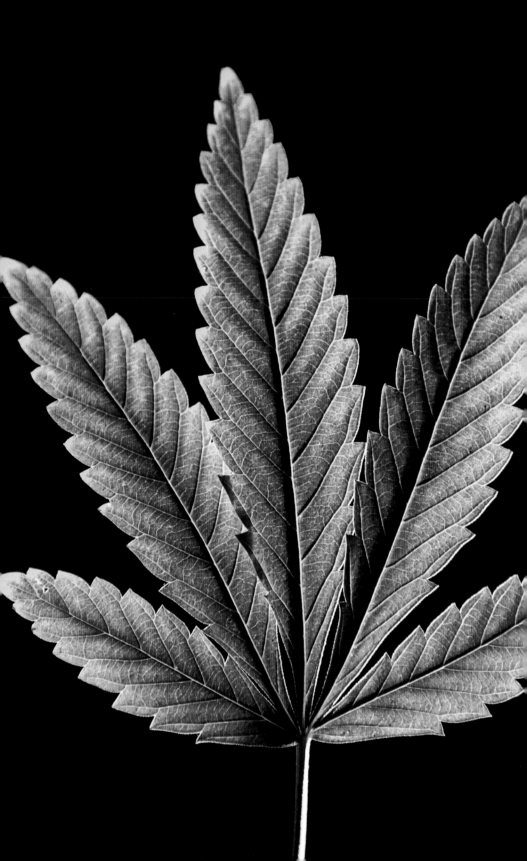

Introduction

The purpose of this book, as the title implies, is to teach you the fundamentals of growing medical-grade cannabis without making the process complicated—my aim is to simplify the procedures, step-by-step; elucidate on the methods needed to produce first-class medical-grade cannabis; and outline the creation and construction of a perfect growing environment from the very first attempt. That said, a basic familiarity with terms and systems is assumed. If you are ever mystified by a reference, please turn to the index of this book.

As long as you follow the instructions and stay within (and understand) the parameters stated, you will be guaranteed to produce a bountiful harvest, superior to anything you have ever grown. And, if this is your first time growing, this book enables you to simply produce incredible marijuana, without having to know exactly why you are doing what you are doing. There are already many books that explain the ins and outs of growing, down to the last detail (see bibliography), but my purpose is to provide only the essential information needed to get you growing successfully.

Growing cannabis has been my only vocation for over 30 years, and in this book I teach the basics: how to do it, when to do it, and so on. You get the benefit of all my years of research and information. After you are acquainted with the basics and understand the procedures,

◀ Some cannabis leaves turn golden at harvest the same as leaves on the trees do in the fall.

Photo: Mel Frank

you can proceed to the information and methods needed to successfully build and operate a medical marijuana supergarden, not to mention how to refine the variables and do it right the first time.

About the Author

K is the owner and president of Trichome Technologies, the grow op chosen in June 1999 as the Best Growroom in the 25-year history of *High Times*. Between

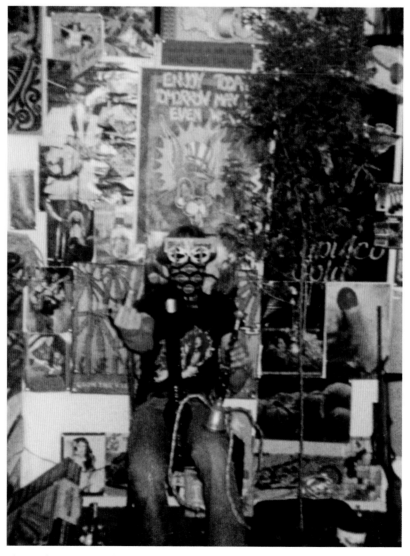

Photos: K

The author at 13, with a Hydropot hydroponic system.

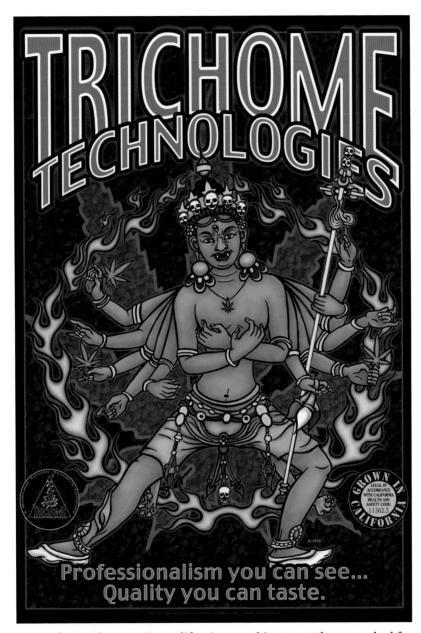

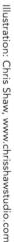

1997 and 2000, he won nine California Cannabis Cups. K has consulted for many of the top activists, doctors, scientists, authors, photographers, publishers, and researchers in the medical marijuana community, and was featured on *60 Minutes* in 1996, the same year he was interviewed by CNN.

The owner of a seed company that holds 200 proprietary cultivars (strains

A Plethora of Unique, Proprietary Genetics

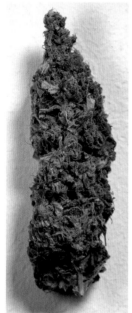 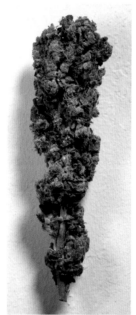 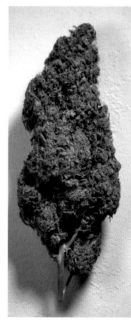

Juicy Fruit, THC 26.2%.   G-13, THC 27.2%.   MIRV, THC 26.8%.

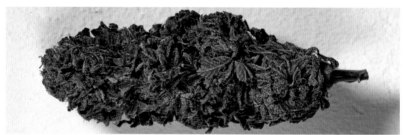

Purple Kush / Ultra Violet, THC 16.1%.

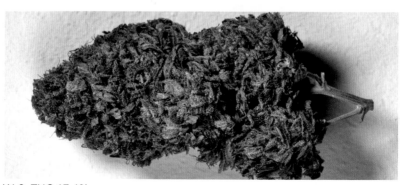

Photos: K

W-2, THC 17.6%.

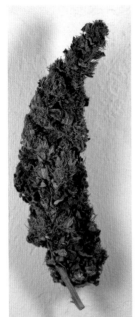
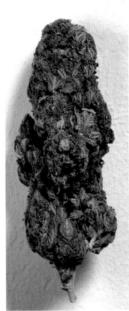
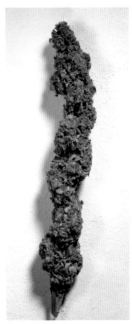

Kryptonite, THC 16.9%.

B1 (Sweet One), THC 13.6%.

NLx6, THC 22.5%.

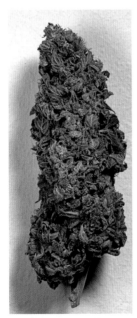
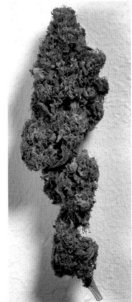
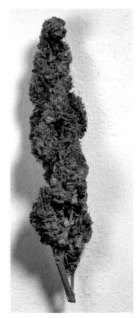

Washington, THC 22.6%.

Blueberry, THC 22%.

Yoshi, THC 11.8%.

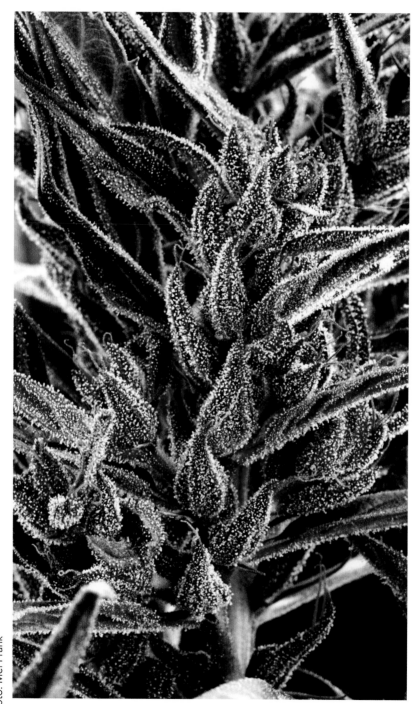

Photo: Mel Frank

The plethora of color in cannabis can range from green to purple.

/ varietals) of cannabis, K has logged thousands of hours of production and genetic cultivar research, and bred and stabilized genetic cultivars that are now world famous. His work has been featured in *High Times* over 50 times in 15 years. He has over 30 years of cannabis research, cultivation, and breeding experience. He has also been a contributing writer for *Red Eye Express* (England) and a photo contributor for *Burst High* (Japan).

Acknowledgements

I would like to thank Connie Parsons for always loving, supporting, and being there for me; Mom and Sonny, R.I.P., for always loving, supporting, and being there for me; Thadra and Family; Grandpa Willis, R.I.P.; Grandma Dalores; and Dad.

My gratitude is also owed to: Jeff Goldberg, Freebie / MG Imaging, R.I.P.; Steve A.; Thomas Alexander at *Sinsemilla Tips*; Andrew; Andy and Liz McBeth; Jack Lloyd; Mike B.; Patrick B.; B-Legit; Etienne Fontan; The Berkeley Patients' Group; Debby Goldsberry; Todd McCormick; Jeffy G; Gloria, Max, and Cavalera Tribe; Winslow / Abe; Jorge Cervantes; Robert Connell Clarke; D.P. Watson; Charlie V; Liana Held and Liana Ltd.; Dye / Zonfrellow / Parsons Families; Brian E.; Felix; Michael Franti; Freebie / MethodSeven; Dale Gieringer; Kenneth Gary Goodson, A.K.A. Thomas King Forçade; MEL FRANK; Ben Hill; Tommy H.; Dr. Cal C. Herman; Michael Horowitz; Sir Albert Howard; Jeff and Dale Jones; George Jung; Michael Kennedy; Baron Justus von Liebig; Frank H. Lucido, M.D.; Dr. Todd Mikuriya, R.I.P.; Naboru; Nick and Zorro at *Red Eye Magazine*; Stephen P.; Ed and Jane Rosenthal; Denis Peron; La Roy S.; R. Dope Connoisseur; Tony Serra; Ray Schrutz; C. Zadik Shapiro; Chris and Alex Shaw; Alexander Sasha Shulgin, R.I.P.; Ann Shulgin and Paul Daley of the Alexander Shulgin Research Institute; Chris Simunek; Danny Danko; Bobby Black; Nico Escondido; Craig Coffey; and everyone at *High Times Magazine*.

The following individuals inspired me during my years of growing and while writing this book: Luther Burbank, George Washington Carver, Galileo Galilei, Nelson Mandela, Gregor Mendel, and Leonardo da Vinci.

The following authors' classics of cannabis literature have proved invaluable:

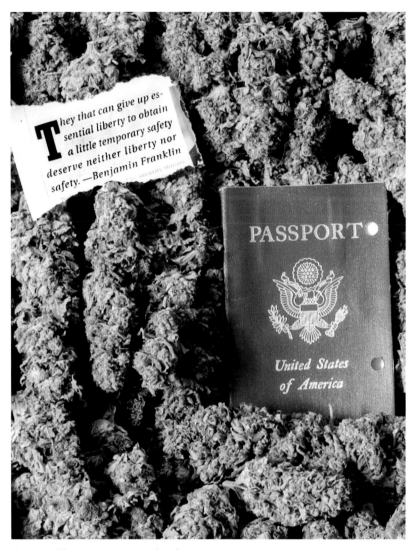

They that can give up essential liberty to obtain a little temporary safety deserve neither liberty nor safety. —Benjamin Franklin

PASSPORT

United States of America

Give me liberty or give me death.

Mel Frank's *Marijuana Growers Guide*; Jorge Cervantes's *Marijuana Horticulture: The Indoor / Outdoor Medical Grower's Bible*; Nick and Zorro's (from *Red Eye*) work; J.M. McPartland, R.C. Clarke, and D.P. Watson's *Hemp Diseases and Pests: Management and Biological Control*; Etienne De Meijer's *Diversity in Cannabis*; Jim Richardson and Arik Woods's *Sinsemilla: Marijuana Flowers*; Robert Connell Clarke's *Hashish* and *Marijuana Botany*; Suomi La Valle's *Hashish*; and Ed Rosenthal's *Marijuana Grower's Handbook*.

Photo: K

Quotes

Narcotics have been systematically scapegoated and demonized. The idea that anyone can use drugs and escape a horrible fate is anathema to these idiots. I predict in the near future right wingers will use drug hysteria as a pretext to set up an international police apparatus.

—William S. Burroughs in *Drugstore Cowboy*

Excellence is attained by those who care more than others think is wise, who risk more than others think is safe, and who dream more than others think is practical.

—Bud Greenspan

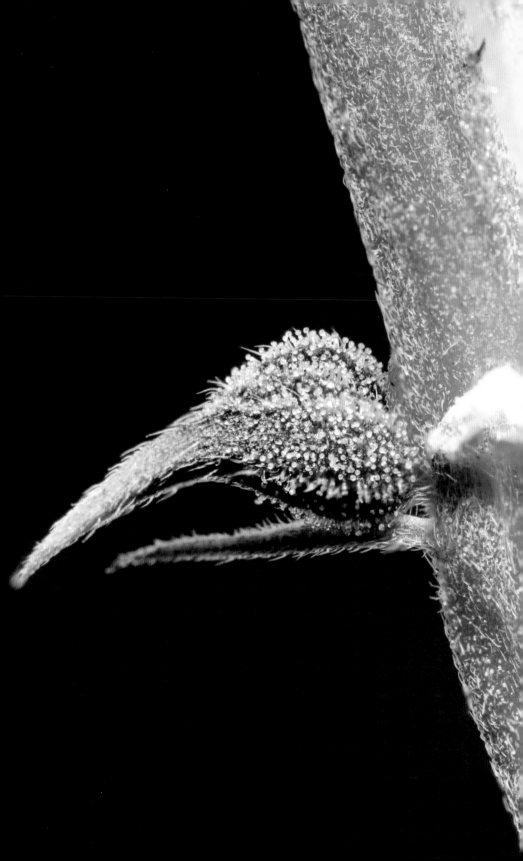

Marijuana Terminology

by Mel Frank

Over the years, authors have used a multitude of names to describe the same parts of the marijuana plant. This inconsistency has led to some confusion, and authors' incorrect use of botanical terms has further muddied discussions. Most of the confusion centers on female flowers, which are the focus of most marijuana growing discussions. In this book, the author, K from Trichome Technologies, strived to be accurate and botanically correct when naming specific plant parts. I hope his effort will encourage consistent use of correct terminology.

Botanists and horticulturalists, speaking generally, correctly use the term *bud* to mean any newly emerging plant part as it first appears as no more than a nub or protuberance, whether it will become a branch, flower, or leaf. However, for those entirely new to marijuana discussions, the term *bud* commonly refers to a *distinct cluster of female marijuana flowers*. This is so universally ingrained in marijuana usage by consumers and growers alike that *bud* is used here also. Botanically, marijuana buds are *racemes*.

Female flowers usually form in pairs that are so tightly bunched together with succeeding pairs that such pairing is apparent only in "running" buds most commonly seen in Southeast Asian cultivars. Much more typically, female flowers grow closely together, forming compact,

◀ Purple and green bracts.

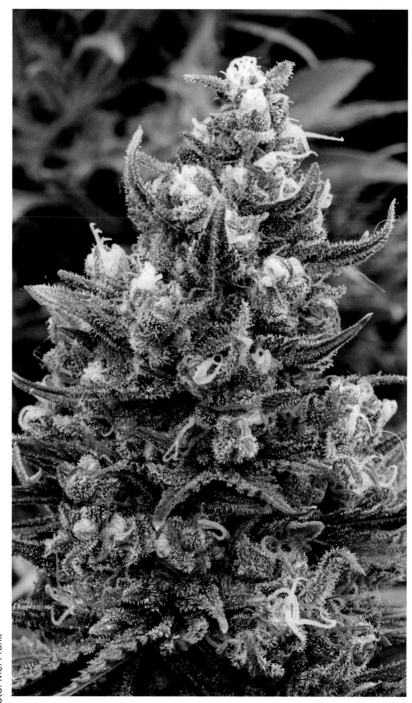

Photo: Mel Frank

Female flowers growing together, forming a compact cluster.

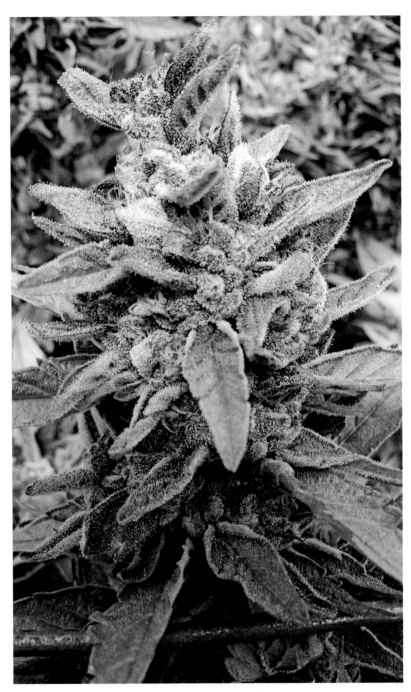

As the lifecycle of the plant ends, many colors can appear, such as purple bracts and sometimes even colored stigmata, i.e. purple and pink/red.

Photo: K

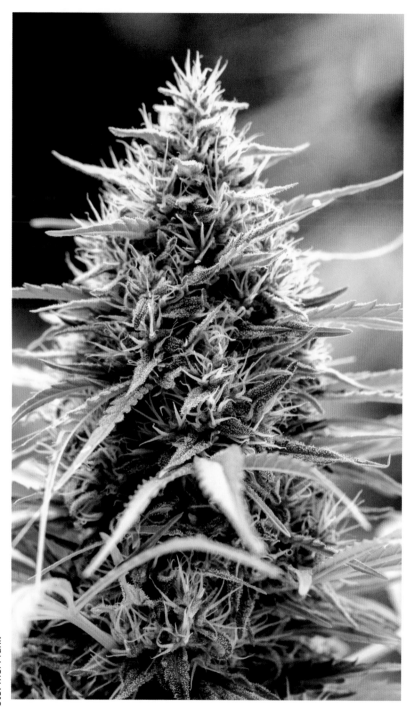

Photo: Mel Frank

This MK Ultra x Sensi Star has a dense cola.

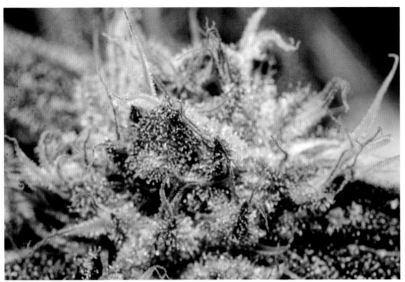

More so than the stigma, the ripeness of the resin gland ultimately determines when to harvest.

egg-shaped or teardrop-shaped clusters, typically about one to two inches long, consisting of dozens of densely packed individual flowers. The oldest flowers are found at the bud's base and the youngest at the top.

Cola, another commonly used term for female flower clusters, more often refers to an aggregate of buds that, having formed so closely together, looks like a single, very large bud. Colas form at the ends of stems and branches and can be well over a foot long. *Foxtail* is another name for cola, but the term is rarely used these days except by those whose history with marijuana goes back to the 1960s or 70s.

Those general terms—bud, cola, foxtail—are easy enough and universally accepted, but when discussing specific plant parts with botanical terms, confusion reigns. Foremost is the incorrect use of either *calyx* or *false calyx*. Growers read or hear about swollen calyxes being a sign of maturity and an indication of readiness for harvesting. What are incorrectly called calyxes or false calyxes are correctly identified as *bracts*.

Cannabis flowers do have a calyx, which few growers have ever recognized since it is barely perceptible without a microscope. The cannabis calyx is one part of the *perianth*, a nearly transparent, delicate tissue that partially encloses the ovule (prospective seed). Each female flower has a single ovule enclosed

Photo: Samson Daniels

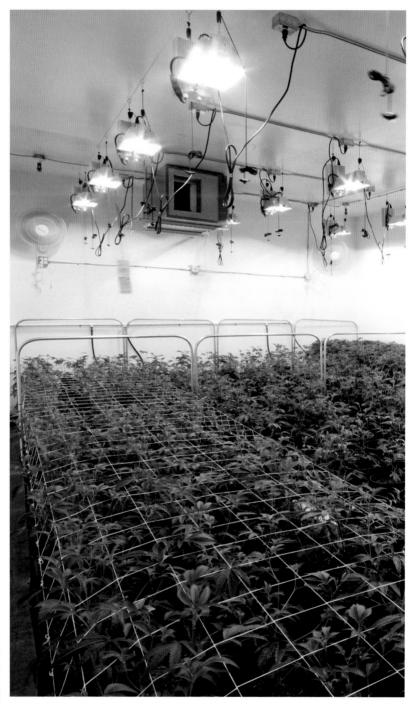

Photo: Mel Frank

A clean, well-organized cannabis grow operation in the vegetative stage.

in its perianth, which is encapsulated by bracteoles, which are covered by a whorl of bracts. The bracts and bracteoles are small, modified leaves that enclose and protect the seed in what some growers refer to as the seed *pod*. The bracts, with their dense covering of large resin glands, contain the highest concentration of THC of any plant part. Bracts make up most of the substance and weight of quality marijuana buds.

By definition, a perianth consists of a corolla and a calyx. In more familiar showy flowers, the corolla is the brightly colored petals we generally appreciate when looking at flowers, and the calyx is the smaller green cup (sepals) at the flower's base. Bright showy colors, large flower sizes, and enticing fragrances evolved to attract insects such as bees and flies, or animals such as birds and bats to collect and transfer pollen to other flowers. Cannabis flowers are not brightly colored, large, or enticingly fragrant (at least to most non-humans); marijuana plants are wind-pollinated with no need to attract insects or animals to carry the males' pollen to female flowers.

The marijuana perianth is only about six cells thick, so to distinguish calyx cells from corolla cells is best left to botanists with high-powered microscopes. This book uses the correct term, bracts, for the green or purple, resin-gland studded, specialized "leaves" encasing each female flower—not pod, not calyx, and certainly not false calyx.

Each female marijuana flower has two stigmas that protrude through the bracts from a single ovule; they are "fuzzy" (hirsute), about $\frac{1}{4}$ to $\frac{1}{2}$-inch long, usually white, but sometimes yellowish, or pink to red and, very rarely, lavender to purple. Stigmas (*stigmata* is another botanical plural) are the pollen catchers. Some authors identify stigmas as *pistils*, and this too is incorrect. The pistil is all of the reproductive female flower parts: two stigmas, a style (tube connecting stigma to ovule), and the ovule. Each flower then has only one pistil but two stigmas. The term is misused in many books and articles that describe a single cannabis flower as having two pistils.

If pollinated, the ovule of each female flower becomes a single fruit (an *achene*) holding a single seed. The perianth, which includes the calyx, tightly clasps the seed and often contains tannins, which give mature seeds their mottled or speckled coat. Between a thumb and finger you can rub the perianth off of seeds. A well-pollinated single bud develops dozens of seeds, a cola easily holds hundreds, and even a small, but thoroughly pollinated female can bear thousands of seeds.

Male Cannabis Flowers

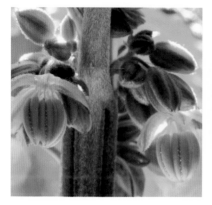

Male flowers.

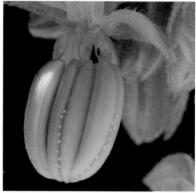

Male Skunk #1 flower.

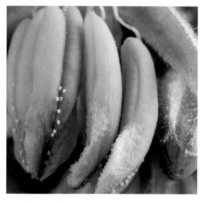

Anther pollen slits opening
magnified X5.

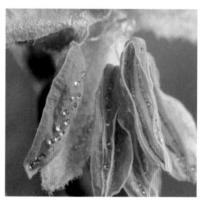

Anthers empty of pollen.

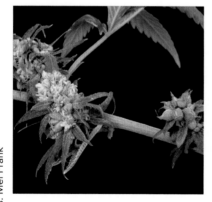

Forced selfing for feminized seeds
on a Grand Daddy Purple plant.

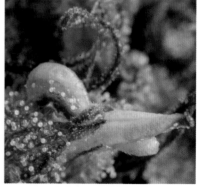

Rogue anthers in buds hold
feminized pollen.

Photos: Mel Frank

Female Cannabis Flowers

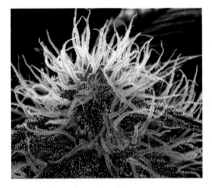

Stigmas on female plant.

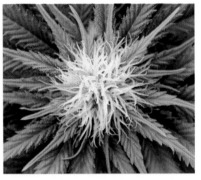

Stigmas on female flower seen from above.

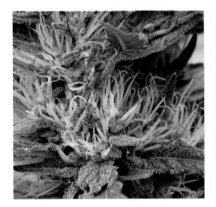

Stigmas beginning to dry out.

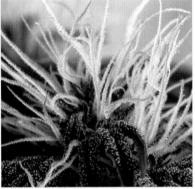

Pakistani plant's stigmas after 4 weeks of flowering.

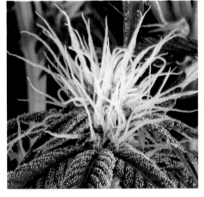

Stigmas can range from short to long. These are considered long stigmas.

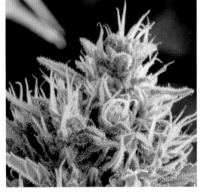

Darkening of the stigmas indicates the onset of maturity.

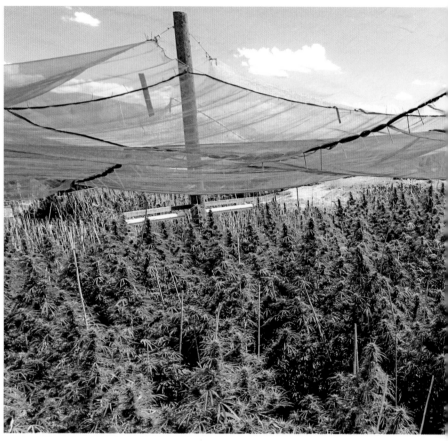

Cannabis being grown outdoors in Southern California by a collective.

The male (*staminate*) marijuana plant gets less attention, because once gender shows most gardeners remove all males to prevent pollination, so females (*pistillates*) will remain seedless (commonly called *sinsemilla* from the Spanish *sin semillas* meaning *without seeds*). Male flowers look more like familiar flowers than the female flowers do, and although they are only about ¼ to ½-inch long, thousands can develop on a large male plant. Most of the flowers develop in loose clusters (*cymes* or *cymose panicles*) or (very roughly) about ten flowers each, borne on tiny branches and their side (lateral) branches. Each male flower consists of five, usually white or greenish, but often tinged purple, *sepals* (sometimes identified as *tepals*) that non-botanists might describe as "petals" and five pendulous stamens that bear pollen in sacks called *anthers*. Anthers hang by a short, thin, threadlike *filament* and

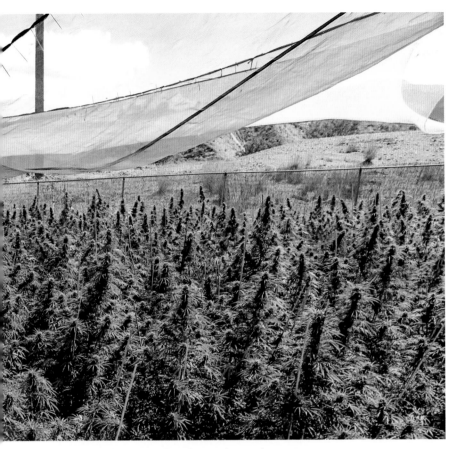

together, filament and anther make up the *stamen*. Once mature, two openings on opposite sides of each other open zipper-like, starting at their base, to slowly release their pollen into the wind, carrying it (hopefully) to stigmas. It has been estimated that the thousands of flowers on a single male can release more than 500 million pollen grains.

Unopened male flower clusters remind some growers of tiny grape clusters, and fresh anthers look like tiny bunches of bananas. Here male flowers are simply called male flowers or male flower clusters, and the pollen holders referred to as either stamens or anthers. Hopefully when writers and growers use botanical terms such as calyx, bract, stigma, pistil, anther, and stamen, they will use the terms correctly. The colloquial terms bud and colas are universally used to represent racemes, as pot and grass are used to represent marijuana, and for these, there is no impetus to change.

— Mel Frank

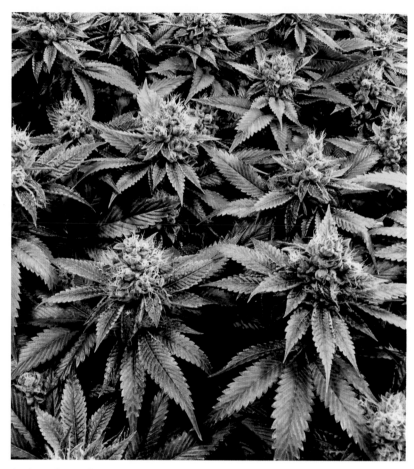

A view of a uniform canopy.

The Definition of "Strain"

The cannabis plant is very diverse and there are many variations. Many people refer to these variations as "strains" and "varieties." For the purpose of clarification and continuity, I will first define these terms, and then explain why the word "cultivar" has been chosen to be used throughout this book.

Strain: (Biology), variants of plants. This term accounts for variations, but not chemical diversity within species.

Variety: (Botany), see "Plant Variety" below. A taxonomic rank below that of species. (That being stated, variety is improper.)

Photo: Mel Frank

Plant Variety: (Botany), a taxonomic nomenclature rank in botany, below "subspecies" but above "subvariety" and "form." (An infraspecific rank, usually a cultivar or hybrid.) "Variety" is an informal, ambiguous, and vague substitute for cultivar or hybrid (Biology). (The term "variety" or "varietal" is improper nomenclature in that it best describes grapes and rice. "Varietal" is not even an official botany term.)

Varietal: for horticultural term, see "cultivar." "Varietal" is normally used to describe rice and grape varieties. It is the improper nomenclature for cannabis.

Cultivar: A cultivar is a plant or grouping of plants selected for desirable characteristics that can be maintained through propagation. Most cultivars have arisen in cultivation by careful breeding and selection for flower color and form, but a few are special selections from the wild. Similarly, the world's agricultural food crops are almost exclusively cultivars that have been selected for characteristics such as improved yield, flavor, and resistance to disease. Very few wild plants are now used as food sources. Cultivars form a major part of a broader grouping called "The Cultigen," which is defined as a plant whose origin or selection is primarily due to intentional human activity. (A cultivar is not the same as botanical variety, and there are differences in the rules for the formation and use of the names of botanical varieties and cultivars.)

All of that being said: for the purposes of continuity, this book will refer to genetic diversities as "cultivars."

For in depth explanations on these terms, as well as definitions of "chemotype," "chemovars," and much more, it is recommended that you read Robert Connell Clarke's book *Marijuana Botany*.

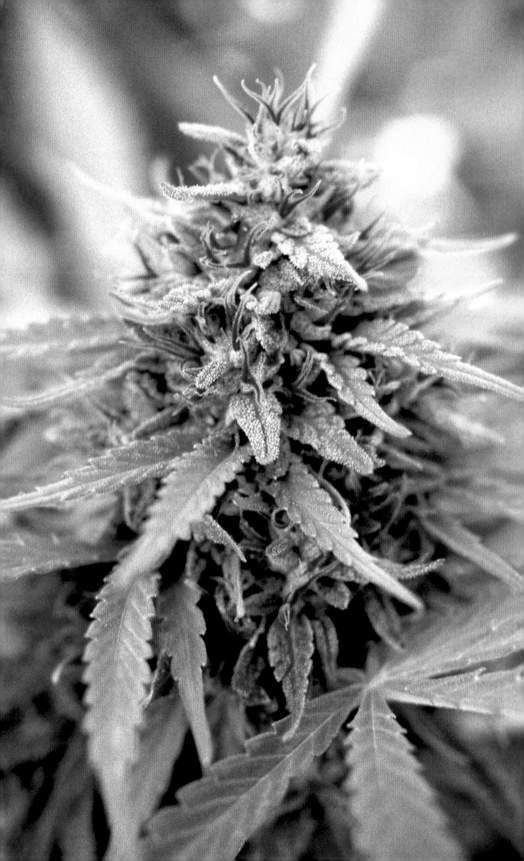

CHAPTER 1

Cannabis Basics and Gender

Cannabis is an annual plant. Defined as a plant that germinates, grows, reproduces, sows seed, and dies within 12 months, cannabis deposits its seeds to replicate its genetics. The next year's crop will continue the evolutionary process.

The needs of the cannabis plant are very basic! Light, air, water, nutrients, and soil / medium are the five main needs, and they must be balanced in proper proportions, adjusted to the correct levels, and scheduled to obtain optimum growth rates, results, and overall perfect conditions.

Inadequate attention to any of these details will result in very poor crop yield and quality, if not complete failure. Depending on the methods and techniques you choose, the life cycle of a cannabis plant can be as long or short as you want it to be. To a point, you are in control.

The cultivar (variety / strain) of plant you grow and methodology / techniques you use will dictate exactly how fast or slow your particular garden's plant life cycle is (e.g., cannabis indica finishes its life cycle much sooner than cannabis sativa). Also, some cultivars root

◀ This is Red Bud, an Original Afghani from 1981.

Photo: Mel Frank

1

Identifying Male and Female Cannabis Plants

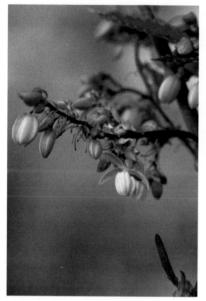

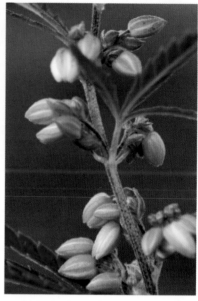

Pollen sacs on a male flower.

A closer look at anthers which will soon open and release their pollen.

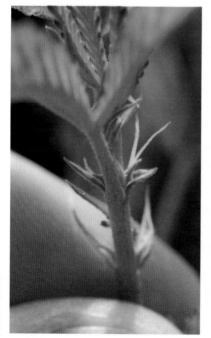

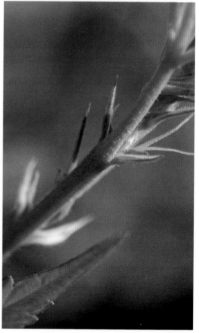

Female preflowers.

Young preflowers on a female plant.

faster than others and some must vegetate longer to produce perfect clone material. In proper conditions, mother plants can be kept indefinitely, ensuring a never-ending supply of clones.

Males

Male plants are used for breeding. They must be examined closely to determine whether or not they possess characteristics or traits that are desirable. For sinsemilla production, no males should be present in the flowering chambers—unless you are hoping to get seeds.

Females

Female plants are grown for their flowers, commonly referred to as buds, and the smaller surrounding leaves that have trichomes on them. Buds develop on the top of the plant and tips of the branches and continue downward, beginning at each internode. The bract is round, teardrop-shaped, and has two fuzzy hairs protruding from its tip. These are the stigmas, and their function is to capture pollen and facilitate pollination / fertilization to produce buds. The stigmas are also indicators of successful pollination when breeding and, to a very small degree, of determining pre-ripeness. Buds, obviously, are used for medicine—to be smoked, vaporized, or manufactured into baked goods and hashish.

Hermaphrodites

Hermaphrodites have both male and female characteristics, determined either by genetics or stress. Improper breeding practices can also produce hermaphrodites. Typically, a plant, male or female, will show hermaphroditic traits in later stages of flowering, and can cause pollination. Because of this, they should be separated or eliminated from your other plants. Environmental stress can also produce hermaphrodites—stress from irregular light cycles, light leaks, chemicals, excesses or absences of nutrients and fertilizers, or erratic / extreme temperatures.

Sinsemilla

"Sinsemilla" can literally be translated into "without seeds." To eliminate the possibilities of pollinating your female plants, there cannot be any males, hermaphrodites, or stray pollen in the flowering chambers. (You would want to include males in the chambers if you're intentionally pollinating for seed

Female, Male, and Hermaphrodite Plants

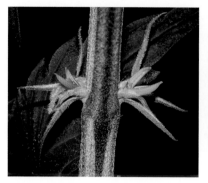

Female preflower with stamen.

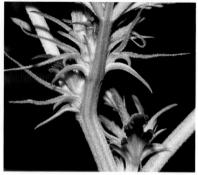

This is what the female preflower looks like.

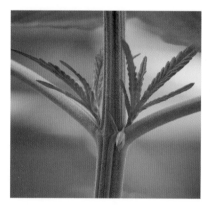

Identify the male by the little sac visible at the internodes.

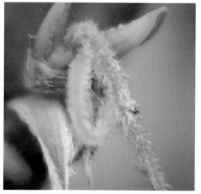

Macro shot of the preflower visible at the internode.

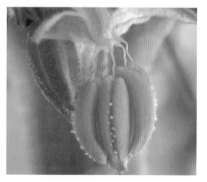

Closeup of a male plant's stamen. The anther / pollen sac is visible.

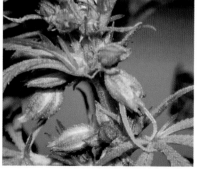

Plants can be forced to produce male flowers / pollen that will produce feminized seeds.

Photos: Jasmin

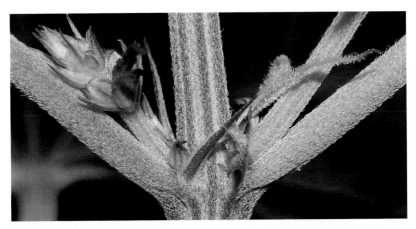

Female and male flowers are emerging from this hermaphroditic plant.

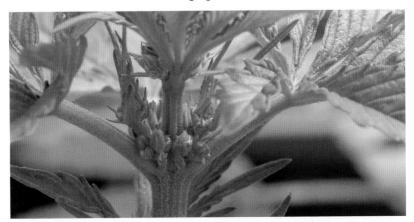

Young male plant. Identify these early if you don't want seeded bud.

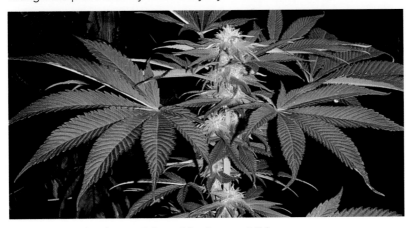

Maturing female plant with broad fan leaves visible.

production.) Seedless marijuana is more desirable simply because (from a purchaser's point of view) a bud that contains seeds weighs more than a bud without seeds, and gives you less bud per gram and thus less smokable product); also, seeded buds require extra preparation and de-seeding / cleaning before being consumed (i.e., smoked, vaporized, etc.). Simply put, seedless buds are better buds. From a market standpoint, seedless marijuana is worth more than seeded marijuana. As of the late seventies / early eighties, all marijuana considered "high grade" is seedless.

That said, it is possible for some cultivars to produce more available THC when seeded because of the increased surface area on the bract. The bracts are made larger by the developing seed. In most cultivars, larger bracts produce more trichomes or at least produce larger trichomes. Again, this only applies to some, not all, cultivars. All of this aside, the fact remains that seedless marijuana is more desirable to the consumer.

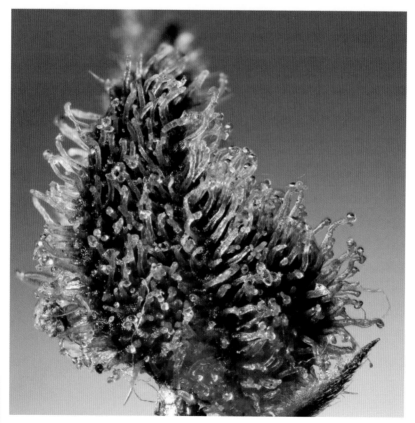

Photo: MoD

This bract is laden with trichomes.

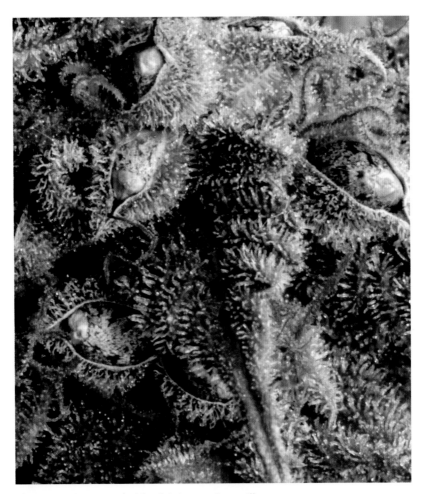

This is a mature seeded bud. It is not sinsemilla.

A Note on Calyx-to-Leaf Ratio

The female sinsemilla flower is comprised of small, trichome-laden leaves and bracts with stigmata protruding from their tips. The bract is commonly (and mistakenly) referred to as a calyx—hence the phrase "calyx-to-leaf ratio," a measurement of bracts / calyx to leaves. The bracts are covered with trichomes, more so than the surrounding leaves. In most cases, the higher the bract / leaf ratio is, the higher the THC levels of the bud are. For example, a 60/40 calyx (bract) to leaf ratio is better than a 30/70 ratio and will produce superior buds / flowers both in quality and quantity of overall flavor, strength, and THC levels. Many seed companies use these ratios when they advertise their strains.

Photo: Mel Frank

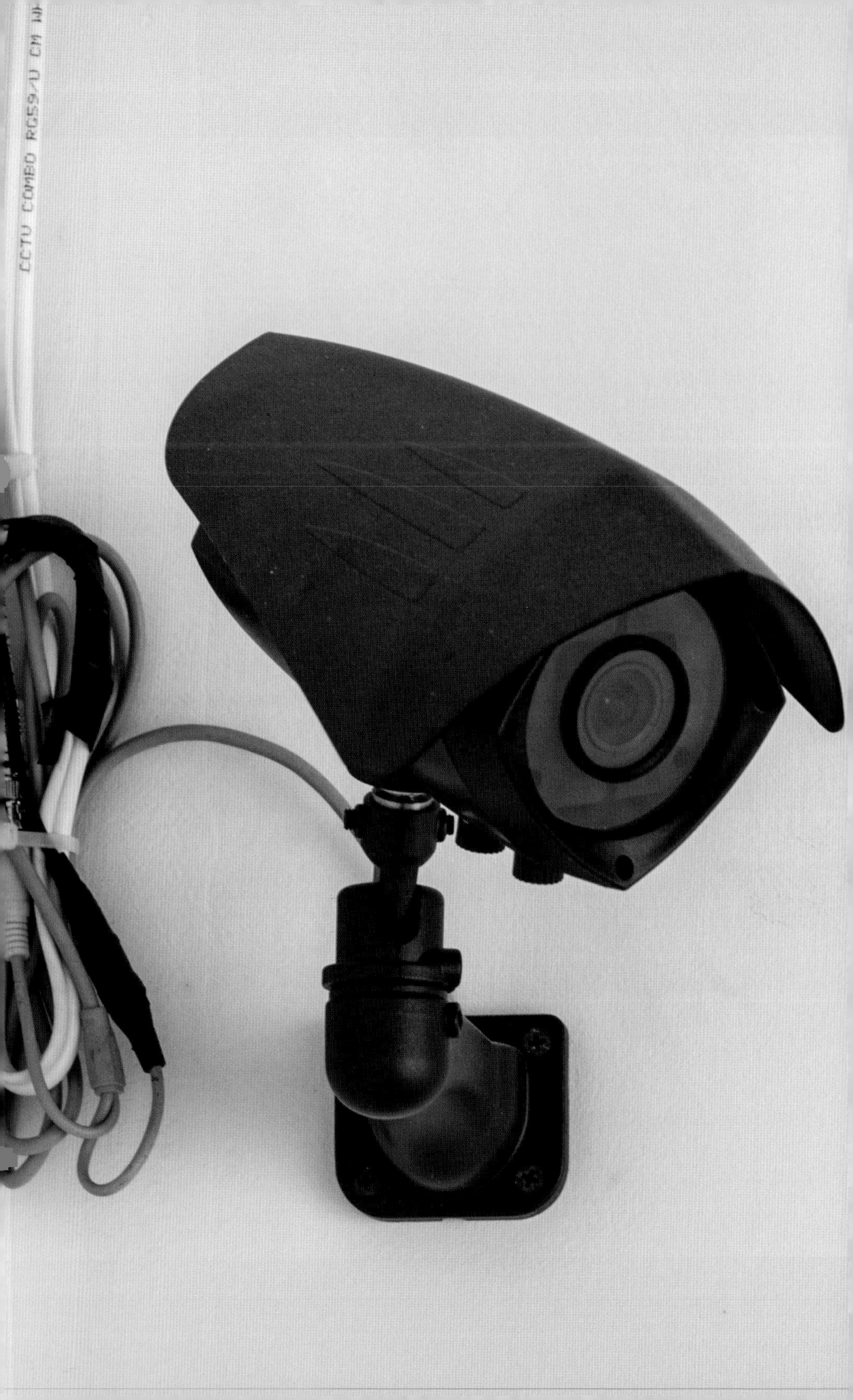
CCTV COMBO RG59/U CM

CHAPTER 2

Grow Security

Legalities

Some states in the USA have drug-free zone laws dictating severe penalties for persons possessing or growing marijuana, medical or otherwise, in a given proximity to schools. Investigate the laws in your location.

Consider consulting a medical marijuana lawyer (consult the National Organization for the Reform of Marijuana Laws (NORML; norml.org) or Americans for Safe Access (ASA; safeaccessnow.org) to find one. It will give you peace of mind and inform you of the law and your plant limits.

Never possess firearms. For "possession of a firearm while committing a felony" you could be sentenced to five years in prison for one gun. Be positive that you have no warrants or unpaid parking or moving violation tickets. Do not have parties, guests, or unacceptable noise at your grow location that might disturb neighbors, causing them to call law enforcement. Sometimes, you are guilty by association. Do not have criminal friends.

Visibility

Whether you choose to grow in your basement, spare bedroom, outbuilding, or outside in your backyard, prying eyes are a serious concern. Being able to bring growing supplies and materials in and out of the location without

◀ Always monitor the perimeter of your grow room.

Photo: Stoned Rosie

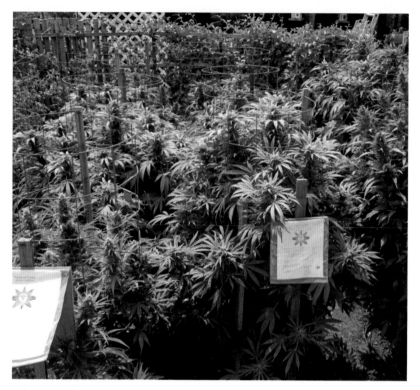

A legal California medical marijuana garden. The posted signs denote that it has been recommended by a physician.

your neighbors or anyone else wondering what you are doing—or worse, knowing exactly what you're doing—is paramount. Preferably, the area should be quiet and private, with a buffer zone between your grow area and public access.

Electricity

Electrical availability is the most important factor in choosing a location. Do not overload circuits and make sure there is more available power than you need. Also, it is imperative that your location have a building code-compliant electrical system. No substandard wiring can be tolerated. All outlets, fixtures, timers, etc. must be heavy duty, grounded, and installed by a professional. If you are not capable, then consult a licensed qualified electrician or educate yourself at your local hardware store and library—look for basic electrical books.

Photo: K

Remember: inspected fire extinguishers properly rated for electrical and structural fires may someday save your life. Buy many of them and place them in the critical areas of the building.

The location of your power meter is also a big issue. You want the meter to be in a secure location away from public view and law enforcement. At the same time, you must grant easy access to the meter reader without having them walking past your growing area, which risks arousing suspicions of your activity and may cause you big legal problems.

Light leaks can tell everybody what you are doing; you can't have the windows of your house, basement, or outbuilding illuminate every time you access the growing area. Stop all light leaks! Keep lights on in the daytime and off at night. If possible, avoid detectable (thermal-imaging) hot spots. If you must keep your lights on at night for temperature reasons (i.e., winter nights get very cold), utilize a good heater to maintain constant temperature and use a thermal shield along with your insulation in your wall construction.

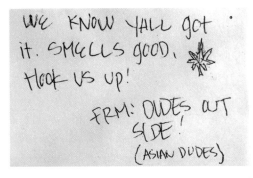

While it seems funny, this note, which was left on the door of a largescale grow in California, caused a complete tear down of the operation which ultimately cost over $250,000 and led to significant delays in production. Keep your work discreet.

Odors

Getting a note like this in your mailbox will cause big problems. A friend received this little note when he showed up at his grow facility one morning! It caused complete pandemonium and a complete shutdown of all growing activities at a cost of $250,000 to the operation. The cause? Smell! Filtration was neglected and trace odors escaped the building during harvest.

You must have excellent ventilation possibilities, ideally access to the roof or areas where you are able to draw in and exhaust vent air—preferably a place not visible to passersby. Do not vent growroom air to an insecure area with public access. All incriminating odors must be eliminated, period! Your growing area must have slightly more air going out than in, creating a negative pressure so errant smells will not escape. All air must be filtered with carbon / charcoal filters (covered in the chapter on ventilation). Ozone generators kill unwanted smells and in return create their own smell; they are sometimes useful outside of growrooms.

Note, however, that you do not want to place ozone generators in the growing area because they will greatly diminish the final smell / flavor of your buds. Also, it is wise to place urinal cakes in the final exhaust duct to eliminate trace odors. *Again, you must eliminate all odors*—many a search warrant has been granted on the grounds of smell alone.

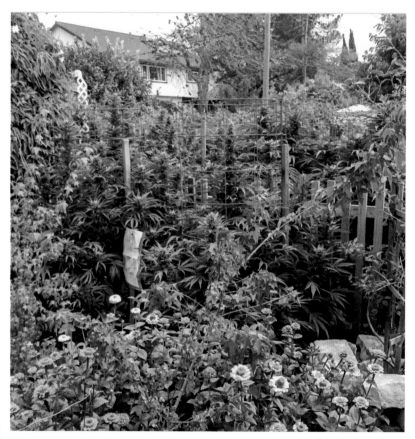

Photos: K

Cannabis is just another crop; it is a great companion to all of the other plants in your garden.

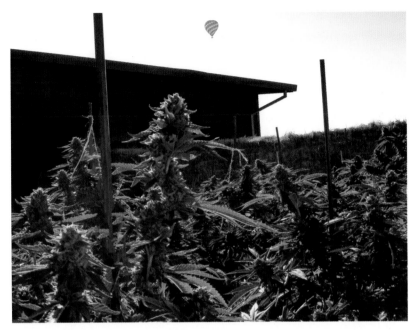

Lofty expectations.

Moisture

Excessively moist or heavily insect-infested areas are unacceptable places in which to grow. Dehumidifying a large area can be difficult and expensive for the beginner, and even if you have taken great precautionary measures, if the surrounding areas are infected with insects and molds it is almost inevitable they will migrate into your garden someday!

Eliminate the possibility of any and all water leaks and spills. Water leaks and spills have been the downfall of many growers. Downstairs neighbors can call landlords. Water can cause electrical shorts, fires, high humidity, and mold.

Many unlikely devices, such as an early-warning water leakage system or a perimeter sensor alarm system, can be utilized for your purposes. There are many out there, and they work for indoor and outdoor settings. Some good ones include the Swann Security monitoring system, the Campers Alert portable detection system, a good quality water detection system, and an all-weather motion-detection camera in either 35mm or digital. These are just three simple things that could help you avoid problems. The first will alert you (but not your neighbors) to a water problem. The others will alert you to intruders, human or animal.

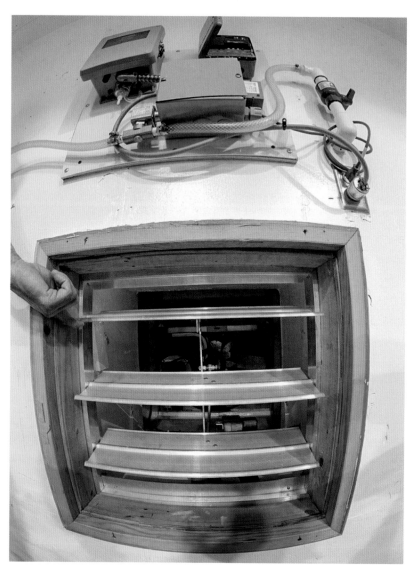

Ventilation intake and controls.

General Advice

Eliminate or minimize all noises. Place rubber mounts on all fans and moving equipment. Place condensed foam under all ballasts to reduce buzzing noise. For small gardens, inline fans are much quieter than others. Place all ballasts in a separate, designated room, vented to avoid heat buildup.

Never steal power or water! This will make you a thief and a criminal.

Photo: Freebie

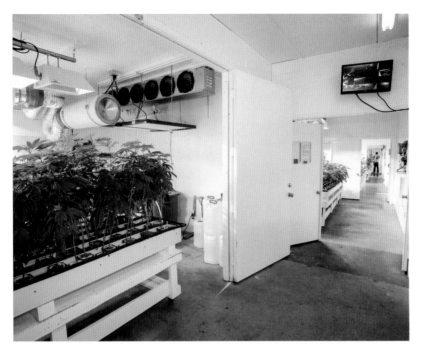

Chambered grow operation with ventilation, air filtration, and security systems visible.

Never show or tell anybody about your plants—trust no one! Do not put marijuana grow-related waste or evidence of it into your garbage; once you place your garbage out for pickup it becomes public property and anybody can search through it to gather evidence against you. This means plastic baggies, stems, rolling utensils, and so on: all of it must be separated and disposed of properly at your local landfill or secure disposal site.

Growing equipment and literature must not be sent to a marijuana growing location and should not be paid for or addressed in your name. Stay away from other growers. Do not telephone growing supply stores. Do not telephone or e-mail other growers or online grow sites. Instead, seek out the information you need online without contacting the sites, and then buy (with cash) what you need from a growing supply or hardware store. Alternately, mail order to different addresses: be creative, safe, and smart.

Above all, use common sense. If your basement floods every winter, don't grow there. If your neighbor is an angry police officer who hates you, don't grow at home! When considering a location, ask yourself if you can withstand

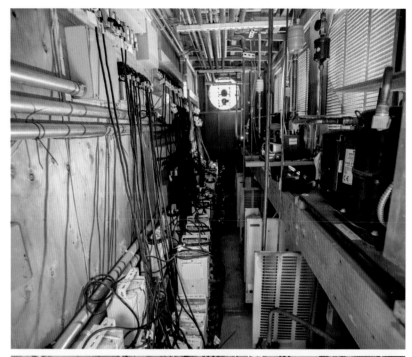

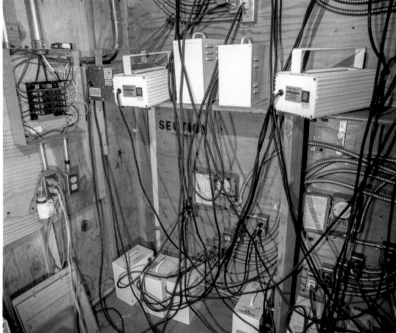

Place ballasts in a separate, designated room, vented to avoid heat buildup.

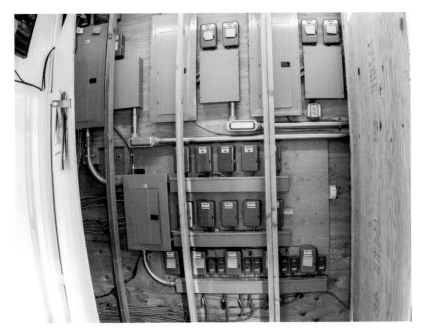

The electrical system controls are located outside of the grow space.

close scrutiny there. Do you belong? Will people who drive past or see you come and go ask themselves what you're doing there? And will they wonder if what you are doing might be illegal? These are some of the many factors you must consider when building your growroom / garden. Every situation and location is different. Each will have unpredictable nuances, good and bad. Ultimately, you must choose! Hopefully, this information will help you make the right decisions.

Think safe, be safe.

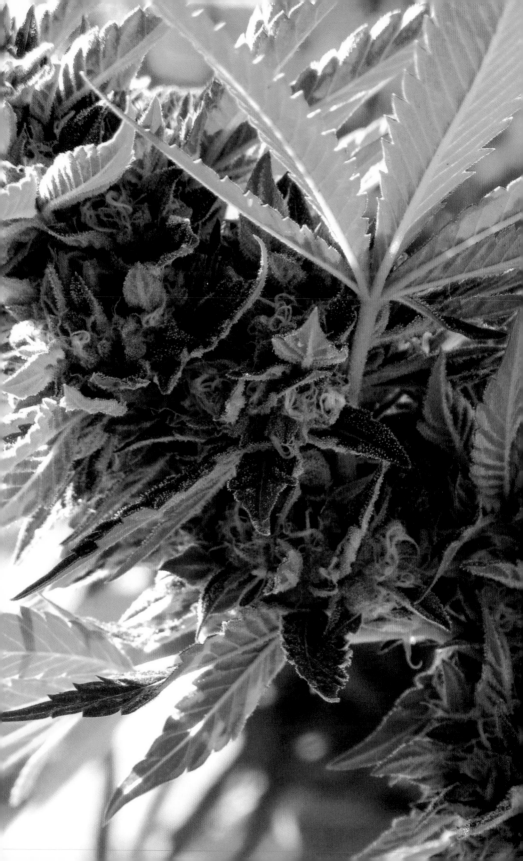

CHAPTER 3

The Symbiotic Rotation Process

For our purposes here, symbiotic rotation is essentially the practice of having all stages of your plants ready exactly when you need them. On the day of harvest you must have vegetative plants ready to install in the flowering room, and your clones must be ready to be moved to the vegetative room. After cleanup and decontamination, the clone room should be ready for more clones, taken from the plants in the flowering room. Empty space is a waste of time, resulting in a diminished supply of bud at your disposal.

For all practical purposes, you don't want plants ready before or after they are needed, but exactly when you want them: thus creating a symbiotic rotation! Refining the variables is key. Catering to the plant's every need is the first priority. Second is maximizing its full potential.

Choosing a Cultivar

Understanding the parameters and limitations of your chosen cultivar is also paramount. You must experiment and investigate all possibilities and options. All plants are different. Here we discuss the two basic cultivars and

◀ Outdoor OG Kush.

Photo: K

their strengths and weaknesses in regard to symbiotic rotation; for their fundamental differences, see the chapter on choosing a cultivar.

Cannabis Sativa

Cannabis sativa typically grows tall and lanky with long internodal spacing, creating long, airy buds. They grow too tall for most indoor situations and take far longer to finish flowering than cannabis indica; sativa can take 8 to 16+ weeks to finish!

The symbiotic rotation style is more labor-intensive if you are growing cannabis sativa. It can be done, but you must skip a vegetative cycle, meaning your flowering sativa plants won't be finished for (probably) 12 weeks or more, so you will have a quandary! By skipping a vegetative cycle the next cycle of vegetative plants and clones will be ready when you need them.

While you are waiting for the flowering plants to finish, your vegetative plants will grow too tall and lanky. The clones will quickly root and deteriorate because of overcrowding and lack of proper lighting, causing internodal (the space between the branches) stretching or slow growth development, and stunting.

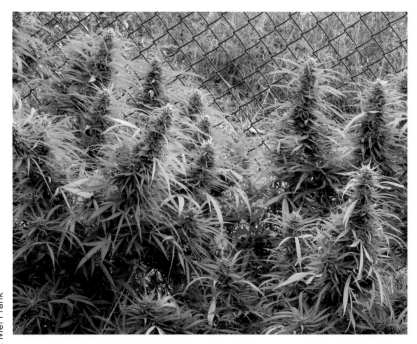

Photo: Mel Frank

This Blueberry Haze is an example of a high-yielding sativa. It eventually produced two pounds of bud.

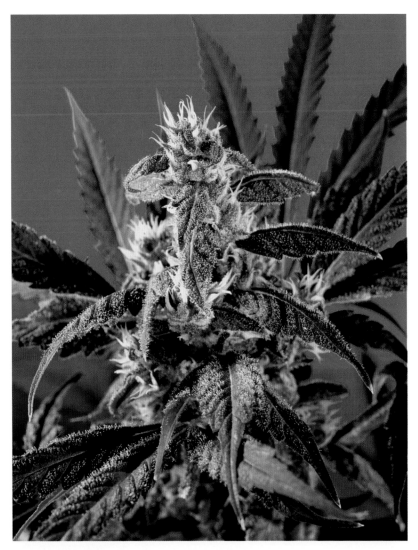

Juicy Fruit in full flower. This wonderful cultivar derives its name from its unique smell and taste. She is sativa dominant.

Photo: Andre Grossman

The way to overcome this situation is to eliminate your vegetative plants after you've taken clones. Wait for clones to root, then install them in the vegetative room. By eliminating the previous vegetative cycle, you have allowed the slow flowering sativa to finish flowering, but still have vegetative plants and clones ready exactly when you want them. Essentially, you are skipping a cycle to wait for the sativa to finish flowering.

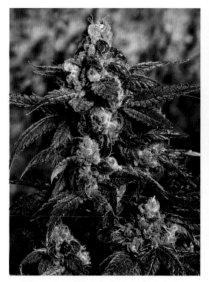 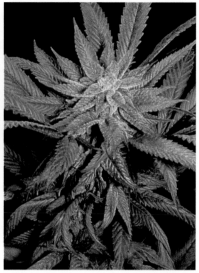

MIRV from Trichome Technologies is a truly fantastic indica-sativa hybrid. It is a highly stable, and very resinous cultivar.

Ultra Violet bud from Trichome Tech has Purple Kush in its lineage. It has a 60 day flowering period.

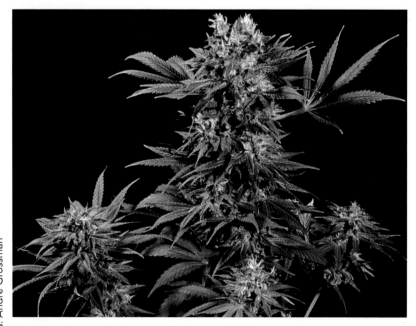

Photos: Andre Grossman

Washington, named after America's first president, is an indica-sativa hybrid stabilized and backcrossed to perfection by Trichome Tech.

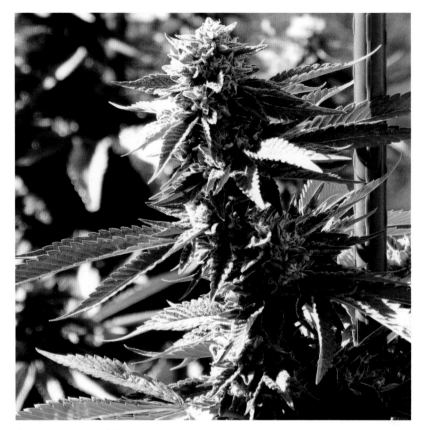

Sun-grown cannabis.

Cannabis Indica

Cannabis indica and cannabis indica / sativa hybrids are perfect adaptations, and so adapt to a symbiotic rotation flawlessly. Starting from seed or clone, you will grow your plants to approximately 10 to 12 inches tall, depending on your chosen genetics / cultivar and internodal length. The plants will have many branches available for clones. Strip the donor plants of all available clones and place donor plants in the flowering room. Clones can take from 7 to 21 days to root depending on environmental conditions and genetics / cultivar. Ideally, you want the plants to finish at approximately 24 to 36 inches tall, so you will induce flowering when plants are approximately 12 to 18 inches tall. So, if you take clones (which take 14 days) and you then vegetate for 14 days, you will have both ready before your other plants have finished flowering. This would create a problem.

Photo: K

23

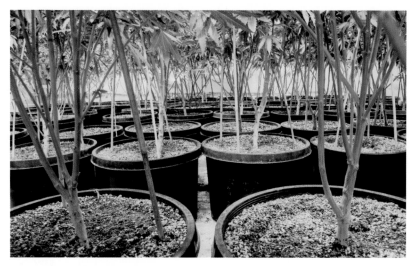

Pruning the bottom branches for rotation garden.

Symbiotic Rotation Timeline

This is an adaptation of Trichome Technologies' schedule for starting new facilities. In this scenario, the grower needs four rooms / chambers / areas: one for clones, one for vegetation, and two rotating flowering areas. Again:

Area 1: Clone area

Area 2: Vegetative area

Area 3: Flowering area

Area 4: Flowering area

(Area 3 and 4 are also used for vegetative growth and for producing more available clone material.)

The rooms / chambers / areas can be a closet or part of a room sectioned off, whatever you like. For simplicity's sake, I'll call them simply "areas" from now on.

Step 1. Start with eight plants from the same cultivar. Grow plants to approximately 12 inches tall and completely strip off any clones. (This process can yield about six to eight clones per plant; about 48–56 total.) Allow 14 days to root each clone.

Step 2. After the clones have rooted thoroughly, 14 days later, install the rooted clones into the area 2 vegetative areas with 18 hours of light.

Step 3. Seven days after installation of the clones, clean plants up. All lower leaves and vegetation should be removed to allow the plants to concentrate all available energy into developing the next batch of available clones. Any unhealthy leaves should be removed. Only healthy clone stock is left on the 6- to 8-inch plants. All healthy upper vegetation and leaves are left on intact.

Step 4. Twenty-two days later, again strip and remove all available clones and eliminate the donors. (This time, you could get up to 400 clones from 64 plants.) Fifty percent of these will later be eliminated; only the best are kept and installed into the vegetation area.

Step 5. Move the remaining half of the plants into the area 2 vegetative room with 18 hours of light. Take only the best plants, and dispose of the other half. This ensures that you only grow the best plants.

Step 6. Clean off all the unhealthy leaves and unwanted lower branches, as in Step 3 above.

Step 7. Twelve days later, transfer vegetative plants to the stage three flowering areas. Put the best one-quarter of the best plants in each room. Keep the lights on at the 18-hour cycle. Dispose of the leftover half of the plants. (In one example, 50 plants were placed in each flowering room and 100 plants were discarded.)

Step 8. Two days later, turn flower area one into a 12/12 light cycle. Area 2 remains 18/6.

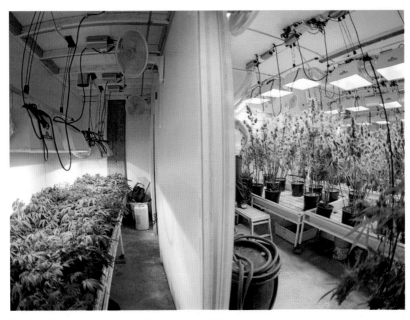

Photo: Freebie

In this photo you can clearly see two different stages of plant development.

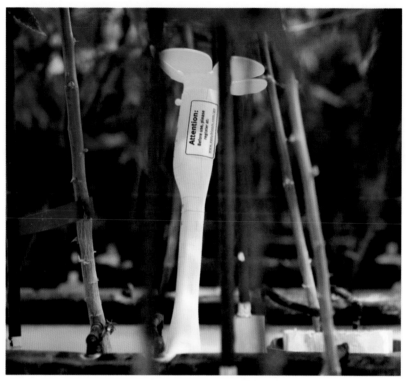

Clean off all the unhealthy leaves and unwanted lower branches.

Step 9. Two days later, take clones from plants in area 1 and 2. The plants in area 4 are topped (the tips taken off to prevent the plant from getting too tall) and only a few branches are left on them while the plants in flowering room 4 are allowed to finish flowering. Light schedules in areas 1 and 2 remain the same (i.e., area one at 12/12 light cycle and area two at 18/6).

Step 10. Twenty-one days later, turn flowering area 4 to a 12/12 light cycle.

Step 11. One day later, transfer rooted clones to area 2.

Step 12. Vegetative plants in area 2 should be grown to approximately 12 inches tall and completely stripped of all available clones—preferably as many as possible. However, leave plenty of viable material to finish flowering.

Step 13. Eleven days later, turn the lights in area 3 to 10 hours on / 14 hours off and significantly lower the ammonium and nitrate nitrogen (nutrient) levels (this process is fully explained later in this book). Eliminate all ammonium nitrate by the end of the growth cycle. (This is the N in the NPK ratio, or the vegetative component in nutrients.)

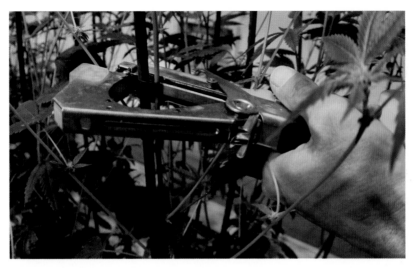

Be sure to stake your plants at an appropriate time so they are prepared for flowering.

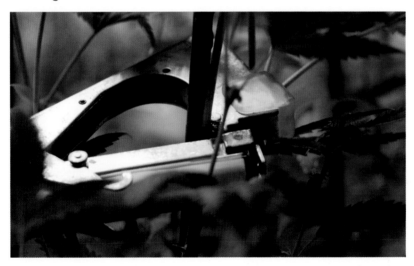

The tool used here is the HT-B2 Tapener Max. It utilizes green gardener's tape for tying up plants.

....

Step 14. Six days later, clean up / strip area 2 (the vegetative room). Remove the lower leaves and vegetation, as well as any unhealthy leaves and material unsuitable for clones, as in Step 3 above.

Step 15. Eight days later, harvest all plants from flowering area 3 and immediately clean and decontaminate the room in preparation for reinstallation.

Photos: Freebie

Step 16. One day later, transfer area 2 vegetative plants to the empty flowering area, changing the light schedule to 12/12. Transfer all area one clones to the area 2 vegetative area. All of this should be done only after a thorough cleaning and decontamination of all empty rooms and systems.

Step 17. Two days later, take the clones from flowering area 3 that have been on 12/12 cycle for 2 days and place them in area 1 for rooting.

Step 18. Fourteen days later, strip / clean up stage two vegetation room. Clean off any unwanted / unhealthy material, as in Step 3 above.

Step 19. Seven days later, harvest flowering room two, immediately clean and decontaminate the area in preparation for reinstallation, and transfer stage two vegetative plants from area 2 to flowering area 4.

Step 20. One day later, transfer area 1 clones to area 2 vegetative area and turn light to a 12/12 cycle.

Step 21. Two days later, take clones from flowering area 4.

Step 22. Eighteen days later, clean up / strip vegetative area 2.

Step 23. Four days later, harvest flowering area 1.

Step 24. Two days later, take clones from flowering area one.

Step 25. Sixteen days later, clean up / strip area 2 of any unwanted / unusable material.

Step 26. Six days later, harvest area 4, transfer area 2 vegetative to area 4 flowering, and turn lights to 12/12.

Step 27. One day later, transfer area 1 clones to area 2 vegetative area.

Step 28. One day later, take clones from flowering area 2.

Step 29. Twenty days later, clean up / strip area 2 vegetative of any unwanted / unusable material.

Step 30. Four days later, harvest flowering area 3 and transfer area 2 vegetative to flowering area 3, leaving the lights at 18/6.

Step 31. One day later, turn flowering area 3's light cycle to 12/12.

Step 32. Two days later, clean up / strip area 2 vegetative of any unwanted / unusable material.

Step 33. Fourteen days later, clean up / strip area 2.

Step 34. Seven days later, harvest flowering area 4 and transfer area 2 vegetative to flowering area 4. Transfer area 1 clones to area 2 vegetative area.

Step 35. Two days later, take clones from area 2.

Repeat this scheduling process over and over again—it is cyclical.

Every step of this schedule was dictated by growing methodologies, envi-

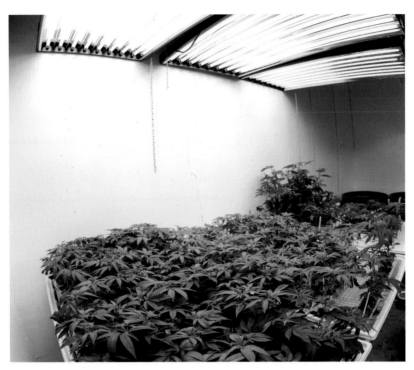

Compact fluorescent lights used in a cloning chamber.

ronmental conditions, and genetics. We used four different cultivars, all indica / sativa hybrids yet each rooted at different times. Each had a different growth rate and pattern, and each finished / matured at slightly different rates also.

All of these factors must be considered when creating a working symbiotic rotation. The same symbiotic rotation cycle can be used for three room rotations or by using mother plants instead of constantly rotating clones and vegetative plants, but in my experience, the above schedule is much more efficient than any other method, period!

The Eleven Steps of Symbiotic Rotation

The detailed instructions above can be boiled down to the following eleven steps. You might not understand every step that follows yet, but by the end of this book, you will. In practice, a symbiotic rotation works as follows:

1. Take clones or start seeds for donor plants.
2. Grow donor plants to a height of 12 inches.
3. Strip off all available clones.

Photo: Freebie

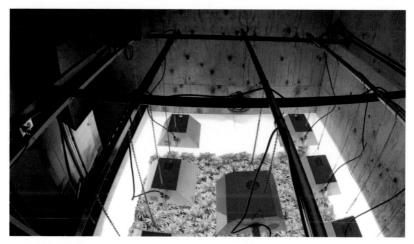

Make sure to have good lights in the flowering chamber.

4. Transfer donor plants to flowering room. Clones will take 7 to 14 days to root.

5. After clones root, hold them in the clone room for approximately 21 more days.

6. Install the rooted clones in the vegetative room for 14 days.

7. On day 12, induce vegetative plants into flowering (with 12 hours of light and 12 hours of complete darkness).

8. Two days later (day 14), take clones from new flowering plants.

9. Move new flowering plants into the flowering room. (The original donor plants will by now have already finished, so the room will be empty.)

10. After approximately 46 to 53 days into the flowering stage, turn the lights to 10 or 11 hours of light, eliminate CO_2, and slightly increase the potassium and phosphorus levels.

11. Eliminate ammonium nitrogen and dramatically decrease nitrate nitrogen or eliminate entirely.

Steps 10 and 11 sound complicated, but they basically have to do with aiding the flowering plants to finish in approximately 50 days, allowing you to install the vegetative plants in the flowering room sooner, thus allowing the installation of clones and the beginning of the process again. They are covered later in this book.

No schedule is set in stone; it is flexible and you must refine it. If you clone and it takes 15 days for them to root, then hold them for 21 days, and vegetate for 14 days; that equals 50 days of vegetative growth and allows the flowering plants to finish in approximately 50 to 55 days. You must experiment and practice to achieve a perfect symbiotic rotation. All the while, make sure you're harvesting your buds at peak potency, and not before.

The same rotation cycle can be achieved by using mother plants. Simply follow the same principles, except take clones from mother plants instead of the vegetative plants. It can sometimes be difficult to get large numbers of clones rapidly from small numbers of mother plants, so it makes more sense to simply clone from the vegetative plants (unless, again, you are only growing a small number of plants with limited space).

Altering Cycles

As stated above, it is necessary to refine the variables and understand the limitations of your chosen cultivar. Working backwards, examine the flowering cycle length. Most cannabis indica and cannabis indica / sativa hybrids finish flowering in approximately 60 days. But, as explained in the cloning section of this book, you can induce flowering in your vegetative plants two days before you clone. You can run lights for ten or 11 hours a day during the last one or one-and-a-half weeks of flowering. Both practices are meant to shorten the flowering cycle. Finishing these plants earlier means being able to induce the vegetative plants into flowering sooner, thus enabling the clones to be transferred to the vegetative room earlier.

After clones have been rooted and installed in the vegetative room, they will grow for approximately seven to ten days (depending again on genetics / cultivar and environmental conditions). On day seven, or whenever they are approximately 8 inches tall, strip off all the lower foliage except the top four leaf and branch sets. If they are not approximately 8 inches tall, wait and then strip them. Four to seven days later, induce flowering two days before taking the next batch of clones—again, shortening the vegetative cycle.

If the vegetative cycle must be lengthened, simply leave them in that stage longer. The clone stage is difficult to manipulate—in this situation you do not want more clones, faster! Because you will be waiting 50 to 60 days for the flowering stage to finish, you want them fast, but also at the exact right time. To achieve this goal, you must be able to hold clones in a form of suspended animation, in perfect health in every way, without them stretching (growing too tall), stalling, or becoming unhealthy. The result is that you will have shortened the flowering cycle to approximately 50 days. If the vegetative cycle is maintained for optimal health, stature, and vigor, plants will be 12 to 14 inches tall, finishing at approximately 24–36 inches tall after flowering.

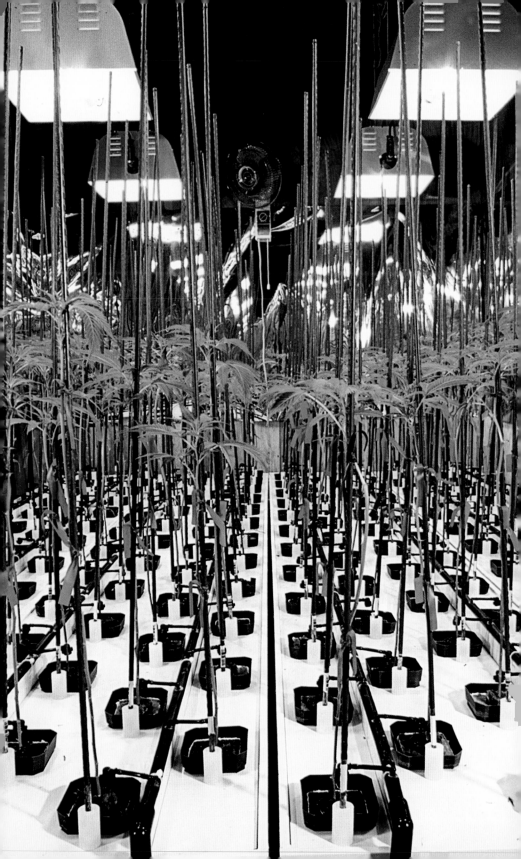

CHAPTER 4

System Basics

The cannabis plant is basically a weed and it will grow almost anywhere. The key trick is to maximize its full potential, to make its yield the greatest possible, with the most flavor and highest THC content.

There are many small- and medium-sized hydroponic, aeroponic, and Nutrient Film Technique (NFT) systems on the market today—some good and some bad. I maintain that simplicity is best for the novice, and recommend an organic soil or soilless mix method of cultivation until you familiarize yourself with the equipment and understand what you are doing. Then, after you completely understand the basic principles of plant cultivation, cloning, vegetative, flowering, and symbiotic rotation, you can progress to one of the units for sale, or even build your own.

Remember, when constructing the cultivation environment, you must consider how difficult it will be to eliminate in a hurry. Do not create a nightmare for yourself. Construct your systems and chambers as if you might have to tear them down and get rid of them as fast as possible. Unnecessary high-tech gadgets can be fun, but too many of them become a quagmire of chaos. Keep it simple: old school, low tech, with as few moving parts as possible, and nothing to break.

◀ Tall plants on the outer edges and short plants in the middle guarantee that all plants receive maximum light.

Photo: Andre Grossman

Construction Examples

Option 1

400-watt light for the vegetative chamber.

8 fluorescent lights for the cloning chamber.

6 600-watt lights in the flowering chamber.

Option 2

2 600-watt lights for a larger vegetative chamber.

6 fluorescent lights for the cloning chamber.

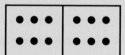

8 1,000-watt light in the flowering chamber.

Option 3

4 400-watt lights in the vegetative chamber.

6 fluorescent lights in the cloning chamber.

12 600-watt lights in the flowering chamber.

Option 4

6 fluorescent lights in the cloning chamber.

2 400-watt lights in the vegetative chamber.

4 600-watt lights in the flowering chamber.

Option 5

A 400-watt or 600-watt light in the vegetative chamber.

A 400-watt or 600-watt light in the flowering chamber.

2 fluorescent lights in the cloning chamber.

Be sure to design all setups with a cleanup area and ballast storage area.

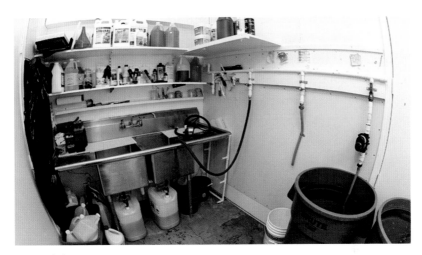

A good cleanup room.

Growroom Basics

Ultimately, you will require five rooms / chambers / areas:

■ Ballast area; must be outside the actual grow space, e.g., adjoining room, a shelf, etc.

■ Cleanup room with a sink, water source, and drainage; e.g., kitchen, bathroom, garage, etc.

■ Flowering area; can be as big as half a bedroom or as small as a closet.

■ Vegetative / mother area; typically half the size of your chosen flowering area.

■ Clone area; the top shelf in a closet is perfect, as minimal space is required.

Ceiling height is usually your limiting factor, so do your best to find or build a high-ceilinged space. If you were to try to grow in an area with a 4-foot ceiling, the lights would hang down 12 inches. The plant containers are 12 inches tall and the tables the plants are on are 12 inches tall (to accommodate wastewater drainage). You can see there would be little growing room left, and heat would quickly build up and cause problems. A 6- to 8-foot ceiling minimum is a must, but the higher the ceiling, the better.

Existing Structures

If you are using an existing structure (i.e., a closet, bedroom, outbuilding, basement, or garage), the shape and size is dictated to you. You will have to work around the design situation you already have. If building a new structure for your growing environment, you will be free to design a perfect situation.

Photo: Freebie

Building a New Environment

If building a new environment, the construction methods you will use are essentially the same ones used in building a house: basic 2 x 4-inch framed ceiling and walls, and so on, with minor differences.

After framing the walls in the dimensions you want, you are ready for the electrical installation (see electrical section). After all electrical wiring, fuse box subpanels, receptacles, and plugs are completely finished, the next step is to install building-code-compliant insulation. This will aid in keeping the environment cool in the daytime or summer and warm at night or in winter. Next, you will place Thermal Shield (available on the internet or at your local hydroponics supply store) over the insulation. To protect you from illegal searches with thermal imaging cameras / devices, wrap all ventilation ducts, too.

After the electrics are done, and once the ventilation (see section on ventilation) is tested and deemed safe and compliant, you will cover the interior walls. Instead of using standard gypsum-type sheetrock, you will want to use a material used in bathrooms called green rock or DensGlass, which is fiberglass faced drywall and very moisture resistant. Walls constructed with green rock and DensGlass withstand moisture—and, when covered and painted with a mold-inhibiting paint (such as Kills primer covered with white paint or sheets of white Fiberglass Reinforced Plastic [FRP]), are the best combination for preventing mold, mildew, and fungi. After the outer walls are completed, you are ready to choose what system to use.

Note: if using an area that does not permit the use of growing trays, a shelf structure is your next best option, custom-made to suit. Ideally, the shelves will be covered with $\frac{1}{8}$-inch thick sheet plastic or waterproof material on top, slightly sloping forward to allow for drainage and eliminating the possibility of stagnating water. Drain this into a collection reservoir, to be dumped by hand or automated with water pumps; whichever you prefer. The shelf must be sturdy and strong, made of metal, plastic, or wood, and, if it's the latter, covered with sealer and mold-inhibiting paint.

Precautions

Whichever system you choose—purchased or constructed, drippers or sprayers, 5-gallon bucket, aeroponic, NFT recirculation, or aerated deep water recirculation in tubes—everything must be sterilized and disinfected.

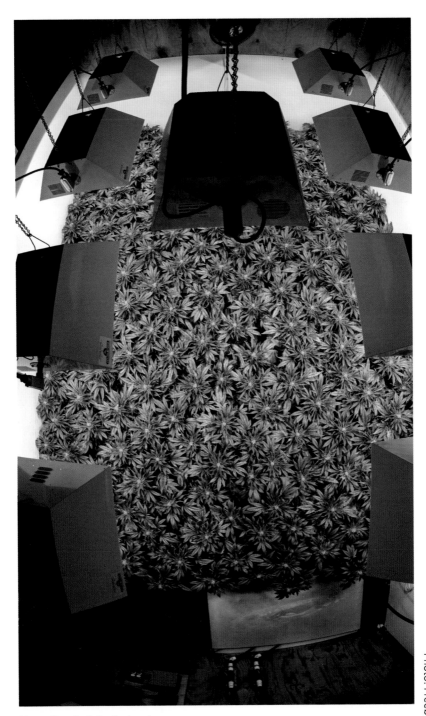

No ceiling height limiter here.

Photo: Freebie

Grow Room Basics

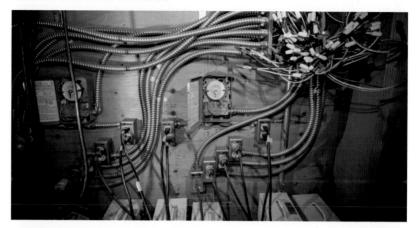

Electrical wiring must be done right.

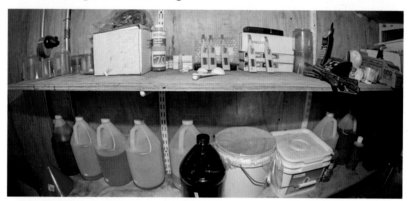

Good organization is key.

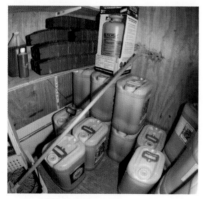

Proper storage for all nutrients.

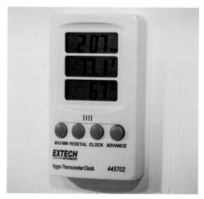

Monitors for temperature, humidity, and PPM.

Photos: Freebie

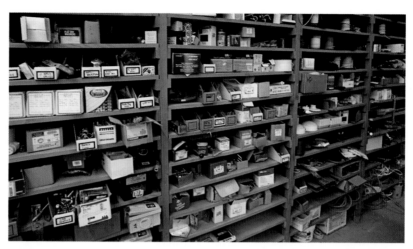

Tools.

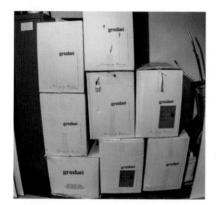

Closet for cloning supplies.

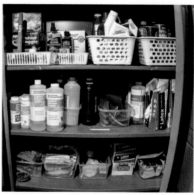

Supply closet.

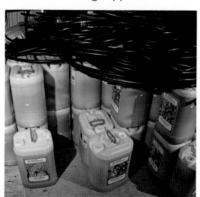

Nutrients and hydroponic system supplies.

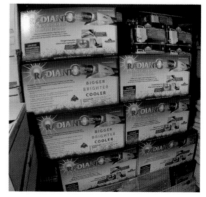

Storage for lights.

Before you introduce plants to a new environment, there are a few precautionary measures to take.

Pyrethrum bombs may be used in your empty chambers to eliminate unwanted pests.

Chlorine bleach, mixed at ten parts water to one part bleach, can be used to clean all surfaces inside the chamber and in hydroponic and aeroponic systems between harvests. Be sure to rinse off all trace amounts of bleach solution after cleaning.

Food grade 27% hydrogen peroxide may also be used to decontaminate growing chambers, mixed at ten parts water to one part hydrogen peroxide.

Note: when undertaking this final precaution, spray either the bleach / water or peroxide / water (Caution! Never mix both!) solution from a 5-gallon pressurized garden sprayer (peroxide does not smell and leaves no harmful residue). Spray walls, ceilings, floors, all cleanable areas and surfaces. Electrical components should be wiped down with a washcloth dampened with the solution. Always wear rubber gloves, a protective breathing apparatus / mask, and eye protection when spraying bleach, and be sure to keep the area very well ventilated. (Flora Kleen by General Hydroponics is a fantastic hydroponic disinfectant. It both sterilizes hydro systems and eliminates salt / mineral deposits.

ONA is a good chlorine bleach alternative. It is used for disinfection and general cleanliness, and does not harm plants or animals. It does not emit toxic fumes. It can be used for sterilizing entire systems and growrooms and eliminating fungi and bacteria even in mid-growing cycle (or, of course, when your grow area is empty). ONA also eliminates mineral deposits.

Greenhouse

Simplistic setups work best, and this greenhouse—a representative setup—demonstrates just that. The medium here is $^1/_3$ Fox Farms "Ocean Forest" soil, $^1/_3$ vermiculite, and $^1/_3$ perlite, mixed with water-retaining crystals. The containers are 2-gallon, and the plants in this picture, at three- to four feet tall in the flowering stage, need to be watered every other day. The nutrients used in this photo were General Hydroponics Flora Series as well as other amendments, as discussed later in the book.

In most environments plants cannot be placed outdoors in mid-Spring because temperatures are still too low for optimum growth. A greenhouse will keep the plants warm, day or night, even in cold or rainy conditions. Greenhouse-grown plants vigorously thrive. The clear plastic covering the greenhouse intensifies the sun and can elevate the temperature inside to roughly 85°F on a day when it is only 65°F outside—a temperature differential of 20°F.

When growing in a greenhouse you can produce three or even four crops per year, rather than one or two, as you can outdoors, uncovered. We place vegetated (approximately 24 inches tall) plants out into the greenhouse on April 20th and immediately induce flowering via light deprivation. (This deprivation is accomplished by using 6mm plastic that is black on one side and white on the other, with which we completely cover the greenhouse.) When the plants are fully mature and harvested, new, vegetated plants replace them immediately, and we repeat the cycle without losing a day of growth. And so on, repeating as we do in the symbiotic rotation process. In this way we get three crops by the first week of October.

When it starts to rain, we place industrial-use large dehumidifiers in the greenhouse to prevent powdery mildew and botrytis (gray bud mold); we also tightly close all of the doors in order to keep out the rain. On overcast or rainy days we augment with supplemental lighting. For example, in a 10 x 10-foot greenhouse we use two 600-watt metal halide and two 600-watt sodium halide lights, as one might indoors, which has the added benefit of raising the interior temperature to desirable levels on cold days. With the doors sealed, the greenhouse must still be allowed to ventilate to keep oxygen and CO_2 levels in proper proportions.

Buds that are produced in a greenhouse are more like indoor buds than outdoors—they are denser, have more THC, etc.—because you have more control of the environment. There are lots of variables. For example, on warm days the doors at each end of the greenhouse are opened and both walls are rolled up and secured using bungee cords. Large oscillating fans are good to mount, to keep the air moving when the doors are closed and the sides rolled down. You must also install intake and exhaust fans.

Cover the greenhouse at night—you must have complete darkness inside to achieve optimum results. Try large sheets of 6mm Visqueen, white on one side and black on the other. The white side reflects heat off of the outside of the greenhouse and the black side absorbs heat on the inside. The cover is what allows you to induce flowering during months of extended sunlight.

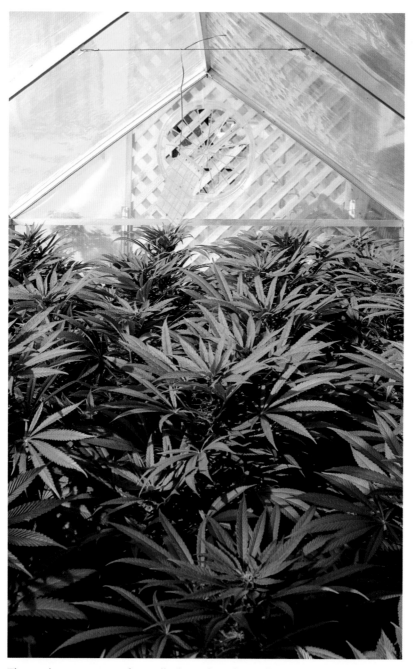

These plants were two feet tall when placed into this 8x10 greenhouse in early August in Northern California. Then, due to fewer hours of available light, they immediately began flowering.

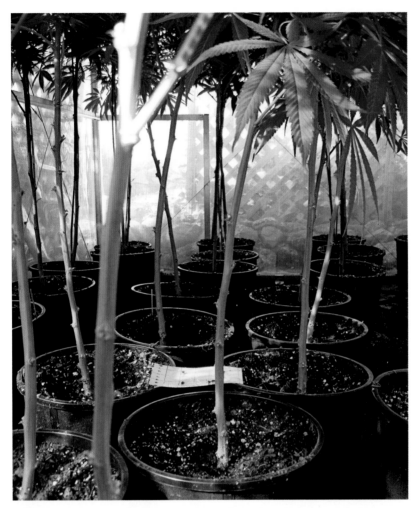

They reach full maturity in early/mid-October. This set-up was easy to produce and maintain.

The plants depicted above were two feet tall when placed outside into an 8x10 greenhouse in early August in Northern California (they began life indoors), whereupon, due to fewer hours of available light, they immediately began the flowering process. The plants reached full maturation in early/mid-October, and thus were in the greenhouse a total of eight-and-a-half weeks. This set-up was easy to produce and maintain. With added ventilation, heat, supplemental lighting, and a a good quality climate controller climate controller, this green-house produced the same quality of harvest throughout the winter months.

Greenhouse Grow Operations

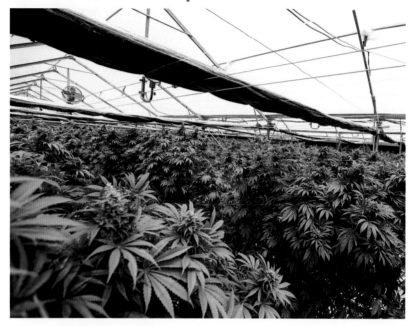

Outdoor cannabis greenhouse with ceiling fans for air circulation.

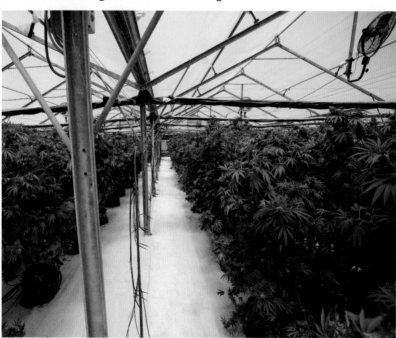

Photos: Better

A roving aisle allows easy access to every plant.

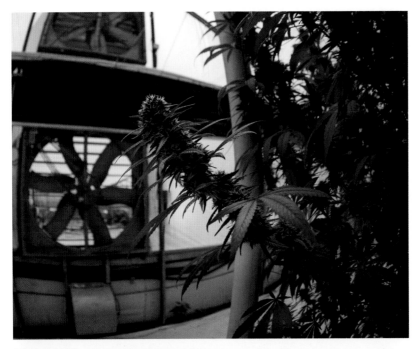

Massive airflow is a must in a greenhouse.

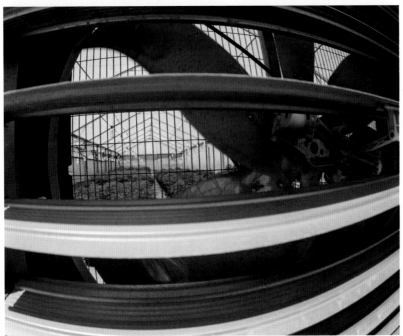

Greenhouse extraction fan seen from exterior of garden.

Greenhouse Grow Operations

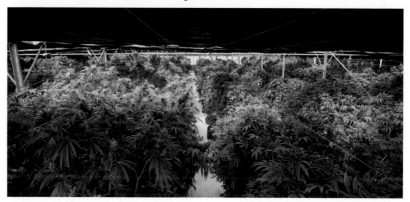

Shade cloths are drawn to cover plants when the sun is at its most intense period of the day to eliminate unnecessary excessive leaf temperatures.

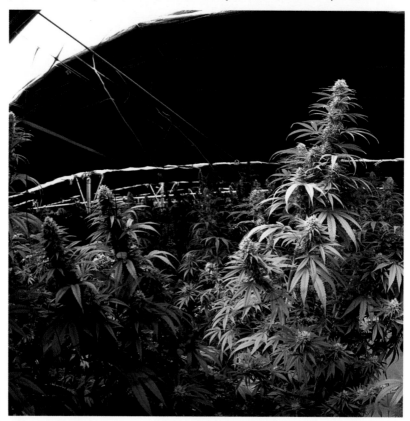

Photos: Better

Elevated leaf temperatures cause unnecessary stress on the plants. Sun shades must be used in excessive light situations.

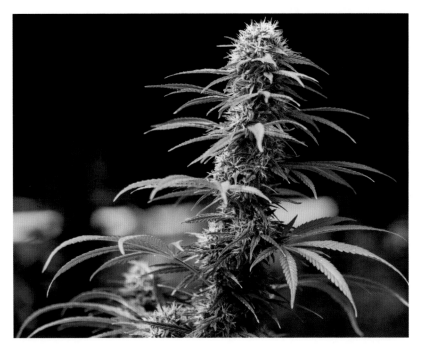

Cola produced in a greenhouse garden.

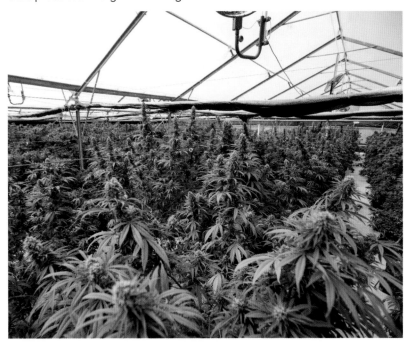

Flowering cannabis in large cannabis greenhouse.

Greenhouse Grow Operations

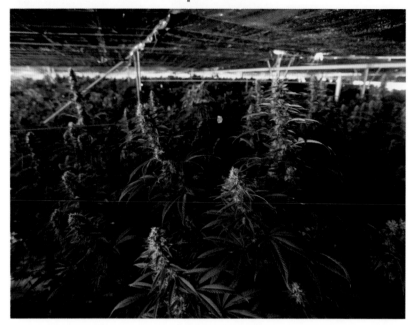

Flowering cannabis in large cannabis greenhouse.

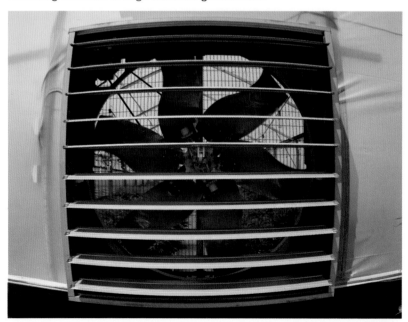

Photos: Better

Extraction fan to keep humidity and temperature levels appropriate in the greenhouse.

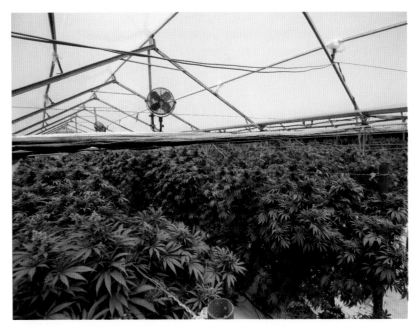

The shade cloth visible in this photo can also be drawn in the evening to keep the plants warm at night and conserve energy on heating.

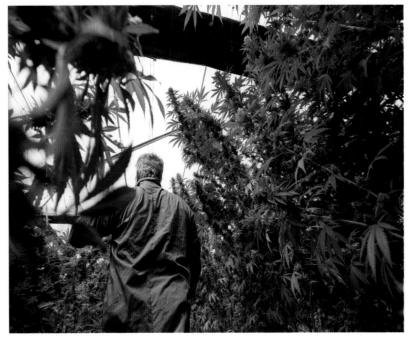

A worker tending to the plants in a greenhouse.

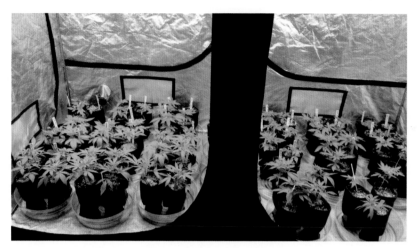

Small grow tents such as this, are perfect for hardening off clones.

Tips for Greenhouse Growing

1. Always fasten thick, weed-inhibiting cloth on the floor of the greenhouse; it is available at any nursery supply store. This discourages weed growth inside the greenhouse that may encourage insect infestation. If growing in containers simply place them on top of the cloth. If growing in the ground, simply cut access holes to the soil through the cloth where you intend on planting. Make sure you clear all weeds and rocks below the greenhouse prior to fastening the cloth.

2. The best position for a greenhouse is to have its longest side run north–south; this will help to avoid excess temperatures in summer.

3. Use anti-hotspot tape to stop heat from the metal frame causing weak spots in the clear Visqueen / plastic. The tape will extend the life of the clear cover by a year.

4. Seedlings and clones that have been started indoors, under artificial lights, require a period of "hardening off" before being planted outdoors. This involves gradually acclimatizing them to outdoor conditions over a period of two weeks. Start by placing them outside in a slightly shaded area during the day and bring them indoors at night. Gradually increase the time that they spend outdoors until they are outside all of the time. Without hardening off, the plants will burn, suffer stress, and growth will be temporarily slowed. With this in mind, it is best to start your plants indoors where the elements are less severe and they have a greater chance of survival.

Photos: K

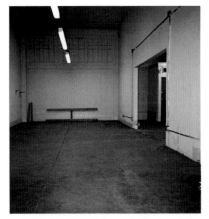 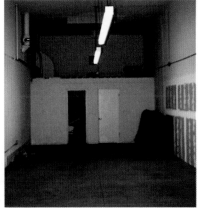

Grow space prior to the installation of a garden.

Indoor Soilless Shelf System

This empty space was used to build an inexpensive, simple, yet very clean and productive (albeit hobbyist) growroom. The ceiling height (16 feet) is perfect for heat dissipation, which is required when using many HID lights. The rest of the space was used for materials for clean up, storage, trimming, etc.

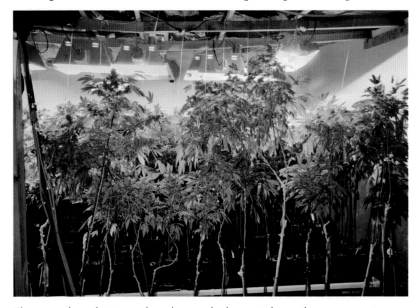

These mother plants produced enough clones to keep the growroom behind them full of plants year-round. The mothers grow in a separate "vegetative room" under 18 hours of light to keep them from flowering.

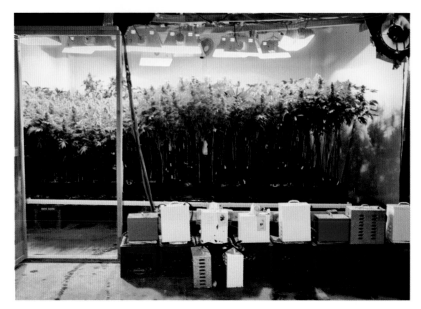

Multiple cultivars in the flowering chamber.

Flowering Chamber

With the mother plants removed you can see the flowering chamber behind them. With simple 2 x 4 construction and white or black plastic Visqueen for wall covering, an efficient, clean greenhouse can be created. In this set-up you'll see a screen door covered in black plastic as an entrance; it creates a roll-up wall that allows easy access during work hours as well as eliminating any unwanted heat or humidity build-up. The ballasts normally sit on top of the structure but in this photo they have been removed to facilitate the take-down of the grow space. The exhaust fan can be seen in the upper right-hand corner of the photo; it is at the top of the room in order to eliminate any unwanted heat and humidity that might build up.

Grow Chamber

Inside the grow chamber we find strong plants and buds ready for harvest. The system here is a soilless mix medium (vermiculite and perlite) in $^3/_4$-gallon containers. The plants sit on a slightly tilted shelf constructed of plywood sheets on top of common plastic milk crates. The plywood is covered with rubber pond liner at the edges to keep water from running off the shelf. At the low side of the shelf is a plastic rain gutter; the runoff water naturally mi-

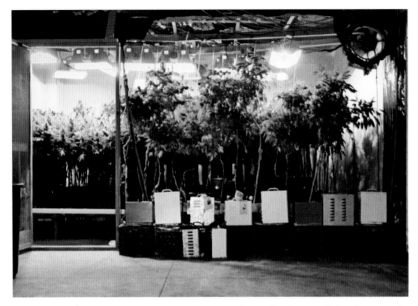

All electrical wiring and components must always be kept off the floor and away from contact with water, for obvious reasons.

grates to the low side of the shelf and runs off into the rain gutter and into a collection reservoir where it is then disposed of with a water pump. The plants were hand-watered every 24 hours in the early stages of development and two times a day in the later stages of flowering.

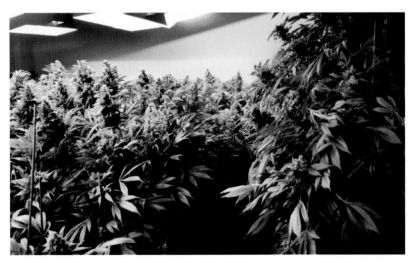

Inside the grow chamber.

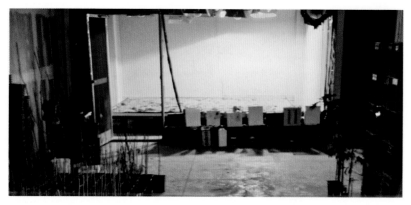

Empty space after plants have been harvested.

Harvest Room and Deconstruction

Harvested and stripped plants are on the left of this picture, with buds hanging in the next room and room deconstruction begun. Another bountiful harvest has taken place and it is time to go build another somewhere else. This location was almost perfect but there is always somewhere better! Always look for that perfect spot.

Organic Soil Shelf System

Here are many healthy, seven-day old plants. This organic media system uses the same shelf system mentioned previously—the difference being the organic media. In this photo you can clearly see the design and set-up of the edges of the shelf. Also you can see that the vegetating plants have had stakes placed in their containers early in life to avoid later root damage. The containers are $^3/_4$-gallon and since these plants, at the time of photographing, will only be in the pots for nine more weeks (10 weeks total), there is no chance of the plants becoming root bound. Furthermore, because small containers are used, more plants can be grown, thus using the space to its full potential. In seven more days the lights will be turned back to 12-hours on and 12-hours off to begin the flowering cycle. The plants will mature between one-and-a-half and three feet tall.

Ten Weeks Later

Ten weeks after installation these plants were ready for harvest: fat, stinky, heavy, sticky, organic buds, and lots of them. There are 11 different cultivars in this room that were preselected so that they all matured at approximately

Photos: K

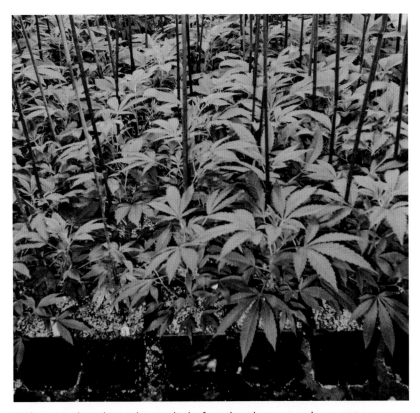

Stakes are placed into the media before the plants grow large so as not to damage the root system.

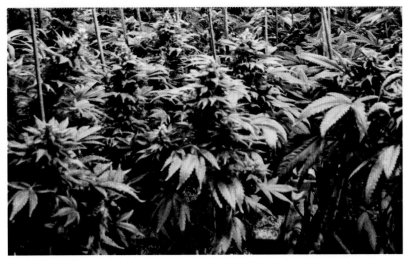

Ten weeks later (same plants as above) the plants are well into flower.

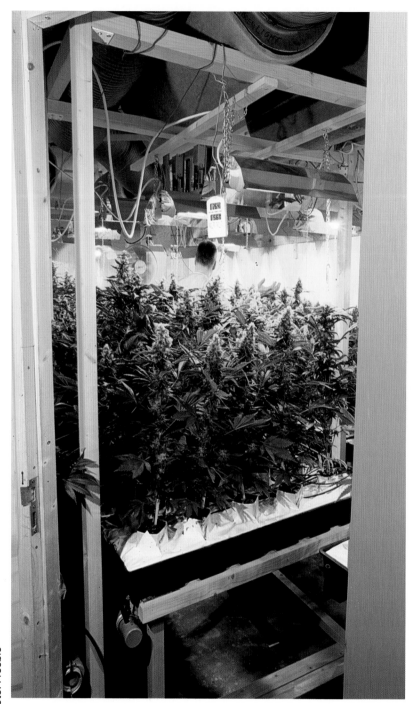

Basic cannabis garden.

Photo: Freebie

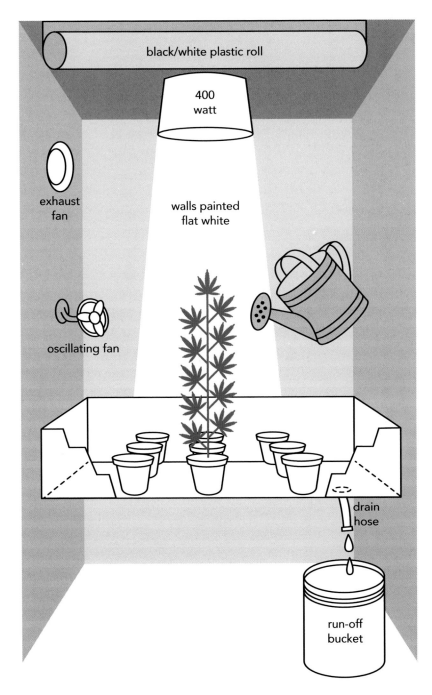

The most common grow system is easy to set up, with no maximization of roots or lights. A sufficient system for a small budget and low yield goals.

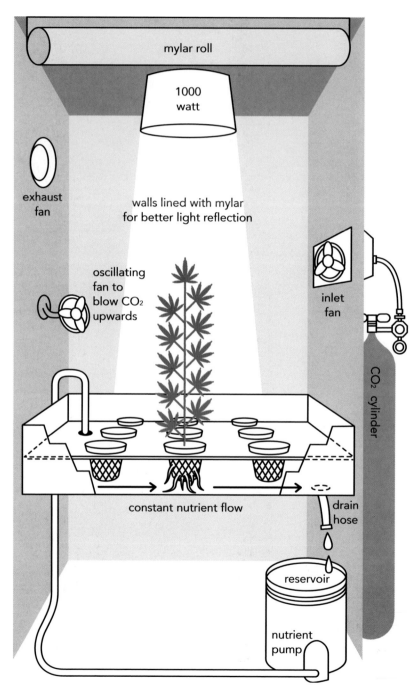

A more ambitious grow system is nominally more expensive to set up, but offers better nutrition, CO_2, light, and root O_2, and ultimately, a better yield.

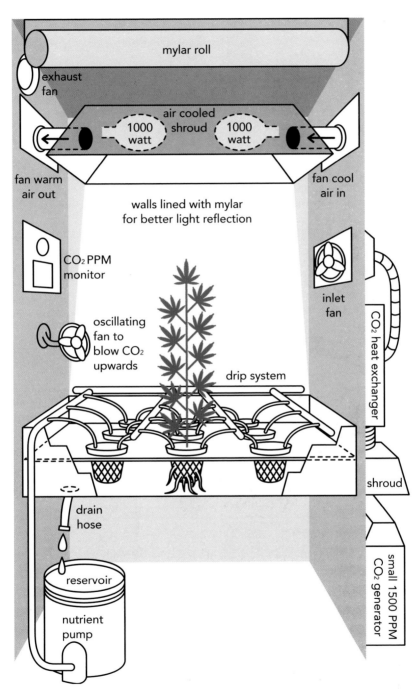

A larger investment for a complex grow system includes features that offer the best nutrition, CO_2, light, and root O_2, resulting in maximum harvests.

the same rate. The same day the plants were harvested, there were more ready to replace them, as per the symbiotic rotation system. Empty rooms only cost you time and money.

Simple, Hand-Fed, Soilless Water System

This is another example of a small, simple system. Rooted clones are placed into three-inch Grodan rockwool cubes and hand-watered every day. The rockwool cubes here are sitting on an egg crate light diffuser atop a common 12-gallon plastic bin, placed to catch runoff water. The bin is emptied after every watering. The plants were allowed to grow for seven days like this under constant fluorescent lighting. After seven days the plants were transferred from the closet to the main bedroom where they were placed in 2-gallon containers and topped off with a soil / perlite / vermiculite mix of media. The plants were then placed on an elevated grow table under a 1,000-watt Halide (HID) light on an 18 hours on / 6 hours off light cycle. The plants will grow like this for 14 days and then the lights will be changed to a 12 on / 12 off cycle. At this point the plants will only require hand watering every three days.

The air conditioner in this photo keeps the room at a perfect 75°F. In the upper right of this photo is a completely blacked-out window (to prevent light-leaks). The garbage can in the photo is used to mix water and nutrients; fresh air enters the room from the open bedroom door. An oscillating fan

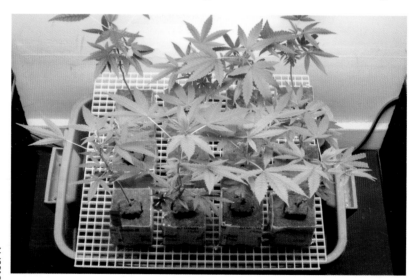

Photos: K

This is a simple, hand-fed rockwool system.

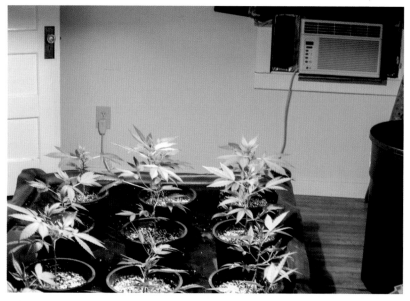

Note the air conditioner for temperature control and the garbage can is used to mix nutrients and water for hand watering.

keeps the air in the room constantly circulating.

Soon there will be buds. After 21 days of vegetative growth the plants required approximately 60 days of flowering growth; 81 days (roughly) total, from root to clone. This is an easy garden to construct and maintain, and best of all, it's inexpensive. Before you buy complicated, expensive pre-built systems you might want to try something basic and straightforward such as this, so that you have a positive first-time growing experience.

Hand-water Rockwool System

This system is as simple as it gets, yet it produced an incredible crop! Plywood tables were constructed with 2 x 4 boards on the sides, to contain runoff water. Again, the table is slightly sloped at one end so that water drains off of it. Clear plastic is placed on top of the table so that water won't absorb into the wood. The runoff water is simply collected at the end of the table in a reservoir and disposed of using a basic water pump. The runoff water is only used once, not recycled.

The 2 x 4s have holes drilled into the end, which will hold stakes that act as plant supports when the cannabis moves into the flowering stage; the

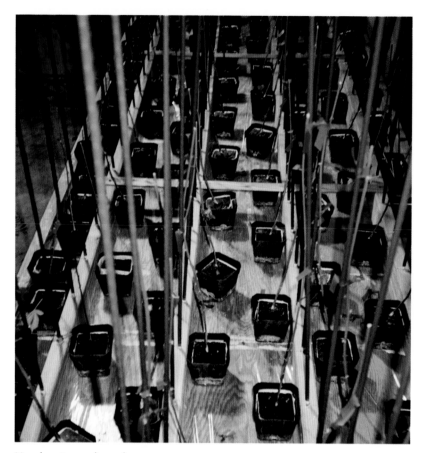

Hand-water rockwool system.

boards are joined together so that they won't fall over. The plants are in 3-inch Grodan rockwool cubes and the cubes are in 4-inch cups. The plants were hand-watered 3 times a day using General Hydroponics Flora Series nutrients (as well as additives and amendments). The plants were kept in the vegetative stage (18 on / 6 off) for 14 days, at which time the light schedule was changed to 12 on / 12 off for flowering.

Harvest Eight Weeks Later

The plants matured approximately eight weeks later and produced an excellent crop—the buds were rock hard, dense, sticky, and the size of a Coke can. The aroma and flavor was incredible. These photos were taken the day of harvest and, because the medium was flushed three days prior to harvest, some

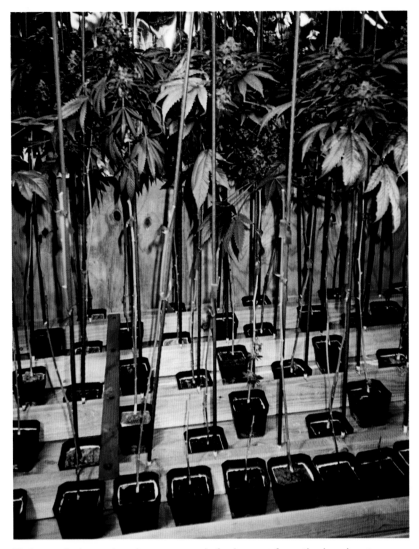

Eight weeks later, the plants are ready for harvest from the hand-water rockwool system.

of the large fan leaves had begun to yellow and die (due to a lack of available nutrients).

A few or many plants can be produced using this method. The choice is yours. The question is: how many plants can you hand water three times a day, every day? If this is too time-consuming for you, then another system is probably best suited for you. This system just shows how simple it can be.

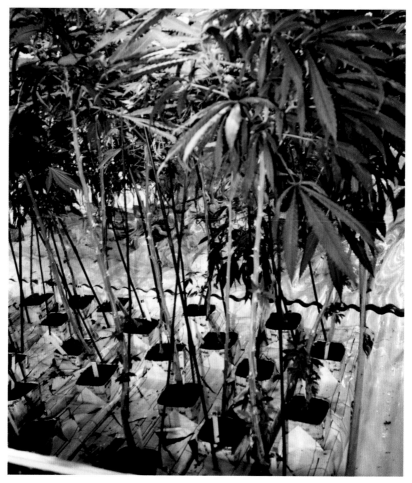

Cube system gardens are another form of run-to-waste system.

Hand-water Rockwool Cube System—Run to Waste

This is another run-to-waste system. "Run-to-waste" means that the system does not recirculate or reuse nutrients or water. This system comprises four-inch rockwool cubes placed on a table on top of corrugated plastic sheets, to enable water drainage. The corrugated plastic directs runoff water to a water-collection reservoir at one end, the contents to be disposed of using a common water pump. As this is only a mother room the plants require hand watering just twice a day; the plants are not allowed to flower or grow because there are clones constantly being taken off them.

Photos: K

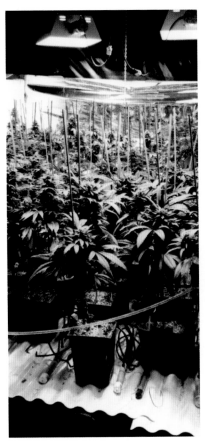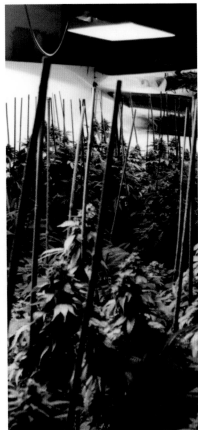

Soilless drip system utilizing ⅓ each of vermiculite, perlite, and potting soil.

Soilless Drip System—Run to Waste

This system uses a soilless medium (a 50/50 mix of vermiculite and perlite). The pots are ³/₄-gallon and the plants are watered and fed using a time-drip emitter system. The plants are automatically watered every day at the same time (first thing in the morning) and the water / nutrient comes from a reservoir under the table with help from a water pump, which pumps water to the drippers and waters the plants. Runoff water drains off the end of the table into a separate water reservoir and is disposed of using another pump.

This system is simple and dependable, as well as fairly inexpensive. You can make it as big or small as you need, and can place new plants on the table as you remove mature plants. It can produce an excellent crop with minimal expended labor or clean up.

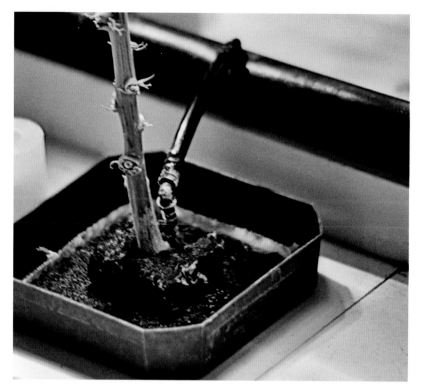

Here is a basic drip system utilizing a ¼-inch drip line. Whenever possible eliminate any light source to the top of the rockwool cube to prevent algae growth on the top of the cube like in this photo.

Basic Drip System

This system uses a ¼-inch drip line and ¼-inch drip line elbow to water a three-inch rockwool cube. The ¼-inch drip line is attached to a ¾-inch feeder line that goes back to a water / nutrient reservoir that has a water pump in it that delivers water and nutrients to the dripper at predetermined times, several times a day. The reservoir is full of filtered, oxygenated, non-chlorinated, nutrient-rich water.

Deep Water Culture (DWC)

This is another good example of a deep water culture (DWC) / nutrient film technique (NFT) system. It is also fairly simple to construct, using only materials from your local hardware store. The system is based around six-inch polypropylene tubes enclosed on both sides and slightly tilted toward the

Photos: K

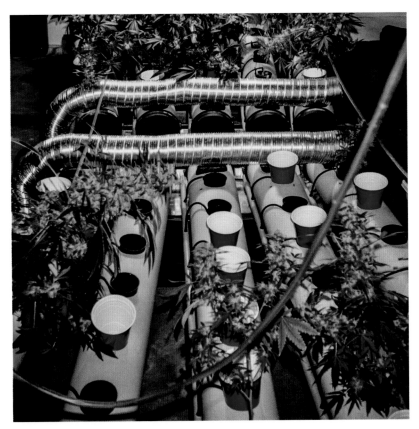

Deep water culture / nutrient film technique system.

center. On the low end of the sealed tube there is a one-inch drain that drains all of the water from the 10 tubes into a water reservoir. A common submersible water pump delivers water/nutrients via $3/4$-inch tubing that connects to a $1/4$-inch drip line, which constantly feeds water and nutrients to the base of the individual plants. The plants are cultivated in $3\frac{1}{2}$-inch mesh baskets covered in clay pellets (Hydroton). Water and nutrients run through the baskets and clay pellets, past the plant roots, to the bottom of the tubes. In the bottom of the tube sits two to three inches of water that is constantly aerated using common aquarium air pumps and air stones. When the water builds up to the desired level (of two or three inches) it naturally overflows back into the reservoir to repeat the process (recirculation). The water flow must be constant and there must always be water present in the bottom of the tubes.

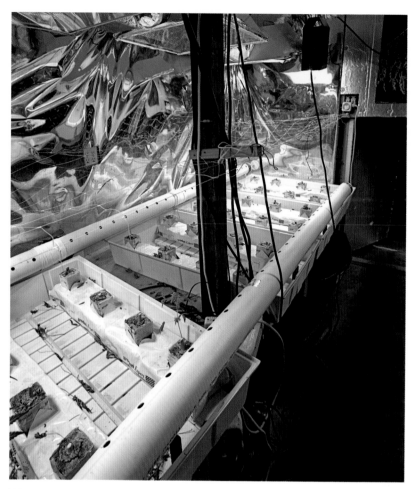

Water temperature is crucial in a DWC/NFT system.

Note that water temperature is crucial in this system. Too hot or too cold and your plants are fucked! Put more technically, this can result in growth stunting, root rot, etc. Heat your water by using titanium aquarium heaters; cool it by using a water chiller. The perfect temperature for this system's water is 72°F at all times, day and night. In this system the water must continually recirculate, 24 hours a day, otherwise the roots dry out or the water gets too hot, causing plant stress.

This type of DWC / NFT system requires the constant watchful eye of someone able to spend a lot of time monitoring the system; mostly this involves checking to see if all equipment functions and plant parameters are acceptable.

Photo: Freebie

This is not a system for someone with little time to spend in his or her garden. Nutrients must be replaced every week to ensure there is no depletion of required nutrients or minerals. That said, it is a fairly simple system to operate—you just have to be vigilant in watching for problems—and to clean, maintain, and tear down for storage. There are many systems like this available on the market but I prefer to build my own.

CO_2 injection tubing surrounds this system and oscillating fans are placed underneath so that air flow and CO_2 levels remain perfect. Reflective Mylar panels also surround this system to reflect any stray light back into the growspace.

The silver aluminum tubing at the center of the system is attached to extraction fans that periodically extract any hot or stale air that may have accumulated in the grow tubes, thus ensuring higher oxygen levels for the root system. Drink cups are placed in empty holes to prevent unwanted algae growth inside the tubes; without light algae cannot grow. This system can be raised or lowered to almost any desired height, which can be an advantage to those with impaired mobility.

Run-to-Waste System

This system is primitive, yet very efficient and low maintenance. It is the same "shelf system" design that has been described previously, except for the

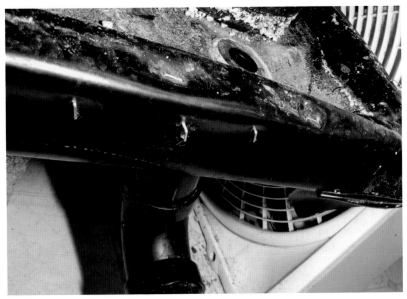

Photo: K

Run-to-waste systems are very low maintenance.

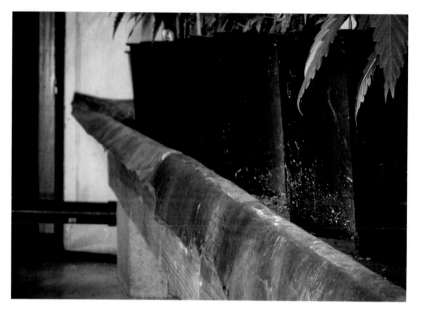

Pots lined up on a run-to-waste system.

drainage. The one-inch drain (for runoff water) is connected directly to a three-inch PVC drainpipe that leads directly to the municipal sewer system, which means no draining of water collection reservoirs. The runoff water simply goes away without you having to do anything, which decreases the amount of work you will have to do every time you flush or water. The PVC drainpipe can be seen at the end of the shelf system in this picture.

Drip System (with Hydroton)

This is another example of a drip system, except that it uses expanded clay pellets (Hydroton) as its exclusive medium. The rooted clones are placed in a two-gallon pot that is $^2/_3$ full of clay pellets, at which point the pot is topped off with more clay pellets and drip feeders are placed at the base of each plant to deliver water six to eight times daily, depending on the growth cycle; plants on an 18 hours on / 6 hours off light cycle require more water than plants on 12 hours of light. A submersible water pump, placed in the reservoir beneath the table, delivers the water and nutrients to the plants; a multi-cycle timer turns it on and off at the desired times each day.

I recommend this system only if you have lots of spare time to decontaminate and clean all of the clay pellets between harvests. This system requires a constant

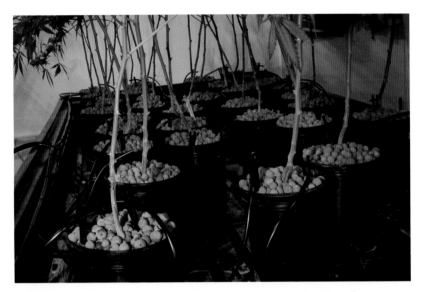

Drip system with hydroton. Keep water temperature at 72°F or else root problems could occur.

water temperature of 72°F or else root problems could occur. A keen eye is required. If the power goes out or the water pump breaks you will have minimal time to repair them or else the plants will die from lack of water; expanded clay pellets hold little to no moisture—their chief purpose is to hold the plants upright and provide ample space for air, water, nutrients, and roots to interact. If simplicity is what you are looking for then this is not the system for you.

Ebb and Flow

This is a classic example of an ebb and flow system. Rooted clones are placed into six-inch rockwool blocks and the blocks are placed into two-gallon pots; the rockwool blocks are then surrounded by expanded clay pellets to add support for the blocks. A water pump is under the table in a reservoir, as described previously; it delivers water and nutrients to the plants by flooding the whole black tray to a depth of 4–6 inches for a period of 5–10 minutes. An overflow drain prevents the water from ever exceeding desired levels. The water and nutrients then drain back in the reservoir for reuse. The cycle is repeated 4–6 times a day depending on plant growth stage. A multi-cycle timer controls the water pump; when the pump stops, the water immediately returns to the reservoir with the help of gravity. The nutrients and water need to be replaced

Photo: K

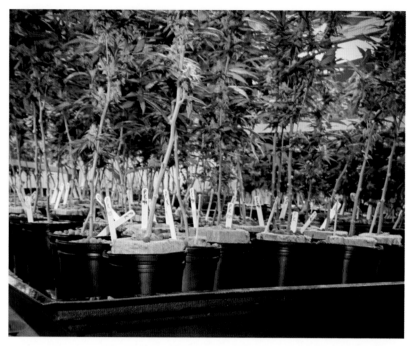

These plants are thriving in the ebb and flow system. It is simple and clean.

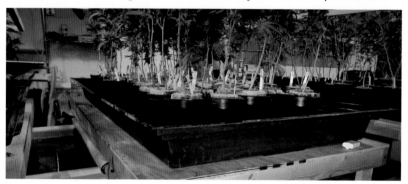

As seen in this picture, multiple trays and tables can be set up side-by-side and use common reservoirs. Another possibility is for each to have its own reservoir.

at least every week in a system such as this in order to keep all the nutrients available to the plants.

A system such as this requires a medium amount of effort and attention, and is best for the intermediate grower. Pathogens and bacteria can rapidly infect systems such as this if proper air and water temperatures are exceeded.

Photos: K

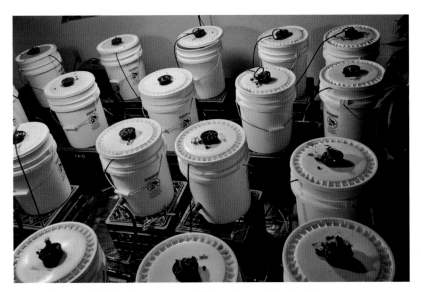

Recirculating NFT bucket system utilizing five-gallon buckets.

Recirculating NFT Bucket System

This five-gallon bucket system works very well, is simple to build and maintain, and is fairly inexpensive. The beauty is that you can plug in and unplug buckets as you want or need them—as many or as few as you desire, quickly and cleanly, and with little effort. Most five-gallon bucket systems require a bucket that is completely filled with clay pellets. This to me is a waste of time and energy, because clay pellets have to be decontaminated and disinfected after each harvest. I would much rather clean and decontaminate a 3½-inch container full of clay pellets than a whole five-gallon bucket.

This system is considered a recirculating NFT drip / deep water culture system. The system works like this: rooted clones are placed into round 3½-inch mesh baskets and covered with clay pellets. The basket is then placed in a three-inch hole cut into the five-gallon bucket lid. A water / nutrient drip emitter is then placed securely on the bucket. The water that comes out of the drip emitter is constantly running through the clay pellets; it exits through the basket and cascades down the developing root system to the bottom of the bucket. At the bottom of the bucket is four inches of water that is constantly draining from the bucket via a half-inch drain at the side of the bucket. Because the buckets are higher than the reservoir (thanks to the milk crates), the water drains back to the reservoir where it is heated or cooled, depending on what is required to keep it

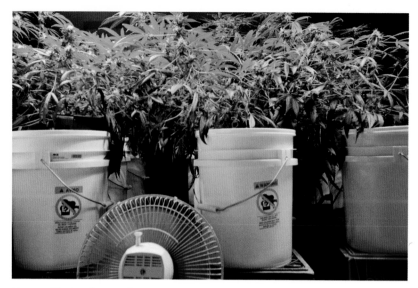

Use oscillating fans to keep air constantly circulating throughout the room.

at 72°F, filtered, oxygenated, and sent back to the base of the plants using a submersible water pump. The water must constantly circulate to keep the plant roots moist or else the plants will die. Because there is so little media, and the clay pellets do not retain much moisture, the water must constantly circulate.

The four inches of water at the bottom of the bucket will quickly fill with healthy white roots relaxing in the oxygen- and nutrient-rich water and absorbing all they need to thrive. Plants are grown vegetatively until they reach one foot tall, at which point they are switched to 12 on / 12 off (the flowering stage). The plants in these photos have been in the flowering stage for approximately two weeks; they will mature and finish flowering between two and three feet tall, requiring no stakes or nets to keep them up because of the shorter plant stature.

All of the materials required to construct this system are available from your local hardware store. There is no need to buy an overpriced hydroponic system unless you really want to or don't have the time or ability to build your own. This system is simple to construct and tear down, as well as to store while not in use. The negatives to using this system are that the water temperature needs to be precisely maintained, as mentioned previously, and that the water must be properly oxygenated to keep the roots from being deprived at the bottom of the large bucket. Furthermore, if the water fails to circulate, plant death will rapidly occur. Plants left without water in this system can die in as little as one

Photos: K

or two hours in hot environments. Growers wishing to plug in a system and leave it unsupervised should not build this type, as it requires daily supervision—not constant work and attention, just somebody to check to see if everything is working properly, i.e., if the water pump is working correctly, whether there are any leaks or clogged drippers or drains, and so on.

After harvest, the clay pellets are placed in a plastic garbage can with bleach and water and allowed to sit for 24 hours, at which point they are rinsed and ready to use again. The mesh baskets are reused as well. The whole system should be wiped off with hydrogen peroxide, and ONA cleaner (a bleach substitute) or Flora Kleen should be run through the drip line system and the rest of the system, allowing the whole thing to disinfect. After everything is rinsed with clean water the new plants are installed—ultimately, a short, hassle-free bit of work when compared to other systems. Remember, you don't have to have an expensive system to get incredible buds.

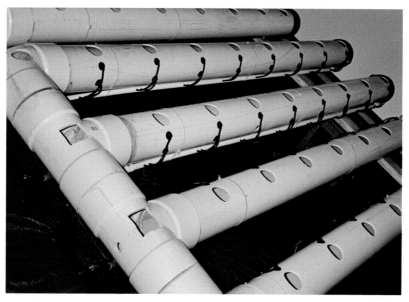

Good example of a home-built aeroponic system from 1991.

Aeroponics

This is a very good example of a typical aeroponic system. Home built, not store bought; anyone can build a system like this, but it requires a skilled grower to make it produce properly and maximize plant growth and yield. Growth rates and yield can be dramatically increased using aeroponic systems, but all environmental parameters and growth controls must be perfect in order to benefit from such a system.

The premise of aeroponics is that air (oxygen) and nutrient-enriched water are misted onto thriving plant roots. The roots absorb any oxygen, water, and nutrients they need at that particular moment and the remaining nutrients recirculate back to a reservoir to be re-aerated, temperature adjusted, and sent back to the plant roots to begin the process again. The mist is sprayed onto the plants' roots with two (in case one gets clogged) four-gallon per hour misters, which are placed directly across from the roots, mounted in the side of six-inch PVC tubing. The tubes are capped at one end and joined at the other, draining into the common reservoir.

This system is not for somebody who wants to plug it in and leave it for long periods of time. It requires constant attention to make sure that misters aren't clogged, the pH and PPM are correct, water and air temperatures are adjusted, and CO_2 levels and water oxygen levels are optimum. This system requires multiple inspections each and every day; no "holidays." Excess water temperature or a broken water pump will result in total and devastating crop failure.

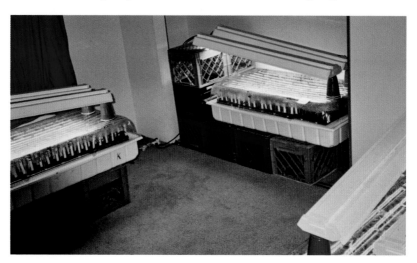

Closet system set up for clone production.

Closet Cloning

Within reason, any space can be used to produce clones, as long as you monitor and control environmental factors such as temperature, humidity, and exposure to oxygen-rich air. In this case, a spare bedroom was used as well as the lower portion of the closet. The clones are under domes that retain moisture and humidity, and the temperature is kept up with a common household thermostatically-controlled air heater. If the humidity or temperature of the room exceeds desired levels, a humidistat-controlled filtered intake and exhaust fan will bring the levels back to acceptable ranges.

For small gardens, just the closet can be used to produce as many clones as you need, anytime you need them. A very small air heater, fluorescent lights, a humidity dome, and a few other items are all that you need. Three or four clones can easily be placed on the shelf on the top of the closet, in a small tray with a humidity dome, if you only need a few clones every once in a while.

Growtubes

Growtubes such as these can be used to construct many completely different hydroponic systems. Place misters in the side of them for aeroponics, or place drippers at each plant site for NFT tubes. You can also fill the growtubes with oxygenated, nutrient-treated water and use them as a deep water culture system. Finally, you can simply place rockwool in the mesh baskets and use the tubes as a periodic drip feed system.

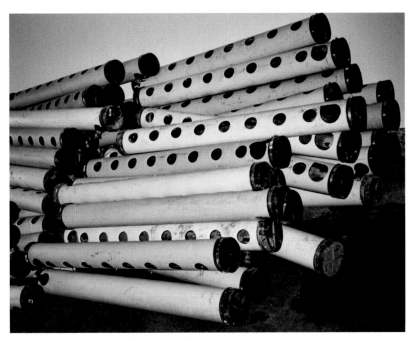

Stack of growtubes to be cleaned.

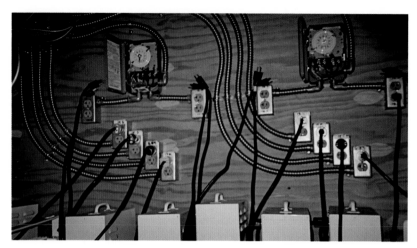

Always have a clean and tidy electrical system.

Timers, Ballasts, Wiring

A professional-quality electrical system is a must! Many growers are displaced or arrested every year because they overloaded electrical circuits or installed inferior wiring, timers, or other electrical components. The example you see here is small, simple, and professional. The ballasts, which are the white boxes at the bottom of the photo, plug into the power outlets that run to Intermatic timers (center of the photo) which are connected to a junction box that houses the main wiring and the wiring that goes to the lights themselves in a separate room. The reason for separating the ballasts and plants is to prevent any unwanted sources of heat that could elevate growroom temperatures and cause plant growth stress or even death.

Drying Racks

This method provides excellent airflow and is inexpensive to construct, but should have Plexiglas underneath to collect any resin glands that may fall.

After harvesting and manicuring the buds, you can gently place them on simple drying racks such as these. For small amounts or irregular harvests, elaborate drying racks do not make sense and are usually not required. That said, for small or intermittent harvests you can stack window or door screens on top of each other with milk crates (see photo above). The screens allow for complete airflow under and on top of the buds. All trimmed leaf, also known as shake, is also placed on a rack. A dehumidifier is placed in the room and

Photos: Andre Grossman

78

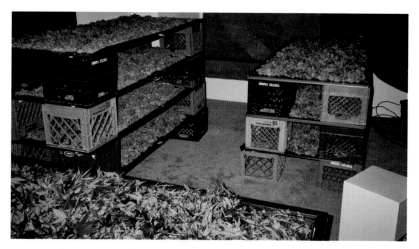

Very simple yet very effective drying rack.

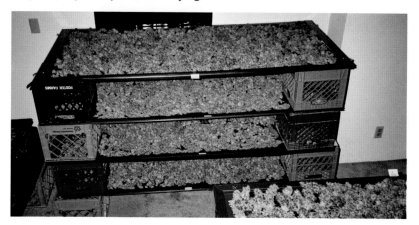

Cannabis drying on improvised racks.

set for 0% humidity; it will need to be drained every four to six hours. A heater should be set to 75°F and placed in the center of the room. Place an oscillating fan in the room to move the air around and facilitate even drying. Rotate the buds periodically (again, every four to six hours) to facilitate complete and even drying. When shake and buds are in the drying stage you must be aware of conditions in the drying room at all times. Slow-drying buds can mold and begin to decompose; over-dried buds burn too quickly and produce a harsh, tarry smoke with diminished odor and flavor. Buds and shake usually take four to six days to dry, depending on conditions. Proper drying is kind of an art—not too fast, not too slow—and even drying is a must.

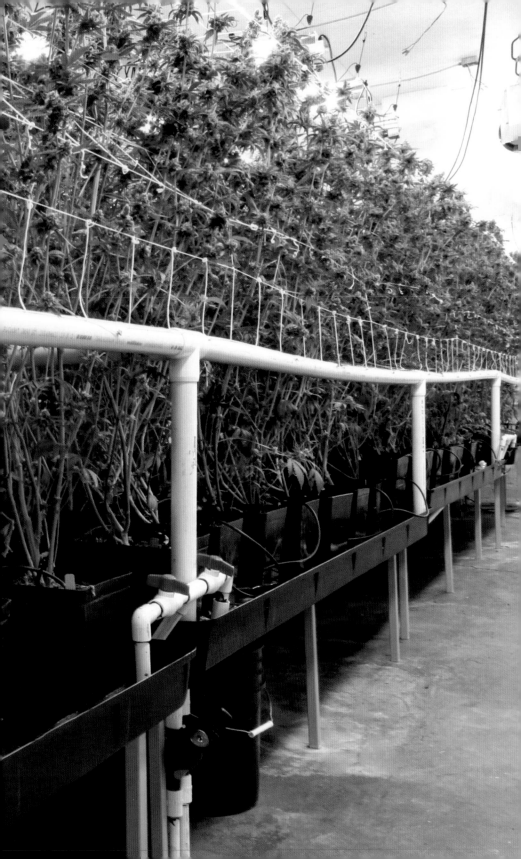

CHAPTER 5

Growing Medium

Soil vs. Hydro

There are some pros and cons of both soil-based and soilless (hydro) growing. Refer to the chart on the following page and compare them to your capabilities and needs, weigh up the pluses and minuses, and make your own choice.

Hydroponic gardening requires careful monitoring of your grow at all times and involves much trial and error when you are first starting out.

Medium / Drainage / Aeration / Container Size and Shape

■ There are many soilless mediums available, coir (coconut fiber), recycled foams, and many others. I prefer a mix made up as follows: $1/3$ inert soil, $1/3$ perlite, and $1/3$ vermiculite with water-retaining crystals (see Soil Mix page).

■ For drip irrigation or ebb and flow systems / low maintenance systems, and rockwool when using hydroponics, aeroponics, or NFT systems: whichever you use, you must have adequate drainage and aeration to the root zone, either by oxygenated water delivery in rockwool systems, or by capillary action in soilless mix systems.

■ The actions of the plant utilizing available moisture and evaporation dries out the media, drawing surrounding atmospheric oxygen into the root zone.

◀ Grow room with nutrient delivery system visible.

Photo: Mel Frank

SOIL

Pros	Cons
1. Stable and very heat tolerant	1. Needs regular changing and is bulky to compost or dispose of
2. Easy to work with	2. Susceptible to pest infestations
3. Does not dry out too rapidly and allows more time between feeding / watering	3. Mildly difficult to monitor nutrient build-up and pH level
4. Available anywhere	4. Less sanitary than hydro (soilless)
5. Reusable for outdoor plants, greenhouse, or garden	5. Lots of water is needed; 25% of every watering must be flushed out to prevent nutrient build-up and pH fluctuations
6. Excellent for beginners or experts on a large scale	6. Observers (neighbors, passers-by, etc.) might wonder why you are always bringing soil in and out of the building
7. Good for indoor / outdoor and organics	7. You need space to mix the soil with with other elements (perlite, water crystals, etc.)

HYDRO (soilless)

Pros	Cons
1. Easy to dispose of refuge	1. Very sensitive to extreme temperatures
2. Easy to clean / decontaminate	2. Susceptible to bacteria and major disease if too hot
3. Easy to maintain nutrient and pH levels	3. Holds little water / nutrients, so must be watered frequently, usually with automated pumps and reservoirs
4. Better for transplanting and moving	4. Medium must be disposed of after one use every time, unless properly sterilized
5. Accelerated growth rates	5. Requires a specialty store
6. More efficient with water and nutrients	6. Demands diligent attention be paid to every detail (pumps, timers, etc.)
7. Once perfected, it is much a less time consuming system	7. Difficult to incorporate organics
8. Not as heavy, so easier to work with	

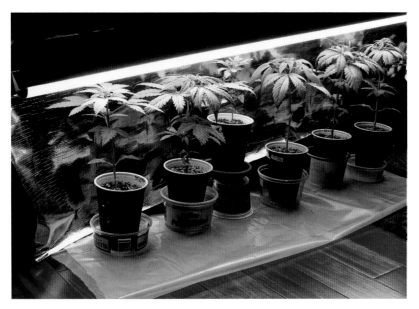

This grower is using a very basic soil medium in cups to start these plants.

■ If growing large container pots outdoors / indoors, you may need 50-gallon to 500-gallon containers. But if you are short cycling your crops, meaning only 10-14 days of vegetative growth and 50-60 days of flowering cycle, you will only need a $^3/_4$-gallon container. In the short time span given, all water and nutrient needs are perfectly controlled and provided, there is no time or need for the plants to become root bound so $^3/_4$-gallon containers are perfect and more than adequate.

■ Simply put, you can fit more square containers into a given area than you can round containers. Efficient use of space is something you must always consider, especially when using sea of green methods, or any other situation whereupon you may have many plants in close proximity to each other.

Note Regarding Container Size: "Potting Up"
■ You cannot place a rooted 2-inch clone into a 50-gallon container (or any other large size container). You must first go through a process called "Potting Up:"
■ 1) You must place 2-inch cuttings into 4-6-inch containers, thus allowing proper oxygenation to the root zone.
■ 2) When the root zone of the cutting utilizes the available soil of the first container, it is to be moved to the next size up container (10-12-inches).

Photo: Mel Frank

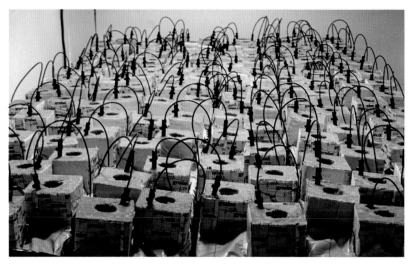

Drip system setup using rockwool cubes. All that is missing are the cannabis plants.

■ 3) After the cutting utilizes the soil available in the 10-12-inch container, it can be left in that container to flower and be harvested, or moved to any larger container size that you desire.

■ 4) The point being, you can't simply transfer a 2-inch rooted clone to a large container and expect it to metabolize and process the nutrients and water that is available without proper amounts of oxygen. The purpose is to incrementally increase the pot size as the size of the root zone of the cutting increases, without the plant getting root bound.

If you do choose to go for hydro, you will need to bear in mind certain time-honored growing rules for using rockwool—the medium that commonly replaces soil. Rockwool is, like fiberglass, a compound made of spun stone; also, as with fiberglass, you need to be careful when working with it. Always wear a particulate mask when using rockwool; wear gloves and always try to avoid working with the rockwool when it is dry. Dry rockwool particles are unhealthy to breathe.

Using a soilless medium expands the possibilities for monitoring. Take note of how much water you add and what the pH balance is; pH stands for "potential hydrates" and it measures alkalinity and acidity; it should always be between 5.8 and 6.5. Remember: never let your rockwool stay wet all the time or get bone dry; don't water at night, and keep to a consistent watering schedule.

Photo: Mel Frank

Hydroponic Grow Systems

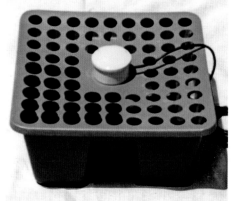

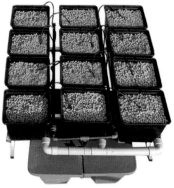

Aeroponic cloning system.

Dutch pot system with hydroton.

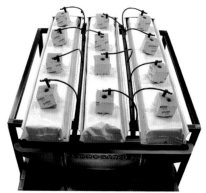

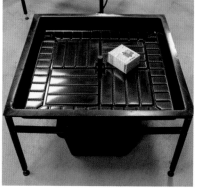

Drip system with rockwool.

Empty ebb and flow table.

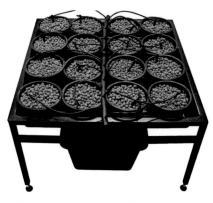

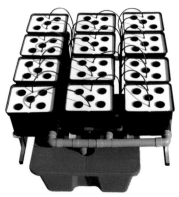

Ebb and flow table with pots and hydroton installed.

Aeropot system with blue reservoir visible underneath.

Photos: Hydrofarm

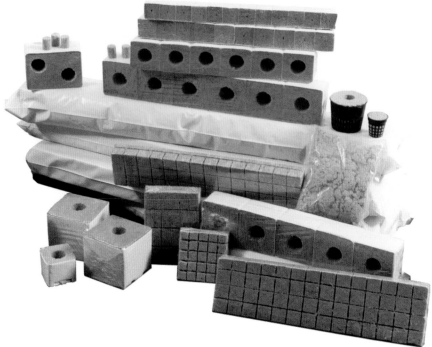

Rockwool collection.

Rockwool Tips

■ Monitor the nutrient and pH levels twice daily

■ When watering, make sure you drain 25% as runoff to avoid salt / nutrient build-up (Note: only when running to waste nutrients, as opposed to recirculating)

■ Keep pH between 5.8 and 6.5, depending on the cultivar you're growing—some like it higher, some like it lower

■ Dispose of all unused rockwool—never allow dry rockwool to sit around

■ Always pre-soak / flush rockwool with nutrient-treated, pH-adjusted water before use

■ Covering the top of the rockwool and eliminating light exposure will prevent algae growth which can inhibit nutrient and oxygen uptake, resulting in poor, unhealthy growth. It also helps discourage fungus gnat infestations

■ Never allow rockwool to completely dry out because it is unhealthy to breathe. Keep it moist, as plants prefer moist, not dry, media: a dry medium will kill a plant

■ Keep medium / rockwool temperature between 70°F and 75°F

Photos: Hydrofarm

Using Rockwool Effectively

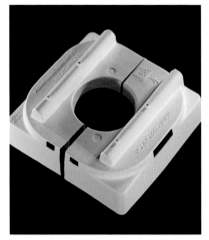

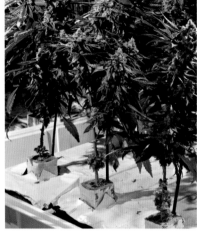

Drip caps available from www.cube-cap.ca are fantastic for water conservation and preventing algae.

A rockwool system like this is more labor efficient than most other systems.

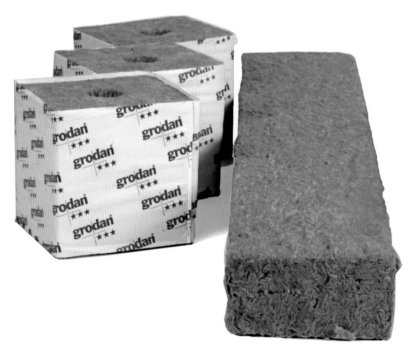

Rockwool is an inert media comprised of heated / molten rock that has been processed similarly to cotton candy.

Top Left Photo: Freebie Top Right Photo: MG Imaging Bottom Photo: Pepper Design

An Example of Hydroponic Nutrients

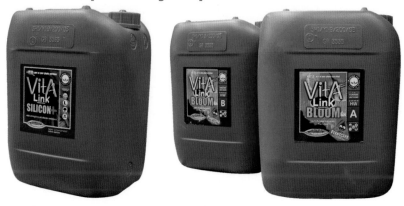

Hydroponic nutrients in containers of this size are generally used in more industrial-size grow operations.

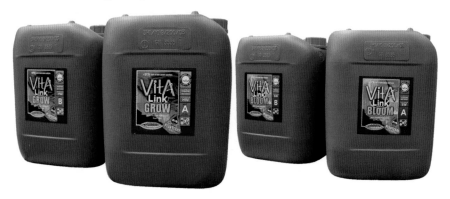

There are many different lines of hydroponic nutrients. Experimentation is the best way to find what works for you.

Advice for the Beginner

In my opinion, a soil / soilless mix medium is the easiest and most tolerant medium you can use. Rockwool systems can be delicate and unforgiving. Unless you use very large cubes, they dry out quickly and you must have an automated watering system or water by hand multiple times a day, every day! Expanded clay pellets, Hydro Corn, and puffed rock, for instance, are even more unforgiving because they hold absolutely no water, so they must be watered almost continually. Automated drip irrigation is easy to construct but must be monitored closely. Regardless of the medium you use, you must have adequate drainage both for the plants and the room itself.

Photos: Hydrofarm

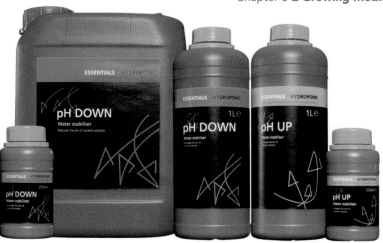

pH Up and pH Down can be used to correct pH imbalances in your nutrient / water solution.

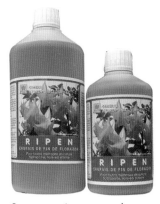

Some nutrient amendments encourage flowering growth.

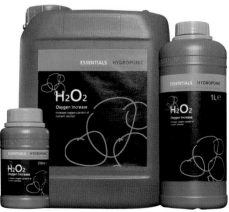

Hydrogen peroxide can help prevent pythium.

Growing in a Soilless Mix

A semi-soilless mix of ⅓ perlite, ⅓ vermiculite and ⅓ Fox Farms "Ocean Forest" (an excellent organic potting soil) is ideal, and it is mostly soil-free. As this medium is basically an inert substance, it doesn't hold large quantities of nitrogen, phosphorus, or potassium, nor for that matter does it supersaturate or hold any water for any long period of time. To counter the eventuality of some plants drying out faster than others, I mix water crystals into the soil: superabsorbent crystals similar to those used in some nursery soil, which is explained in more detail later in this book. Ideally, watering should take place every two to four days. I want the pots to

Hydroponic Nutrients

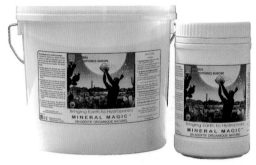
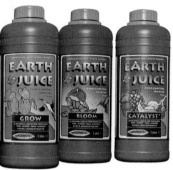

There are many organic options available to you.

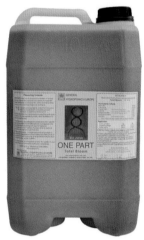
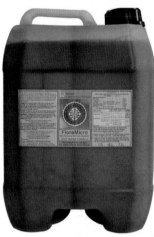

Many companies formulate products specifically for hard water situations.

dry out somewhat on the fourth day, while staying moist on the bottom, so that I can give them a new nutrient mix.

Nutrient Mix and Salt Buildup

With a soilless mix, approximately one quarter of all nutrient-enriched water going into the pots must be run off in order to wash out the last salts from the previous watering, together with any nutrient buildups. It is very important to check the pH and nutrient levels of the water going in, against the pH and nutrient levels of the runoff water coming out. If you send your mix in at pH 6.2 and nutrients at 1,200 PPM (PPM stands for parts per million, and measures the amount of nutrient in the water), and it comes out at pH 6.0 and 1,650 PPM, then you know right away you have a major nutrient buildup. At this point,

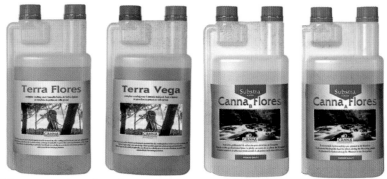

More examples of nutrients.

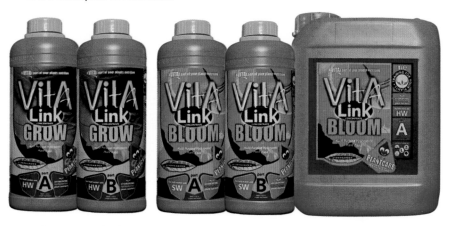

Multi-purpose hydroponic plant food. Experiment to see what works for your garden.

you must flush out your soil pots with pH-adjusted water and test again until such time as what goes in the top matches what comes out of the bottom, within 100 PPM, at a pH of 6.2. This is extremely important because if the pH is extremely higher or lower than 6.2, the plants will take in less of some nutrients and more of others or completely stop uptake of nutrients and water.

Note: Synthetic fertilizer users can also use a 50/50 mix of vermiculite and perlite as a substrate (in containers) for NFT, drip, aeroponic, and fogponic systems.

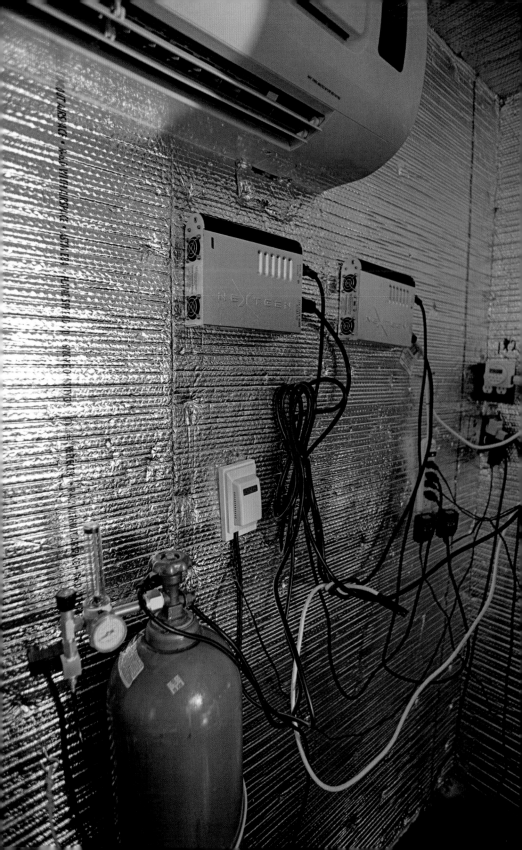

CHAPTER 6

Ventilation, Heat and CO$_2$

Ventilation

The number one mistake most growers make is underestimating and undersizing the ventilation in their growrooms, causing major heat and humidity problems. Your ventilation system is literally the lungs of your grow system. It must be, at the very least, adequate for your needs, allowing for more than sufficient movement of air going in and out. To calculate what size ventilation fans to use, first find out the cubic footage of your grow chamber. Use this formula: height x width x length. Fans are sold using cubic foot per minute (CFM) as a measurement. Oversize your fans—get something bigger than you need. Ultimately, you want to be able to completely exchange and evacuate all air in 3 to 5 minutes.

For safety, you must filter all incoming and outgoing air. Filtering incoming air decreases the risk of airborne contaminants. Filtering outgoing air is simply necessary for odor control. This is very important. I can't emphasize this enough: you must control and eliminate all odors of cannabis!

Urinal cakes (the white, hockey puck sized, odor-eliminating cakes you see in urinals) are one option. Placing them in your final exhaust air ducts masks and eliminates

◀ You must keep all electrical cords and wiring tidy and clean, unlike this photo. In this photo also visible are air conditioning unit, CO$_2$ delivery system, and ballasts.

Photo: Freebie

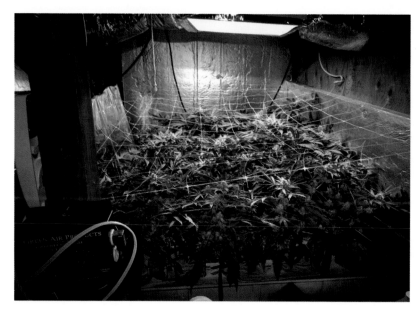

Environmental controller visible in lower left hand corner.

any residual trace of cannabis odor. They are inexpensive, readily available, and work well for a long time. Placed in the duct after the filter masks any odors, they make it seem as though the vented air is coming from a bathroom, not a growroom.

Charcoal filters can be used for outgoing air, and are available at most grow stores in many sizes and for many different applications. However, for incoming air, charcoal filters will not eliminate mold or mildew, so you must get air scrubbers, which are widely available.

In-line fans are perfect for moving air in smaller chambers, and roof ventilators are great for medium-sized chambers. For large chambers, you will need industrial-duty exhaust fans with motorized dampers. Evaporative coolers can be used in the vegetative chambers, but not in flowering rooms, because they increase humidity, which can cause mildew and mold.

There are standard equations for calculating the exhaust rate in a given room; one of them is to multiply the area of the room (think back to grade school: (length x width) by height). The resulting figure is the number of cubic feet per minute (CFM) you will need to evacuate. Fans are provided with these measurements, so all you need to do is match the correct fan up to your figure. Remember to oversize, as you never want to overload the fans. They should come on and evacuate all the air while replacing with new in just three to five minutes.

The opposite of exhaust is intake, and unless you have access to fresh, filtered air in your growroom, you'll need to set up some form of intake fan. The general rule is that for every one CFM of exhaust, you need one CFM of intake to replenish the exhausted air. Note: all intake air should enter at ground level and exhaust air should exit from the top of the room at the opposite ends of the room, creating a complete air transfer.

Preferably, you should have slightly more air exiting the growroom than entering, to create a negative pressure situation in order to stop errant odors from escaping into the surrounding environment. To achieve this, use a fan speed controller (available from grow stores and some hardware stores) and simply plug the intake fan into the speed controller, then plug the controller into a power outlet. Turn on the fan and adjust the dial so that the speed of the intake fan is slightly less than the exhaust fan—thus ensuring that no odors escape the room without going through the charcoal filter. If you don't care about escaping odors, a positive pressure is preferred. It is difficult for mold spores and pests to enter a positive pressurized greenhouse or growroom. This is how legal plant producers operate their ventilation systems.

Air movement within the chambers is also very important. Oscillating wall-mounted fans keep air and CO₂ moving around the chambers perfectly. Don't force too much wind on the plants—a nice, even breeze is the goal, not a hurricane.

Heat

Heat around plants can be a problem. The more lights there are, the more heat is being generated. Heat is measured in British Thermal Units (BTU). To give you an idea of how much heat is produced, a 1,000-watt light gives off approximately 3,400 BTU per hour, which could boil approximately 2 gallons of water in an hour. The larger and more lights you use, the hotter your environment gets.

Temperature is the most easily manipulated factor. Heat will cause or aid internodal stretching / stem elongation, root borne disease, molds, and mildews; it will also stop plant development. The perfect temperature for cannabis is between 70 to 75°F, and 80°F if using CO₂-enriched air. These are acceptable parameters. Every cultivar of cannabis prefers a different humidity and temperature range: experiment and find the perfect humidity and temperature

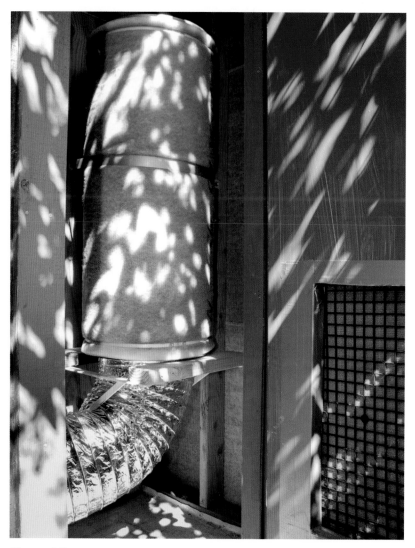

Charcoal filter.

range for your specific needs. As a guide, humidity must be kept at 74 to 80% in the cloning chambers. In the vegetative stage, chambers should range from 60 to 70%. The flowering chambers require from 50 to 60%.

Window air conditioners are fantastic growroom refrigerators (again: oversize, not undersize). They are also rated in BTU capacity; for example, two 1,000-watt lights generate 6,800 BTU per hour, requiring at least a 12,000-BTU air conditioner.

Photo: Samson Daniels

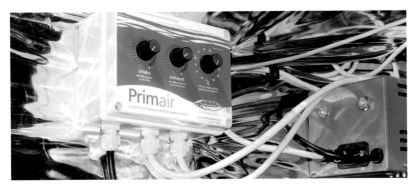

Air intake, exhaust, and temperature controllerX.

Heaters

Cold winter days and nights can cause growroom temperatures to drop to undesirable levels—excessively cold nighttime temperatures will slow plant growth and sometimes stunt the plant completely, resulting in diminished yields. You must monitor these temperatures. A thermostat-controlled heater will rectify this situation—either place the thermostat to your desired temperature and let it come on and off automatically as needed, or plug the heater into a good quality climate controller and let it maintain ideal temperatures for you. Grow stores sell inexpensive digital hi/lo temperature displays with a sensor probe you can place where you want in the medium.

Note: Remember there is a difference between ambient temperatures (surrounding air in the growroom) and radiant heat (heat directly under the lights). You must also measure the temperature at the plants' canopy, as excessive radiant heat will burn plants, dry out their leaves, and diminish the potency of your buds by destroying resin glands at the bud tips (or whatever is closest to the heat source). Never place lights close to plants; use the digital temperature display's probe to monitor temperatures at the canopy.

Caution: Do not point heaters at plant reservoirs or any combustible materials or surfaces. Simply let the heater warm the air. Don't point it at anything that will melt or burn! Don't point it at anything, period! Be safe.

Basic Grower's Tip: Always keep oscillating fans on at night to keep air circulating

Photo: Hydrofarm

Grow Room Monitoring Systems

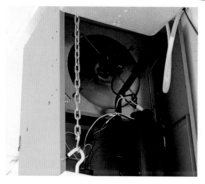

Inside of a dehumidifier.

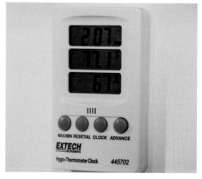

Monitor both high and low temperatures as well as humidity.

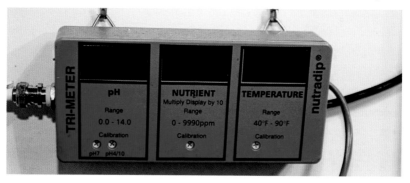

A monitor that keeps track of pH fluctuation, nutrient PPM, and reservoir temperature.

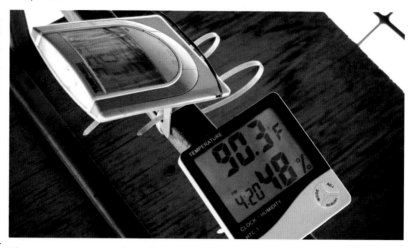

Top Photos: Freebie Bottom Photo: Stoned Rosie

There are many recording devices available to you.

Thermostats and Humidistats

These are utilized for temperature and humidity control, and work by turning fans on and off when either level exceeds pre-set points. Regular air changes are required for optimum plant health. A combined humidistat / thermostat and a speed controller allow you to control the airflow and the number of air changes per hour. They also compensate for hot and cold outside climates by increasing and decreasing the air exchange rates. Fans will run faster / slower, yet continuously reach full potential when needed to control temperature and humidity.

CO_2

Carbon, hydrogen, and oxygen make up approximately 90% of the dry material in a finished bud. CO_2—or carbon dioxide, which is made up of both carbon and oxygen—in the air supplies all of the carbon to a plant. Thus, it makes perfect sense that you can accelerate your plants' growth by increasing the amount of available CO_2. Like humans, plants breathe air—the only difference between our respiration and theirs is that their roots take in oxygen and the leaves take in CO_2 and expel oxygen, whereas we take in oxygen and expel CO_2. A plant utilizes CO_2 gas to produce sugars needed for photosynthesis. At night, the plant expels any unwanted CO_2. The CO_2 gas is the carrier source of the carbon that plants manufacture into organic compounds. Thus, increasing CO_2 levels will accelerate plant growth dramatically.

The introduction of CO_2 can accelerate growth by as much as 30 to 35%. The more available light there is, the higher the PPMs of CO_2 must be utilized to compensate. A plant at two months requires approximately ten times the amount of CO_2 than that of a clone / seedling. Simply put, the more light there is, the more CO_2 must be utilized to expedite manufacture of sugar via photosynthesis and, thus, increased cellular division / plant growth.

Besides inadequate ventilation, lack of CO_2 is the biggest mistake growers make concerning air quality. Also, you must employ oscillating fans to keep air / CO_2 moving across the plants' leaves to properly reap the benefits of CO_2 injection; pure CO_2 is heavier than air. You must supply large amounts of air and CO_2 for maximum growth and production. Larger environments need CO_2 injection via air tanks and regulators, but small areas can use massive air-in and -out ventilation systems.

The more light available to a plant, the more CO_2 it needs for photosynthesis.

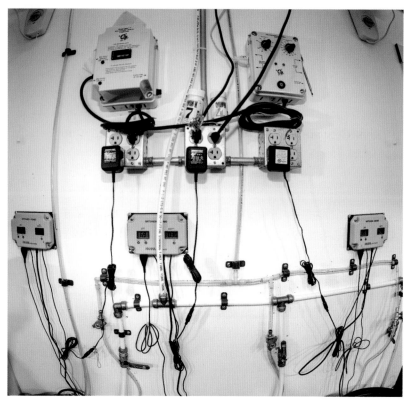

The wiring here is acceptable, although on an industrial scale, hardwiring is preferred. Equipment visible here includes reservoir monitors and environmental controllers.

Atmospheric CO_2 levels can be as high as 400 to 450 PPM. If you ensure that your growroom has very good ventilation and good circulation fans, the plants should have more than enough CO_2. Depending on the size of your chambers, your needs can range from 500 to 2,000 PPM. However, more than 2,000 PPM of CO_2 does not do the plants any good. Extremely high light densities require 2,000 PPM of CO_2. Work up to the higher levels slowly, because all other factors must be in excellent working order for the plants to photosynthesize these higher amounts.

Your plants do not need CO_2 in the dark. Switch on the CO_2 half an hour after the lights come on—after the fans' intake and exhaust go off (they should be turned on first thing in the morning) – and shut it off half an hour before the lights go off. This ensures that the CO_2 is used up before the lights go off. Cease CO_2 injections 7 to 14 days prior to harvest, to ensure complete ripening of flowers/buds.

Oscillating fans must also be placed at the floor level to circulate the heavier CO_2 to the plants. Some growing chambers may need a complete air change every hour to make sure that CO_2 and air are constantly being exchanged. Weather-stripping on doors can eliminate CO_2 loss and leakage. You must circulate CO_2 up from the floor or inject it directly into the fan to ensure good coverage among the plants.

Again, if your garden is not completely fine-tuned, 2,000 PPM of CO_2 can be toxic. Increase levels slowly until you completely understand how it works. If you do not get a 25-30% increase in plant growth, examine the levels of light and root oxygen available to your plant. Higher levels of CO_2 require higher temperatures—80°F. Be aware: this will dramatically increase the water and nutrient usage.

CO₂: Distance / Level

Lights	Distance From Plant	CO₂ Needed for Sugar Production
HID Lamps	4 feet (120 cm)	Ambient*
	3 feet (90 cm)	400 PPM
	2 feet (60 cm)	1,000 PPM
	1 foot (30 cm)	2,000 PPM

Note: these figures are based on running all plant resources available at maximum and at a temperature of 80°F. Also note that you would never place a plant within a foot of a light unless it was air-cooled.

* Ambient CO_2 in the cities is between 400 to 450 PPM.

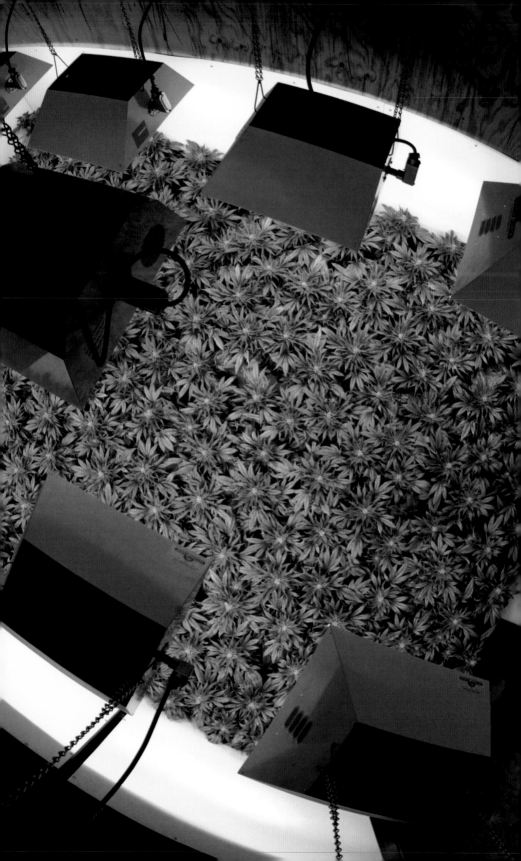

CHAPTER 7

Lighting

Artificial or supplemental lighting is an essential part of indoor cultivation. Plants do not grow without light. Provided in the following text are some examples of different lights and charts to show the appropriate distances between your plants and the lights. In greenhouses, simple incandescent light bulbs can be used to extend the light cycle so that plants won't begin to flower prematurely. All lights must be hung securely, preferably from properly anchored eyelets connected to adjustable chains or adjustable yo-yos designed for this purpose. These are available online and from grow stores. Always make sure all lights are as level as possible, not tilted to one side or the other, and never allow ballast or light cords to sit on the ground where they may get wet or damaged. Always use top-quality, heavy-duty timers.

The choice of lights is endless. There are so many different manufacturers, and they all claim to be the best. Today, there are many high tech lighting options available. Growers can utilize compact fluorescents and induction lights, as well as LEDs, for cloning and vegetative growth for the purpose of heat reduction and savings in cooling costs.

There are many HID lights available, as well. GAVITA Lighting, ePapillon growlights, and Solis Tek all make great HID lights.

Some growers prefer to use plasma lighting. While the costs of a plasma light is high, they have a long life expectancy, and are very, very efficient. All of these lights offer the most usable light spectrums for marijuana—

◀ A special overhead view.

Photo: Freebie

Air-Cooled Lighting Systems

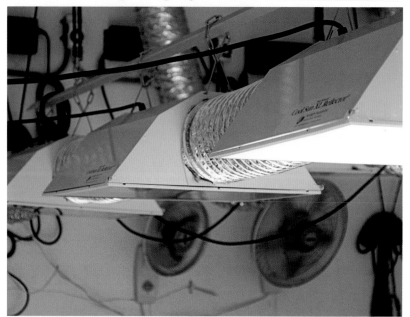

Air-cooled lights.

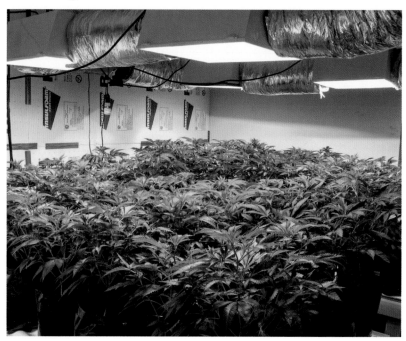

Air-cooled lights in a grow room.

Bottom Photo: Cannanetics

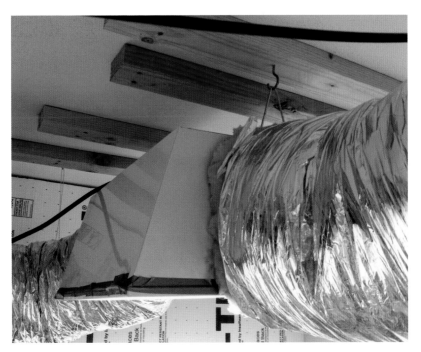

Insulated ducting on the air-cooled lights.

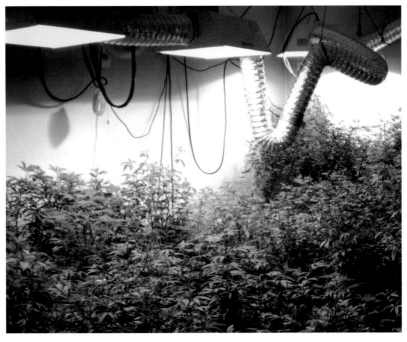

Air-cooled lighting setup in clone mother room.

red, blue, and so on. Don't be tempted to use low-cost, substandard lighting equipment. It is inefficient and could be dangerous. Jorge Cervantes's *Grower's Bible* explains everything to do with lighting, and if you have further inquiry into this subject, I would direct you there.

Air-Cooled Lights

In addition to fans and cooling systems (see chapter 6), air-cooled lights are a smart purchase. A good example is the Radiant Hood AC 8" ducted hood with a hinged sealed reflector and eight-inch air-in and -out flanges, which is available at your local hydroponics supply store. This enables maximum airflow through the hood without any CO_2 loss. It can decrease the heat in your rooms substantially, which in turn reduces the amount of ventilation you need, which in turn keeps your precious CO_2 where it should be. Remember, your average HID light can increase the temperature directly around it by as much as 300°F! Air-cooled lights are the answer.

> **Tip:** The Equalizer Hot Spot Diffuser will prevent hot spots from forming in the canopy and prevent leaf burn.

Light Coverage and Layout

These are examples of different ways to utilize and spread more light using multiple lower wattage fixtures. For small chambers use 400-watt lights for vegetative growth. Medium chambers utilize 600-watt lights. For large chambers such as the ones designed by Trichome Technologies, only use 1000-watt lights.

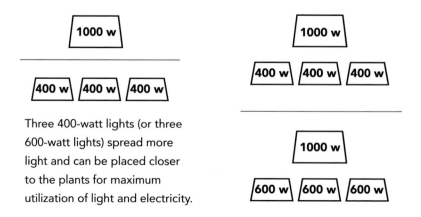

Three 400-watt lights (or three 600-watt lights) spread more light and can be placed closer to the plants for maximum utilization of light and electricity.

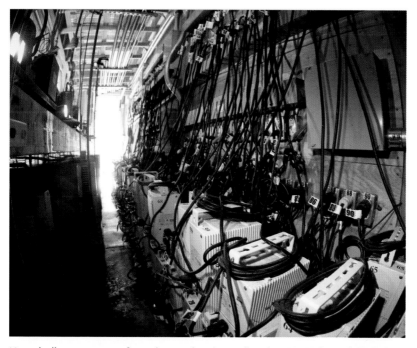

Keep ballasts separate from the garden, but still within 20-40 feet of the lights.

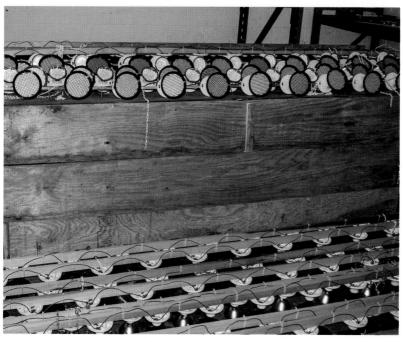

Large bank of LED lights for a grow room.

Top Photo: Freebie Bottom Photo: Dr. Dog and Blackra1n

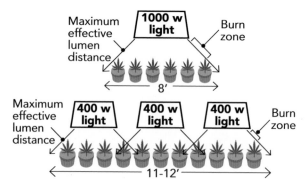

While a single 1,000-watt light could burn plants if placed too low, three 400-watt lights can be placed closer to the plants for maximum utilization of lights and electricity without damage.

Light Distance from Plants

If lights are placed too close to plants, radiant heat from the bulb will burn the plants. Below is an approximation chart depicting light vs. distance for a given area. Note: air-cooled lights can get slightly closer than standard, non-air-cooled lights. The chart below is for standard, non-air-cooled lights.

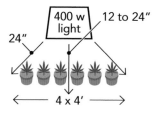

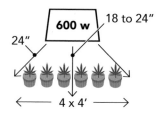

400-watt light at 12–24" away from plant 4' x 4'

600-watt light at 18–24" away from plant 4' x 4'

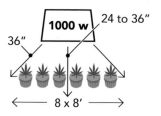

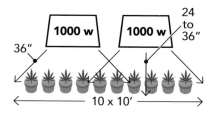

1,000-watt light at 24–36" away from plant 8' x 8'

Two 1,000-watt lights at 24–36" away from plant 10' x 10'

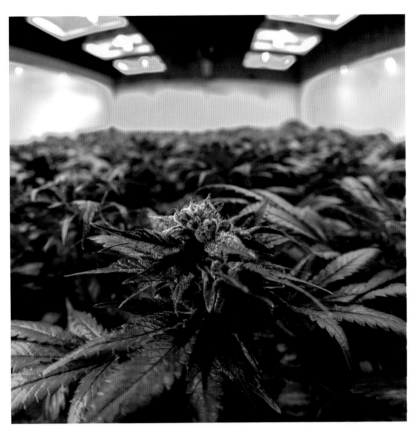

This will help you when you are feeling blue.

Light–Ballast Distances

With the high-powered lights you'll be using, you need to be careful about the distance of the light from the ballast. Here are a few general rules, but it is always wise to consult an electrician or, as a second choice, a manual.

MHs (Metal Halides) are ordinarily safe at up to 40 feet. Any longer and you'll want to use 240 volts.

If you need to go longer distances, 12-gauge wire should be used in place of the standard household 14-gauge.

SHs (Sodium Halides) are ordinarily safe at up to 20 feet. Any longer and you should use 240 volts.

240-volt ballasts typically run cooler and use less power, and therefore are preferred if your electric system permits; most only permit 110 volts. Also, 240-volt ballasts usually last longer than 110-volt ballasts.

Photo: Freebie

Basic Bullets

■ Clones receive 24 hours of light. Vegetative growth requires 18 hours of light and 6 hours of uninterrupted, complete darkness. Flowering growth requires 12 on / 12 off.

■ The name for this division of light and dark is the photoperiod.

■ If you must enter or work inside the chambers in the night cycle, use a flashlight or light with a green filter or bulb. This will keep you from interrupting the cycle.

■ To maximize light, walls or panels must be painted flat white to reflect stray light back to where it is needed. Gloss white is easier to clean, but reflects less. Mylar is the best reflective material available, but is hard to clean, hang, and maintain. At Trichome Technologies, we use plastic polypropylene panels to reflect the light to where we want it. These are easy to clean and maintain.

Plant Rotation for Maximizing Light

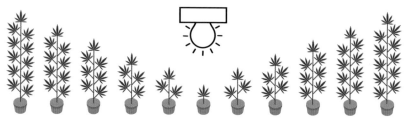

Rotate plants so they receive the maximum light. The smallest plants should be closest to the light, and the tallest plants should be incrementally further away, like stadium seats. Plants should be close together, but not so close that they throw shade on each other.

UVB Light

Knowledgeable scientists have published many articles pertaining to the benefits of UVB light rays on plants, and cannabis plants in particular. Many acknowledge that plants grown at high altitudes produce more THC via larger trichome heads. If you took two identical plants and grew them under identical conditions, except one was grown at a 5,000–6,000-foot elevation and the other at sea level, the plant that was grown at high elevation would be superior to the sea level plant in terms of THC content. Some attribute the difference to the drastic temperature differential between day and night at

Types of Lights: LED Lights

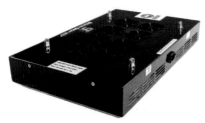 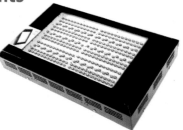

Back side of an LED light. Hooks for hanging LED from ceiling visible.

Front of the LED light. The light emitting diodes are visible.

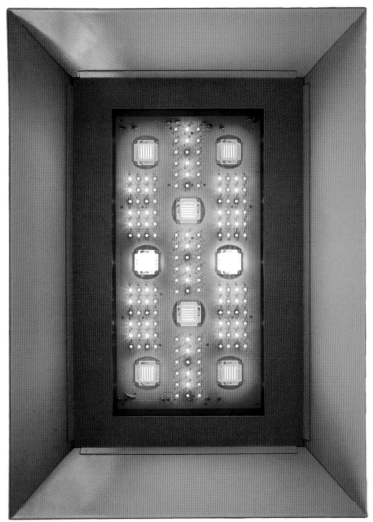

This LED has a light spectrum mix optimized for growing cannabis.

Photos: Stealth Grow LED Lights

Types of Lights: HIDs and Fluorescents

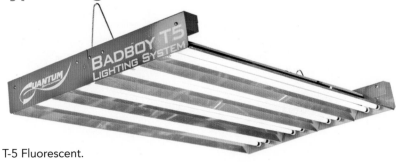

T-5 Fluorescent.

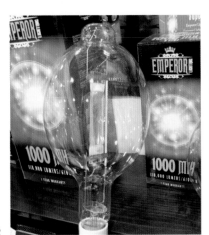

Metal Halide.

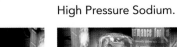

High Pressure Sodium.

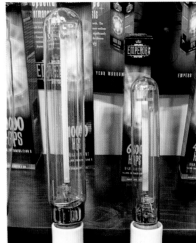

600-watt HPS.

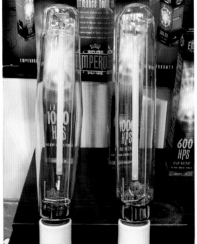

1000-watt HPS.

Top Photo: Quantum Horticulture Bottom Photos: Stoned Rosie

HID Lighting and Fluorescent Lighting

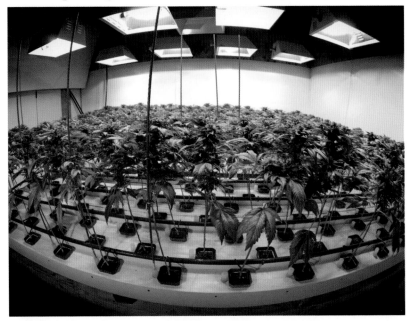

Uniform canopy on a garden beneath a bank of 8 HID lights.

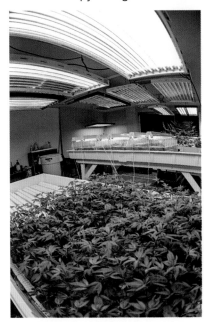

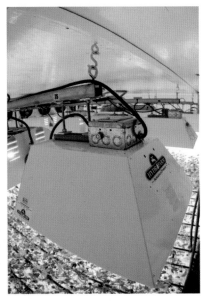

Banks of fluorescent lights above clones.

HID lamp hanging above garden. Note the sturdy chain holding the lamp in place.

Photos: Freebie

HID Lighting and Fluorescent Lighting

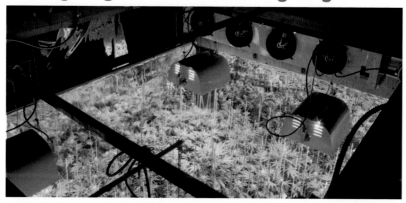

Evenly spaced HID lamps above a Trichome Tech grow room circa 1996.

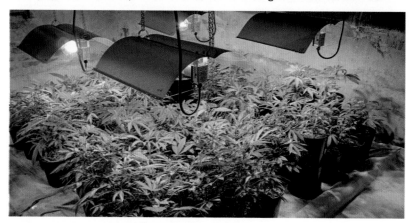

Plants vegging under metal halide lamps.

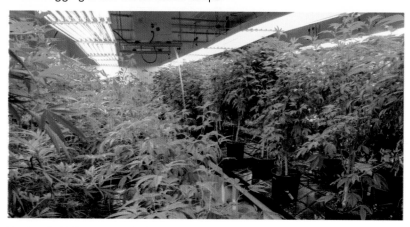

Photos: Mel Frank

Banks of T5 fluorescent lights in a mother room.

such altitudes; I do not believe this to be so. This no doubt has something to do with it, but I believe the increased UVB exposure is the primary cause of the plants' increased THC productivity.

Increased UVB exposure triggers the plants' survival responses and it responds by producing more oil and resin, which are then pumped into the glands in an effort to make the trichome heads larger and so act as a form of sun screen. The bigger and more resin glands there are, the less UVB, UVA, and UVC will be exposed to the plants' surface.

Black lights emit ultraviolet (UV) light but are unacceptable for plant growth, as are UVB enhancers added to existing lighting.

Note that there has been no formal compilation of scientific data to confirm this theory regarding UV light as true, and it is only mere speculation at this point. Hopefully in the future we will compile true data on this subject and either prove or disprove the theory once and for all.

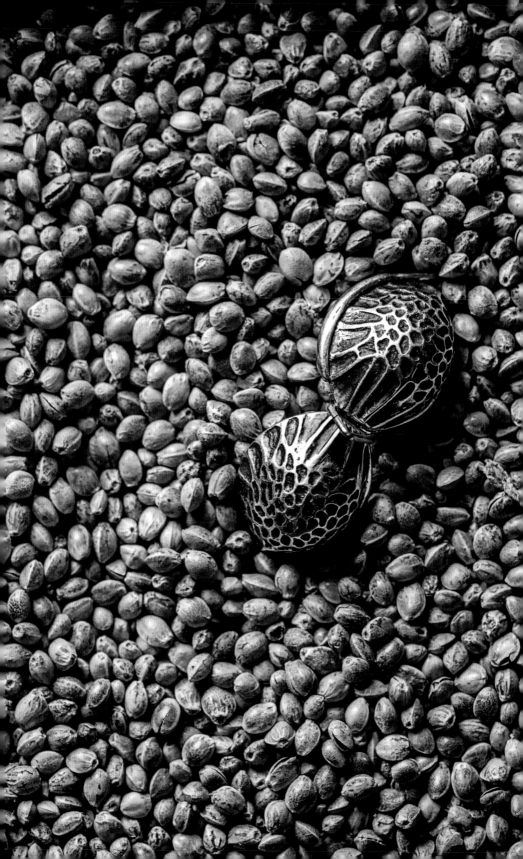

CHAPTER 8

Choosing a Cultivar

Choosing what type of cannabis to grow is a decision only you can make, but it must be an informed decision. You need to know the ins and outs of the cultivar you are growing: its characteristics, idiosyncrasies, and cultivation needs and methods; essentially, its pros and cons. Be sure to choose the right genetic cultivar for your specific environment.

Cannabis Sativa

Sativa is a fantastic subspecies of cannabis and grows outstandingly outdoors. However, it is very problematic indoors and has many negative, undesirable characteristics; it can be particularly difficult to work into an indoor symbiotic rotation (but it can be done; see chapter 3). Sativas grow tall, with large internodal distances that produce airy, loose flowers that can take 8 to 16 weeks to mature.

Cannabis Indica

Indica is also an incredible subspecies of cannabis. It can be finicky and sometimes slightly difficult to cultivate to its full potential, and usually yields low to medium harvests, but is very high in tetrahydracannabinol (THC).

◀ Landrace cannabis seeds from Afghanistan. Note the variety of shape, size, and color.

Old School Genetics

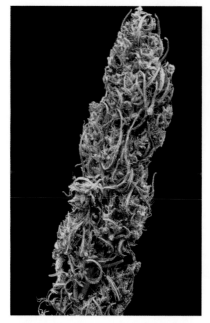

Dried cola from an Afghani Red.

Nug of Purple Plum.

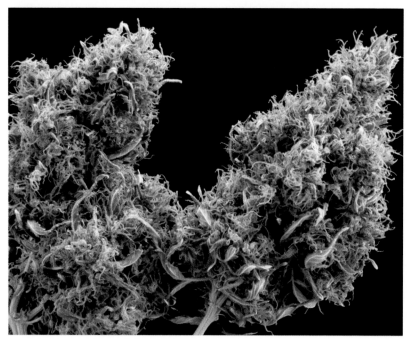

Photos: Mel Frank

This cultivar is called California Red Head, circa 1996.

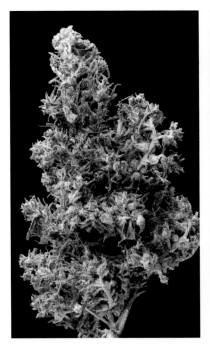

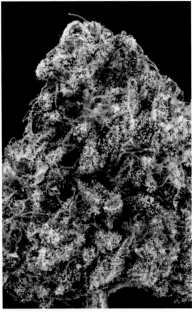

Dried bud of Haze.

Orange pistils visible on a bud of Blackberry.

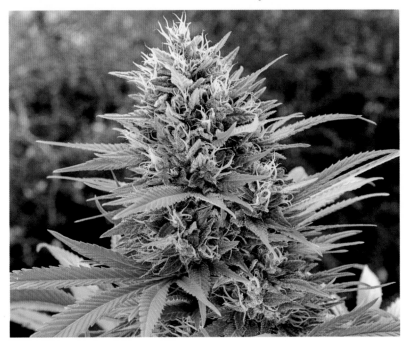

Maui #4 flowering and healthy.

Old School Genetics

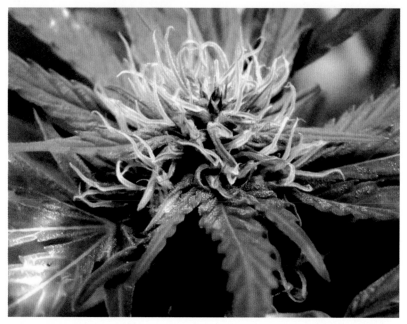

Lovely flower on a Pink Bud Afghani plant (Afghani x African), circa 1982.

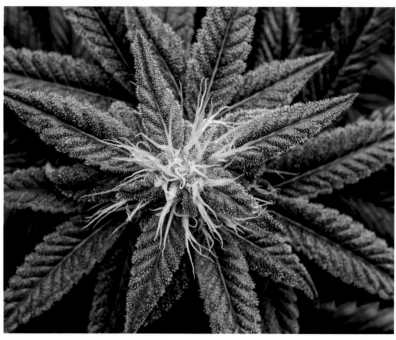

Photos: Mel Frank

Flower from a Garlic (Old Timer) cultivar growing under an LED light.

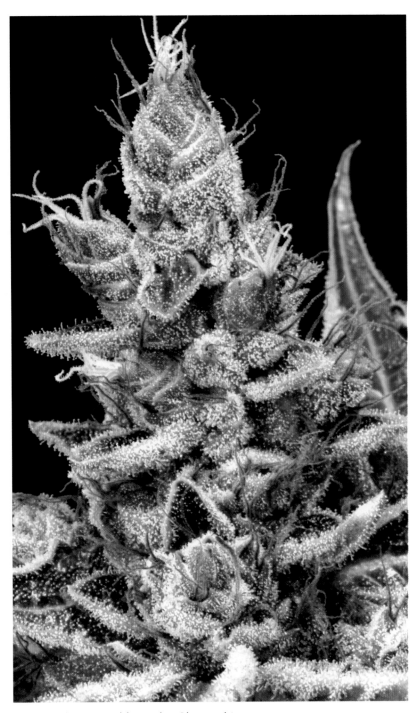

Frosty trichomes visible on this Ghost cultivar.

Landrace Genetics

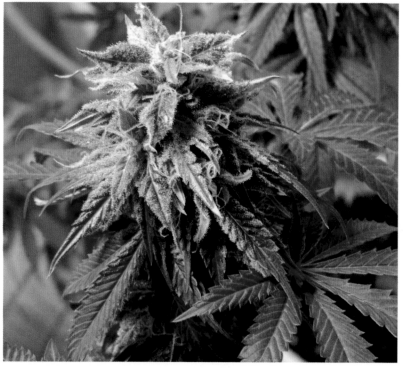

Leaves from landrace Afghani plant known locally as "Afghani Mountain Black."

Landrace Afghani from Kandahar in flower.

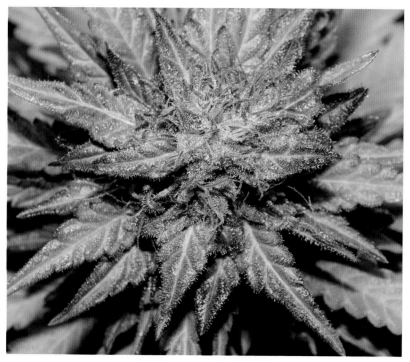

Landrace Afghani Mountain Black plant in flower.

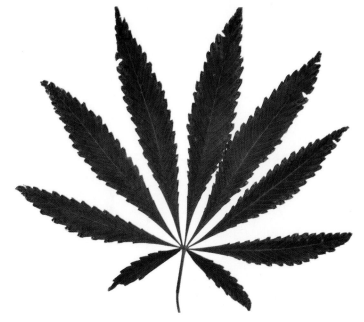

Leaf from a landrace plant from Himachal Pradesh.

Landrace Genetics

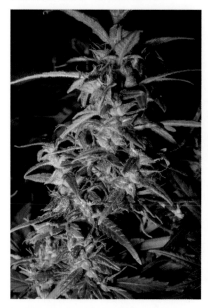

Landrace plant from Himachal Pradesh in flower.

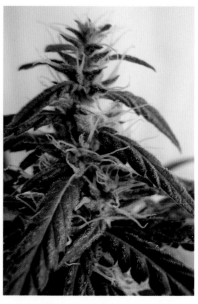

Landrace Thai in flower.

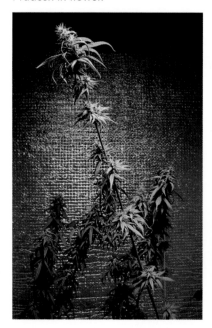

Landrace plant from Mazar-i-Sharif.

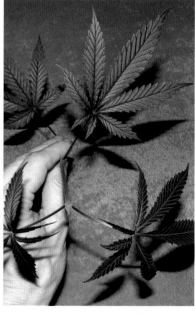

Leaves from a landrace plant from Russia.

Trichome Technologies' version of indica-dominant cultivar G-13 was tested by the University of Mississippi's Mahmoud ElSohly (ElSohly Laboratories, Inc.) and he found 27.2% THC. I love pure indicas—the potent smells and flavors vary from spicy to fruity and are excellent for producing hashish and hashish oil.

Cannabis Indica / Sativa Hybrids

Cannabis indica / sativa hybrids are bred from the best of both worlds; ideally, the best parts of indica and sativa parents. Many of the best cultivars available from seed breeders today are indica / sativa hybrids. There are dozens of seed companies offering the world's best cultivars and phenotypes that are bred for high yield, high resin production, and high THC, cannabinol (CBN), and cannabidiol (CBD) content.

Getting Seeds

Research and isolate the exact cultivars for your specific requirements and desires. Good quality seeds are available through many online merchants, some reputable, some not. It is recommended that you purchase direct from the breeder the cultivars you desire.

Beware! It is illegal to import and cultivate cannabis seeds, or plants, for that matter. The American government aggressively continues to pursue its

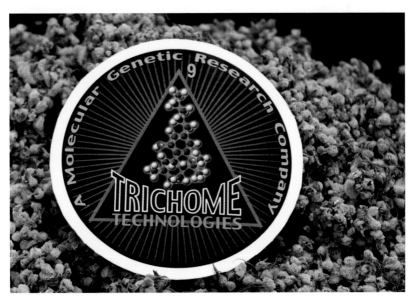

Photo: Samson Daniels

Company logo on a bed of ripe bracts.

Australian Sativas

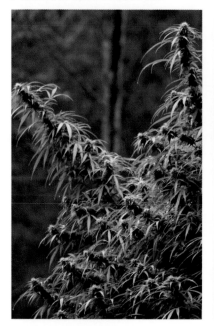

Australian sativa at dusk.

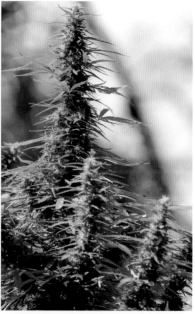

Pure sativa in Aussie sunshine.

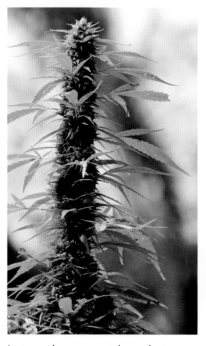

Large cola on an outdoor plant.

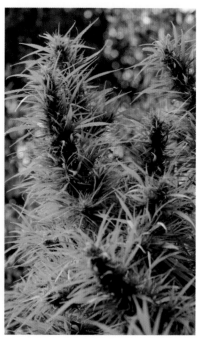

Thin leaves and big colas.

Photo: Kangativa

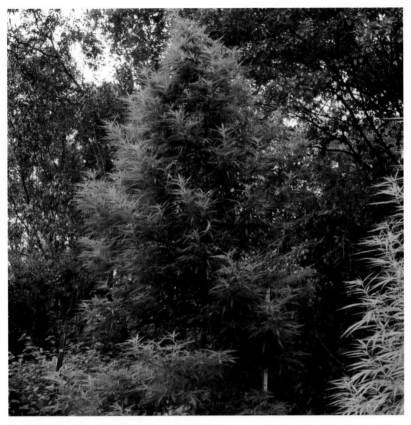

This cultivar is a Hmong Thai sativa cultivar grown in Oz to over 15 feet in height.

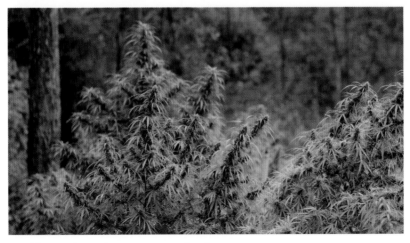

Healthy outdoor plants grown under the sun.

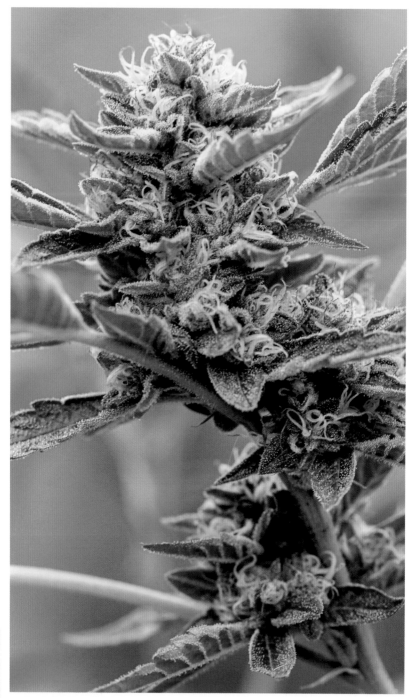

Photo: Mel Frank

Flower on a landrace Pakistani plant.

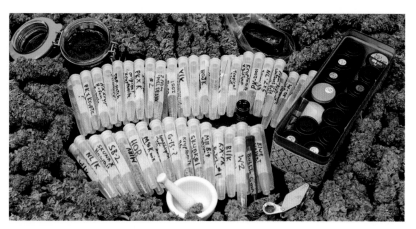

A selection from K's enormous seed collection.

crusade against international seed merchants that distribute seeds in the U.S.A. and the rest of the world. Only accept or purchase clones from a trusted, qualified professional or a reputable grower / cannabis club. Do not buy seeds from disreputable online sources or places such as eBay!

Storing Seeds

Store seeds in a cool, dark place to ensure future viability. Keep the humidity as low as possible; refrigeration or freezing is not recommended. Seal the seeds in an airtight container with a packet of silica gel and store someplace like a dry basement or the bottom of your closet. They can be kept for five to ten years if properly stored, although the longer they are retained, the less viable they become.

Clones

Clones are perfect for accelerating the production process given that they are clean (insect, mold, and mildew free), guaranteed female, and of known origin and genetic background. Install new clones in the vegetative chamber for 14–21 days and re-clone from the originals. This will dramatically increase your numbers and advance your growth cycle rotation. This saves you the time and the process of starting from seeds.

Some landrace cultivars and current genetics are only available as clones. Clones are perfect when installed in outdoor gardens—by cloning in late winter or early spring, your plants have a long growing time and a head start on spring and summer.

Photo: Samson Daniels

129

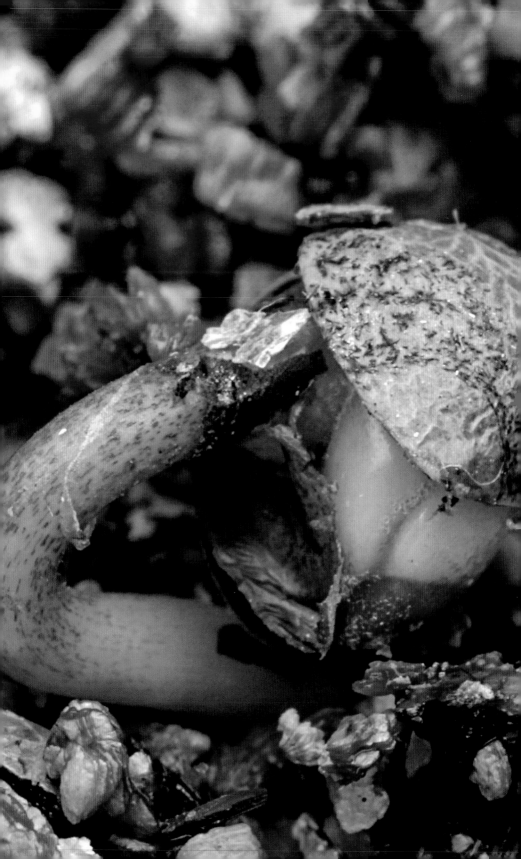

CHAPTER 9

Seed Germination

At Trichome Technologies, we use two basic seed germination techniques: for small seed germination needs, say 100 seeds or less, we use large 24 x 36 x 8-inch clear Tupperware containers. We drill one $1/4$-inch hole for drainage in the bottom and two $1/4$-inch holes for airflow in the lid. We place light diffusers in the bottom of the container, which allows 3-inch rockwool cubes to drain. With the lid closed, it is the perfect environment.

A light diffuser is a plastic sheet of small $1/2$-inch squares. It is used in overhead lighting to direct light straight down. They are available from most hardware and lighting stores, but do not use chrome-plated plastic diffusers—only white. The chrome will come off when exposed to nutrients, etc.

Germinating pads are placed underneath to provide heat—the temperature should be kept at 78°F. Some cultivars prefer higher or lower temperatures, ranging from 70–80°F, but whatever the temperature, it must remain constant. Anything higher or lower than these parameters is not ideal for seed germination. Place a thermometer or digital temperature probe in the medium so you can constantly monitor the temperature and keep it exactly where you want it.

◀ Sprouting seed emerging with the seed husk still attached to the cotyledon. Leave it to fall off on its own as seedlings are quite fragile.

Photo: Mel Frank

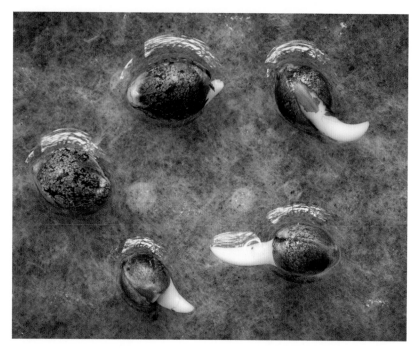

Seeds germinating with the white taproot emerging. Plant the taproot facing down when the time comes and be gentle, they can be easily damaged.

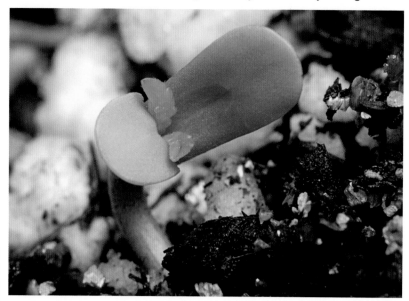

Seedling emerges. The two broad leaves are called cotyledons, and the two small leaves emerging are the first true leaves of the baby cannabis plant.

Photos: Mel Frank

Determining Cannabis / Marijuana Plant Sex

Determining plant sex early is important for good growing. You must identify plant sex as early as possible during the vegetative stage. Males must be quickly removed and destroyed / properly disposed of before they produce pollen or else your crop will go to seed. If you've started from clones of a known female sex, then you're assured that the plants will be female (unless plant stress causes hermaphrodites).

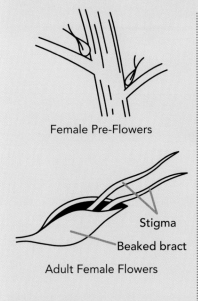

Female Pre-Flowers

Adult Female Flowers

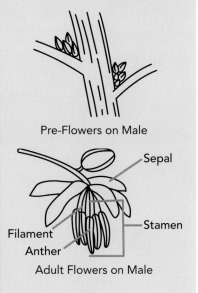

Pre-Flowers on Male

Adult Flowers on Male

Female pistillate flowers have a teardrop shaped bract with two tiny, thin, white stigma protruding.

Male staminate flowers form tiny oval ball-like clusters that extend from the stem on their own stem like micro bunches of bananas.

For lighting, 4-foot cool white fluorescent fixtures, with 2 bulbs per fixture and 2 fixtures per propagation chamber, are used. We prefer 3-inch Grodan rockwool cubes with 2-inch diameter pre-made plug holes in the center. We place a soilless mix of equal parts fine sifted potting soil, perlite, and vermiculite, with a little horticultural sand mixed in to aid drainage and oxygenation. Instead of using rockwool cubes for germination, use the same soilless mix in small 3-inch containers. Seeds are pre-washed in a 2% bleach solution for one minute to eliminate fungal attacks, and then dried off. We then lightly score them on the edge

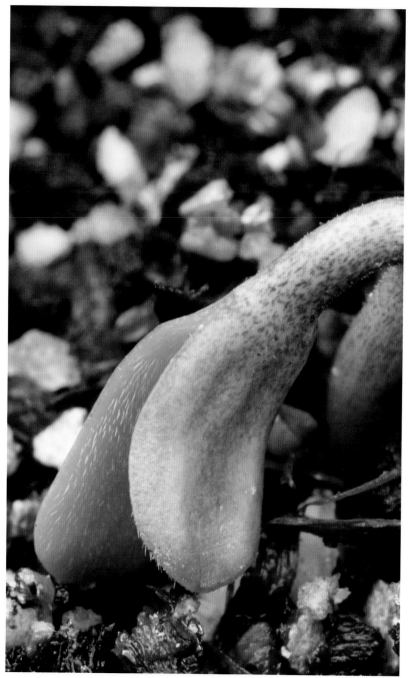

Photo: Mel Frank

Cotyledon visible on a seedling that just emerged. It produced 3 pounds six months later.

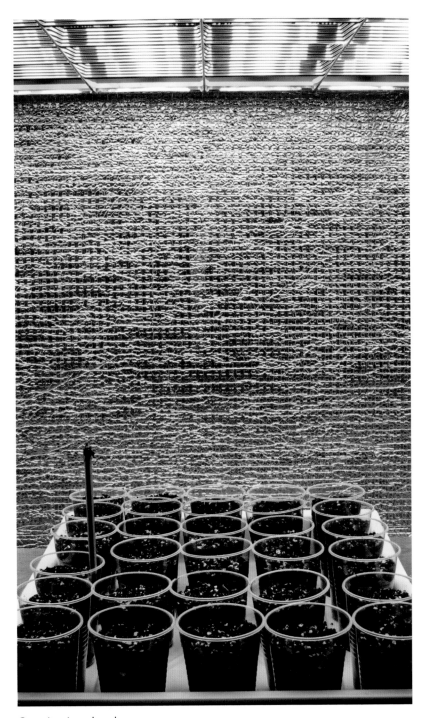

Germination chamber.

with a nail file and place them in a jar of distilled water (at 78°F) for 24 hours. Seeds are then placed between 4 folded paper towels and moistened with distilled water. Finally, they are placed onto Pyrex plates with Pyrex lids on top. The plates are placed in chambers to maintain a constant temperature utilizing germination / heat mats (keep temperature approximately 78°F).

The seeds will germinate in 2 to 7 days. There are some cultivars that take up to 14 days, but this is rare. Water them daily, but do not soak, and never let them dry out—always keep them moist. After sprouting, decontaminate a pair of rubber-tipped tweezers with alcohol, dry thoroughly, and gently place sprouts, with the white tip pointing down, $1/4$-inch into flushed, pH-adjusted, and pre-moistened soilless mix in rockwool cubes. Carefully cover them with medium and water them with distilled water only. After 7 days, water with $1/4$ strength fertilizer—vegetative mix.

Place the chambers over germination / heating pads to elevate temperature inside, then raise or lower the chambers to achieve optimum temperature. Try to keep the temperature at 78°F. Seedlings need oxygen, so monitor moisture levels several times a day and open chambers to allow fresh oxygen in. The cubes are now ready to be placed in the decontaminated chambers. Chambers can then be placed over, not onto, germination pads and under lights.

When the sprouts start to appear, take the covers off the chambers. Continue to provide 16–18 hours of fluorescent lighting, kept at approximately 6–8 inches above seedlings, for 2–3 weeks. Use $1/4$ then $1/2$-strength nutrients or fertilizers until the average seedling is 4–6 inches tall; then transfer them to 600-watt, MH HID lighted chambers. For the first 24 hours, the MH HID must be kept 3–4 feet from seedlings, then lowered to the proper height of about 1–2 feet. Throughout the seedling stage, all lights must be on for 16–18 hours and off for 6–8 hours, depending on your chosen lighting regimen.

Propagating Clones / Germinating Seeds Intended for Outdoor Growth

When propagating clones or germinating seeds intended for outdoor growth, you must germinate using a 12-hour on / 12-hour off light cycle for the first 30 days. Then, you can switch to a 16-hour on / 8-hour off light cycle. Clones must be taken from a plant that is on a 16/8 light cycle and kept on that cycle until they're ready to be placed outside. After that, the light cycle must be adjusted to approximate outside lighting conditions and the plants must be hardened

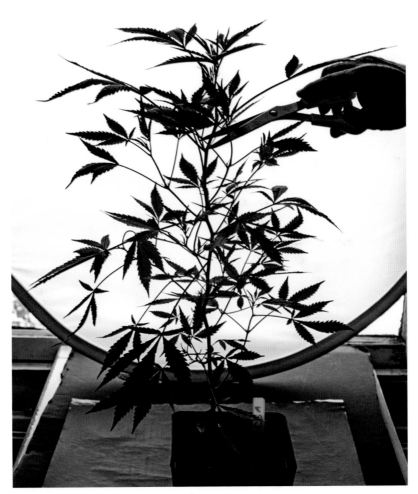

When cloning for sex, you take a single clone from an early veg plant like this, and then flower the clone in your flowering chamber to get an early determination of the veg plant's sex.

off before finally being placed outside permanently. This terminology is explained further in the cloning chapter. The purpose of all this is to simulate springtime lighting conditions. If you placed the clones / seedlings that had been acclimated to an 18-hours on / 6-hours off photoperiod directly outside, they would immediately begin to flower for a couple of weeks before reverting back to vegetative growth, which is a waste of limited, valuable time. However, if you want short plants, you can place them directly outside after an 18/6 photoperiod late in the growth season, and they will begin to flower immediately

Photo: Ed Borg

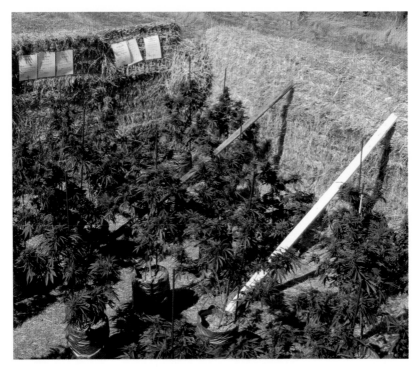

Hay bale garden.

and continue until they are finished. In other words, they won't revert back to vegetative growth, thus allowing you to harvest earlier in the summer, rather than waiting until fall. The goal is to replicate the springtime light cycle that exists outside at the time you are planting, after hardening off. This principle applies to both clones and seedlings to be placed outside. You are trying to replicate true daylight hours, not sunrise / sunset. The best way to achieve this is to add two hours to the time of your local official sunrise and sunset.

Determining Plant Sex

Cannabis is a dioecious plant, meaning that the female and male flowers develop on separate plants. That said, monoecious plants—those that have both male and female flowers on one plant, also known as hermaphrodites—also commonly exist. It is often difficult to determine a marijuana plant's sex in its first seven weeks of vegetative growth. Male plants can grow taller and more rapidly than females, but as a rule there is no way of differentiating between male and female in the very early stages. Under normal conditions, cannabis

Photos: K

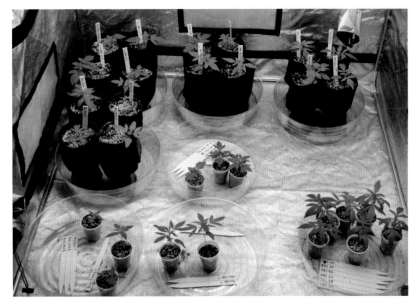

Grow huts such as this one are perfect for cloning or starting seeds, and are readily available and easy to put up and take down.

seeds produce an approximate ratio of 50% male and 50% female plants.

Determining a plant's sex requires close visual inspection using a jeweler's loupe and good lighting, or a loupe with a built-in light. You must understand where preflowers form and exactly what male and female preflowers look like. Typically, the first preflowers appear eight to ten weeks after seed germination with the formation of undifferentiated primordial flowers along the main stalk at the nodes (also known as "crotches" or "intersections,") where the fan leaves, petiole, and branches stem from and meet at the nodes, behind the stipule (leaf spur). If you are lucky, upon first inspection you will find a preflower tucked in among these plant parts.

When the primordial flowers first appear, they are undifferentiated sexually. The tiny preflower is typically 2–10mm in length and is a determining indicator as to whether the plant will be found to be male or female. Males can sometimes be difficult to identify for a novice, but you must be vigilant and eliminate all males at the first opportunity (unless you are breeding).

Male preflowers are typically very small, ranging in size from 2–7mm. They develop in multiple forms. According to Mel Frank, one variation is flat, spade-shaped, and raised on a short stalk; another is pod-shaped and extremely tiny

(2–3mm), either with or without a stalk; and a third variation is teardrop-shaped, stalkless, and easily confused with the female preflower (without its stigmas). Any plant expressing the third type of preflower should be kept for later reinspection.

Female primordial flowers appear as normal (albeit very small) female flowers / bracts / stigmas, the exception being that they form singularly, and never in multiples or as buds. Occasionally only the bract casing (protective seed pod) appears without the V-shaped fuzzy white stigmas present. Upon inspection, if you see a well-developed female flower with the stigmas (pollen-catching appendages) extended to form a V-shape at two or more nodes toward the top of the plant, this is the first indicator that the plant is female. Once you have experience examining, identifying, and interpreting preflowers you will see that if the preflower is raised or has a stalk, it is a male; female preflowers are without stalks.

If you have never identified preflowers you should wait another one or two weeks before discarding the suspected male plants, allowing time for a second inspection. If the first sexing is proved correct by the later preflower formation, you can then begin to eliminate males as and if you wish. If you are unsure of your determination, you can label all of the plants and wait until the flowering cycle begins to make absolutely sure, but you must eliminate the males as soon as possible to prevent seeded buds.

Cloning for Sex

Your next option is to clone for sex (see the full explanation of this in the cloning chapter). This works very well for indoor and outdoor plants. Simply remove a branch / clone and place it in proper propagation conditions under a 12/12 photoperiod. Preflowers will form, along with roots, and indicate plant sex without subjecting the original donor plant to the undue stress of having light prematurely reduced. You must always check and recheck the plants throughout the flowering cycles. Females can sometimes become hermaphrodites and form random male flower clusters within the female flowers. The male flowers can pollinate the female flowers and will produce seeds.

Important: as stated before, if this is your first try at plant sexing, it is recommended that you label all plants either male or female and learn from any misidentification, rather than by mistakenly eliminating any females. Learn from trial and error. Be vigilant. Check and recheck.

Environmental Influences on Plant Sex

It has been scientifically proven that plant sex can be influenced during the early stages of vegetative growth. The sex of your seedlings is predisposed to gender chromosomes encoded in its DNA. While certainly not a golden rule (each cultivar reacts slightly differently), nor with a 100% effective success rate, the following explanations and steps are to aid you in producing the sex of plants you desire (male vs. female). Some seed companies use a simple technique with gibberellic acid sprays to produce feminized seeds. The sprayed female plants produce male flowers / pollen. That, in turn, is used to produce feminized seeds. However, factors such as the environment can also influence gender. Environmental stresses—i.e., erratic lighting schedules, excessive heat or cold, over- or under-fertilization, etc.—will produce a high percentage of males and hermaphrodites. It is important that you introduce these environmental changes at the three-pairs-of-leaves stage and continue for two to three weeks before returning to normal conditions. Other methods of producing pollen from a female plant are: 1) erratic lighting schedules, 2) excessive heat or cold, and 3) over- or under-fertilization, all of which will produce hermaphrodites that will produce pollen that will then produce feminized seeds.

In order to improve your chances of getting the desired result when germinating seeds, follow this table:

Factors For More Males or Females

More FEMALE plants	More MALE plants
Increased moisture in the growing medium (*not* over-watered or constantly soggy)	Less moisture in the growing medium (*not* dry)
High humidity	Low humidity
Lower temperatures	Warmer temperatures
Fewer hours of light (14 hours)	More hours of light (18 hours)
Increased levels of blue light spectrum	Increased levels of red light spectrum
Increased nitrogen levels (N in NPK ratio)*	Lower nitrogen levels
Lower potassium levels (K in NPK ratio)	Increased potassium levels

*E.g., an increased level of nitrogen and lower level of potassium for the first two weeks increases the number of female plants.

Seed Germination with Landrace Hindu Kush

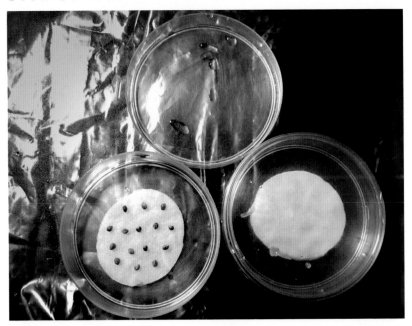

Step 1: Use your chosen germination method.

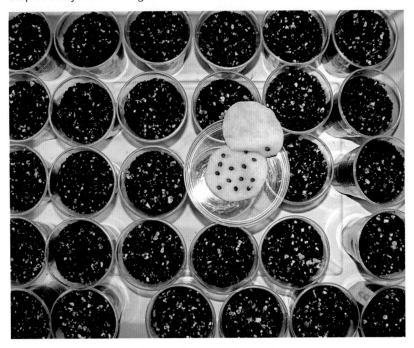

Step 2: Once seeds germinate, plant them in seed cups.

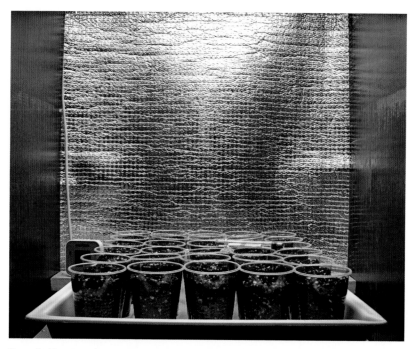

Step 3: Keep a close eye on temperature and humidity.

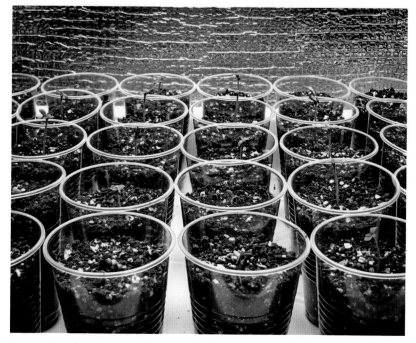

Step 4: Seedling emerges.

Seed Germination with Landrace Hindu Kush

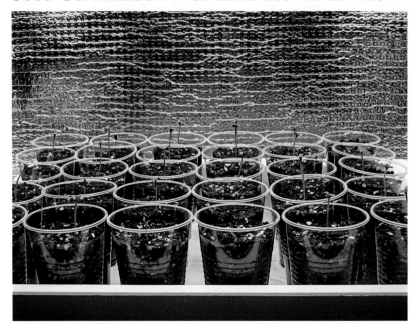

Step 5: Seedlings grow towards the light.

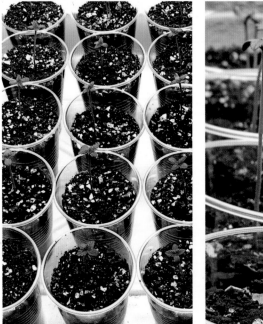

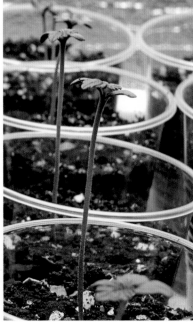

Step 6: Cotyledon and first true leaves are visible.

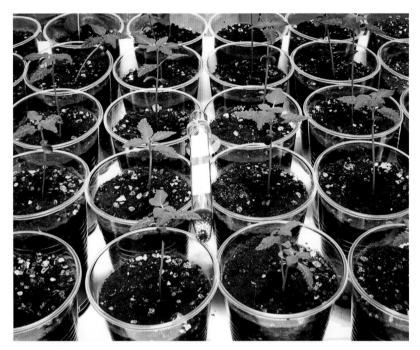

Step 7: More growth and more leaves.

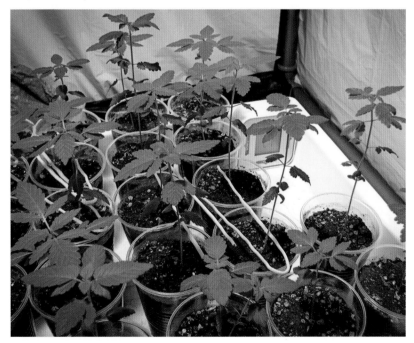

Step 8: Two weeks later.

Seed Germination with Landrace Hindu Kush

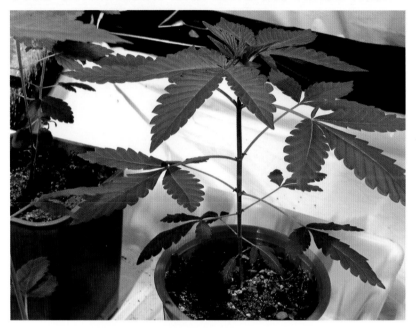

Step 9: Two-and-a-half weeks later.

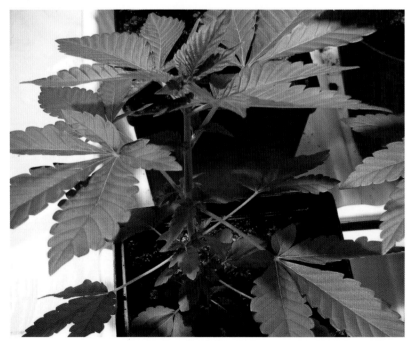

Step 10: Entering the vegetative stage.

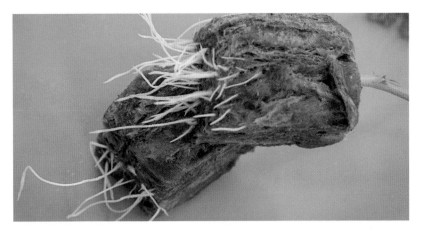

Young roots.

Temperature Guidelines

■ Keep medium at optimum temperature of 70–78°F

■ Keep air temperature at 75°F

■ Do not exceed 80°F for either the medium or the air temperature

Watering Guidelines

■ Do not over- or under-water

■ Do not dry out the growing medium

■ Never have standing water under cubes

■ Keep cubes moist, yet maintain good drainage

■ Beforehand, pH balance your medium: adjust rockwool cubes and soil to 5.8 to 6.8

Tips

■ Remember: young roots are very delicate

■ Keep records and label all seeds and seedlings

There is more to successful germination than getting a seed to sprout. Know the complete germination cycle for your cultivar. When accelerated growth occurs at 3–4 weeks, the vegetative stage of growth has begun.

If you want to know our other methods, for large scale cultivation / production, you will have to wait for the next book from Trichome Technologies which will cover major industrial-scale grows.

Photo: Samson Daniels

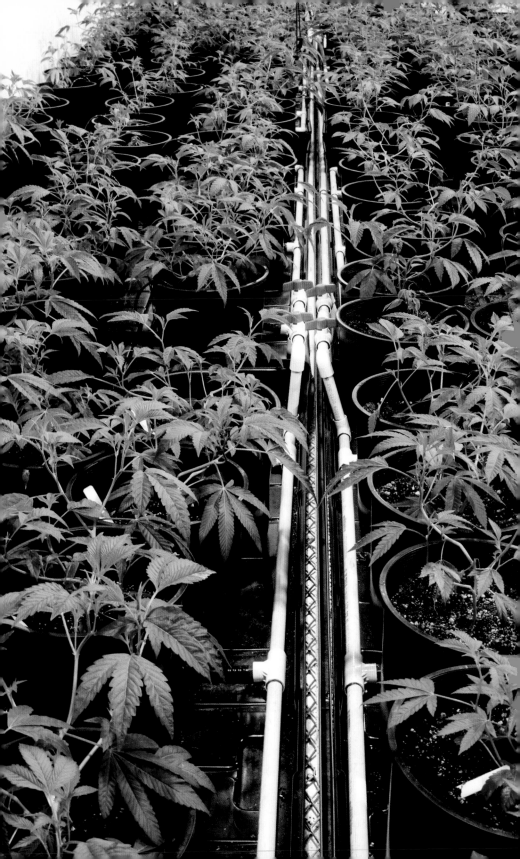

CHAPTER 10

Vegetative Growth

The vegetative stage is just as important as the clone and seedling stages. This stage can be as long or as short as you want—and by altering the photoperiod, flowering can be induced whenever you wish.

Beginnings

The vegetative stage begins as soon as clones or seedlings start rapidly producing leaves and roots. Both seeds and clones can be used to start the cultivation process, but clones are sometimes preferred to seeds, because they are of known genetic origin and are guaranteed to be female. You must know the growth pattern of the cultivars you are working with before you induce flowering: how fast or slow do they grow? In order to reach an ideal height when fully matured and finished, you should decide how tall you want the plants to be, and predict when to begin flowering accordingly.

At Trichome Technologies, we want fully matured, finished plants to be 36 inches tall, so we induce flowering when vegetative plants are 12–14 days in, or 15–18 inches tall. If you extend the vegetative cycle you will get tall plants, and if you shorten the vegetative cycle you will end up with short plants. To force or induce flowering, simply change your light cycle from 18 hours of light

◀ The drip system is feeding these vegetative plants.

Photo: Mel Frank

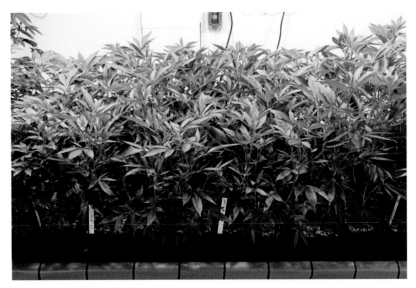

These very healthy plants have survived the clone stage, the hardening-off stage, and are ready for the vegetative stage.

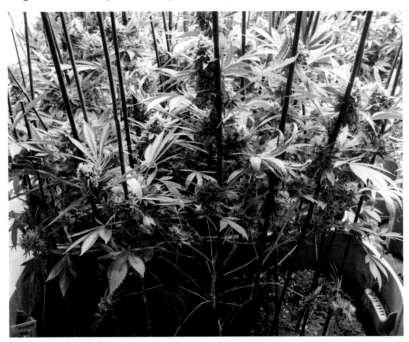

Photos: K

This plant has been grown all wrong. Too much media / soil has been used; it has no drainage; and it has way too many stakes that ultimately increase the cost of production because of the time it takes to tie and untie all the plants.

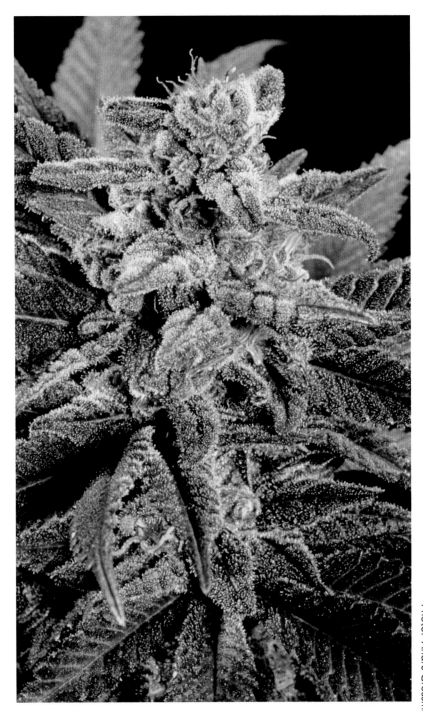

The true Kryptonite.

Photo: Andre Grossman

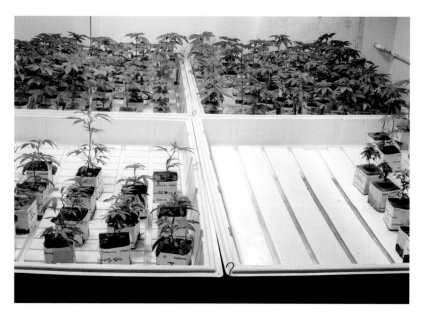

Plants just starting the vegetative cycle.

and 6 hours of darkness, to 12 hours of light and 12 hours of darkness. Out-doors, the photoperiod is dictated by nature, with shortening daylight in the late summer and fall, but indoors, artificial darkness can be created. By covering a greenhouse with blackout covering, you can create complete darkness to control the photoperiod.

At Trichome Technologies, finished clones are placed in the vegetative chambers when they are fully rooted and 4–6 inches tall. We place them under 1,000-watt MH and SH HID lights for 18 hours on and 6 hours off. The lights are kept 48 inches away from plants for 24 hours, then 36 inches for 24 hours, and finally 24–36 inches away, depending on the needs of the plant. Do not put lights too close to plants, because they might dry out, burn, or worse, die. Lights too far away will increase internodal stretching / spacing, and create spindly, leggy plants with light, airy buds. Both are unacceptable.

During the vegetative stage, plants grow rapidly for 5 to 7 days, and are completely stripped of all lower vegetation to re-stimulate vegetative growth. Over the next 5 to 7 days, the plants accelerate growth, producing the next batch of available clones. On vegetative days 10–14 (depending on cultivar), lights are changed to 12 hours on / 12 hours off. To induce flowering, 48 hours later, clones are taken from the plant.

Hindu Kush: Vegetative Stage (Grown for Seed Production)

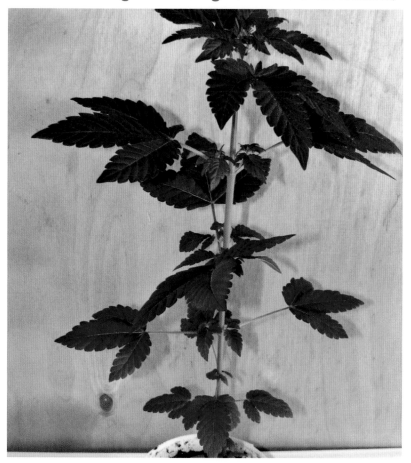

Here the Hindu Kush seen in the Germination chapter has experienced another week of fast vegetative growth.

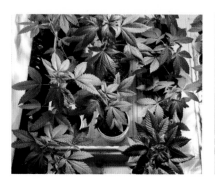
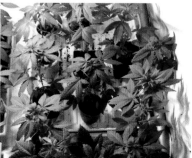

All the seedlings are now in the vegetative stage, week 2.

Hindu Kush: Vegetative Stage (Grown for Seed Production)

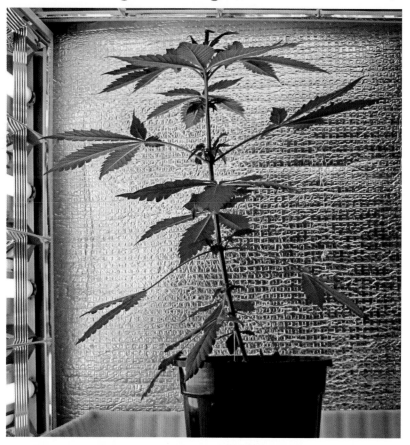

Another week older. Note the growth.

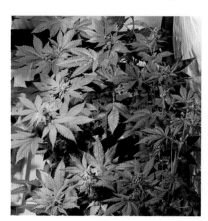
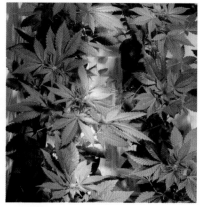

Full garden with breeding males for seed production.

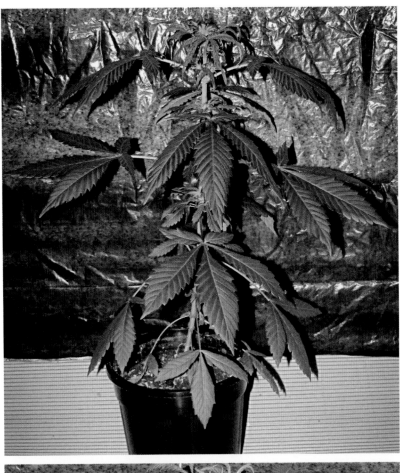

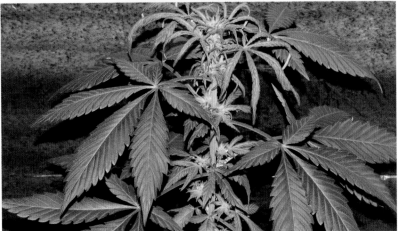

Ten days later and the plants are ready to enter the flowering stage.

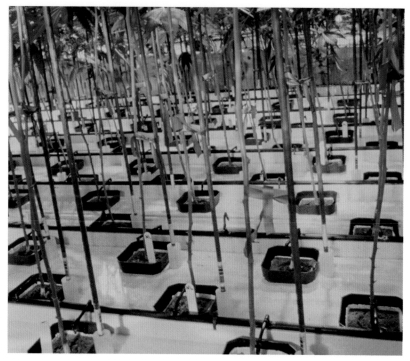

Tip: Strip the lower vegetation as seen here.

Preparation for Flowering

After all available clones are removed, the plants are again stripped of all lower vegetation, transferred to the flowering chambers, and staked and tied to prevent them from falling over. The same process occurs in a soilless mix situation.

Tip

If you happen to bend or break a stem or branch accidentally, you can repair it by using a short section of a drinking straw, approximately two to four inches long. Cut the straw down one side, then slide it over the bent or broken area of stem, and close the ends. Tape the straw around the area that needs repair. For large branches or large outdoor plants you can use a large diameter piece of tubing split down one side and zip tied around the affected branch.

Lower vegetation is stripped off so that all of the plant's energy and nutrients are redirected towards producing stronger clones and bigger, fuller buds. Lower branches are less useful, as they are light-deprived and produce airy, loose buds that are time-consuming to manicure. Remove any branches

Photos: Mel Frank

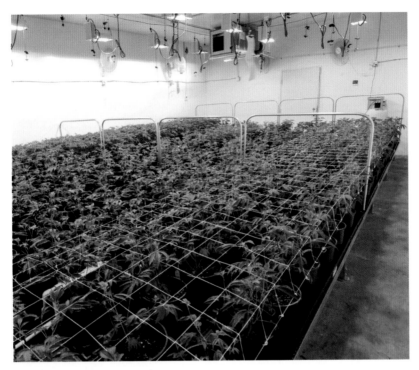

Vegetative plants in growth.

that do not receive direct light. Leave the fan leaves on, except for the lower fan leaves. For the most part, fan leaves should not be removed. They are essential for photosynthesis.

If the fan leaves become old, necrotic, sickly, or just more dead than alive, remove them. Do not keep dead leaves on plants or even lying around the growing environment—death is never a good thing to have around! Cleanliness is a top priority; debris and dead leaves decay in grow chambers, and can host mold and diseases. Keep your environment and chambers spotless! After harvest, all refuse and unusable material must be eliminated as quickly as possible, since they can also cause mold and diseases.

The health and vigor of the vegetative plants carry over to the flowering stage. Healthy vegetative plants make healthy flowering plants. You must pay close attention and watch closely for signs of nutrient deficiencies, over-fertilization, and nutrient build-up, which can raise or lower pH and lock out available nutrients—see the section on 'flushing' in the nutrient chapter of this book for more information.

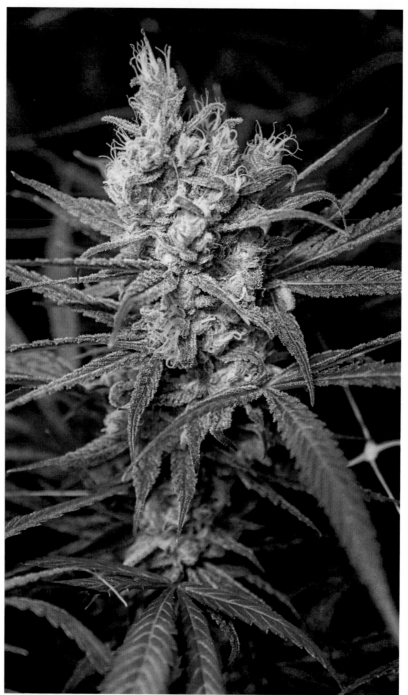

Photos: Dru West

Healthy plant from the West Coast Masters.

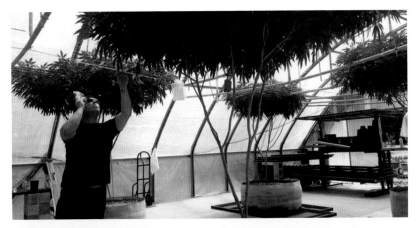

Dru West monitoring the leaves.

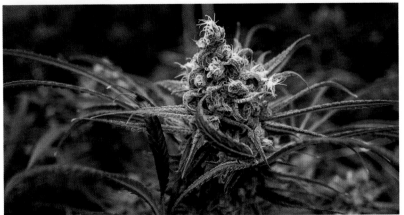

Beauty grown in massive SCROG garden by Dru West.

SCROG (Screen of Green) / Training Your Plants

It is possible to get the same amount from one large plant as it is to get from 10 smaller plants by training and spreading the plants out to maximize light by utilizing a uniform canopy.

An entire book has been written about this method by Dru West. The title of this book is The Secrets of the West Coast Masters: Uncover the Ultimate Techniques for Growing Medical Marijuana. You can purchase a copy of the book from Dru's website: www.westcoastmasters.com

There is no need for me to delve into an entire chapter devoted to this grow style since it has been written about so eloquently in Dru's book.

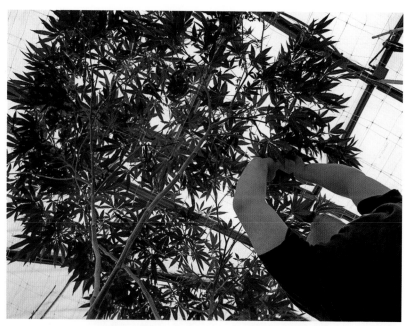

Careful training allows this SCROG plant to yield an insane amount of bud.

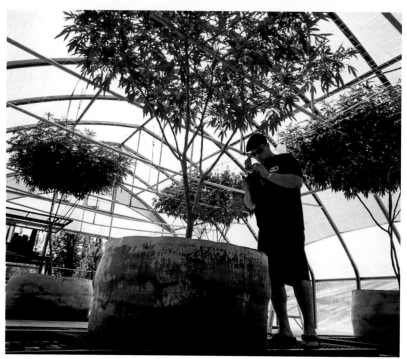

Photos: Dru West

These plants are absolutely massive. This is the power of SCROG.

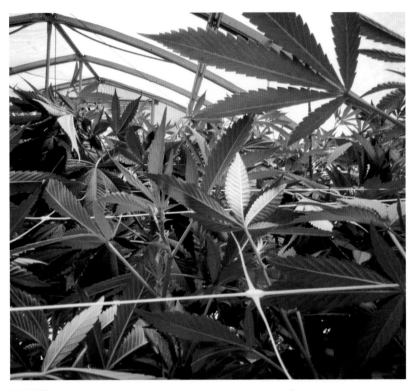

SCROG canopy.

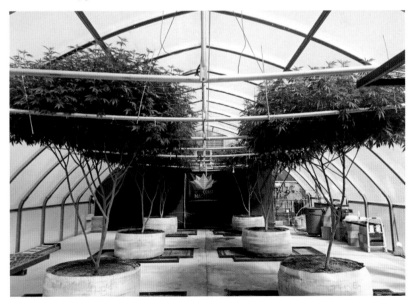

West Coast Masters greenhouse. Amazing.

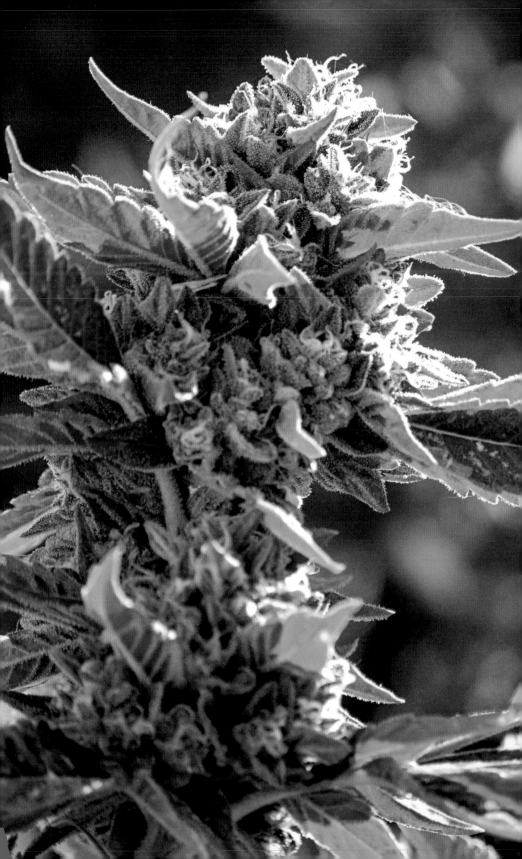

CHAPTER 11

Water and Feeding

Water Quality and Preparation

At Trichome Technologies, before we begin using a new facility, we first analyze the municipal utility district water supply and call the supplier to ask for an annual water quality report. Depending on the water quality results, we decide whether or not to filter. If you have unusually high levels of anything—50 PPM or above—you must filter the water. If using well water, send water samples to a water-testing laboratory for analysis. Water and soil test kits are available from online retailers or you can ask at your local grow supply store. In most circumstances, well water will need to be filtered. High levels of calcium and magnesium—a.k.a. hard water—can damage plants and inhibit healthy growth; furthermore, hard water prevents absorption of some nutrients. Schedule regular water quality tests, using the report's results to fine-tune your water preparation. Any water source over 50 PPM of hardness needs to be filtered/purified.

Reverse osmosis (RO) systems filter almost everything out of the water, including chlorine. However, RO water tends to be unstable as far as pH is concerned. For this reason, we filter 2 batches of water; the first is RO filtered, and the second is filtered through common charcoal filters. Both filtered waters are then mixed evenly at 50/50.

◀ Close to harvest.

Photo: K

This ensures a stable pure starting water source. Quality RO units are available online, and it is recommended that the unit you purchase have a chloramine pre-filter to eliminate chloramine before it gets to the RO filter.

■ Cities / municipalities do not use chlorine anymore. They use chloramine.

■ Chloramine damages membranes of RO systems.

■ Therefore, the chloramine must be removed via charcoal filtration prior to the RO membranes.

■ This will extend the life of the membrane, and limit replacements of membrane filters in your RO system.

The water is then left to sit for 24 hours. During this 24-hour period, we utilize a UV (Ultra Violet) sterilizer, then we massively oxygenate the water by using air stones and an air pump. These are available at any aquarium supply store. They are sized according to gallons to be aerated and sterilized. Note that chlorine and chloramines are different; chlorine dissipates, but chloramines must be filtered out. For decontamination purposes, we also put $^3/_4$ teaspoon of 27% food-grade hydrogen peroxide in 45-gallon tanks of water and let it sit for 24 hours, during which time the water oxygenates. Whether we are using this water for hydroponic, soil, or soilless mix, the methods are the same. Also bear in mind that the water should be approximately the same temperature as the room it is destined for. Plants don't want water to be too hot or too cold. At 72°F, water has the most oxygen-holding capacity, so this is the perfect temperature.

Feeding

The most misunderstood aspect of growing is the constitution and use of nutrient solution. Poor yields and scraggly plants can be linked to mismanagement of the nutrient solution. There is no absolute nutrient formula; growers must experiment with their own systems, observing, testing, and adjusting until the balance of nutrients and needs of the plant are met. Growers must be aware of the issues and provide adequate but not excessive levels of all essential elements. Even with the best management practices, nutrient problems can occur. Nutrient deficiencies are described in the chart below.

After filtration, decontamination, and aeration we mix in the fertilizers. We use General Hydroponics Flora series Micro, Gro, and Bloom and mix accordingly (see the section below on Nutrient Enhancers). Follow the manufacturer's mixing information. Thoroughly stir, shake, and mix in the Micro, then the Gro, and then the Bloom to your desired ratios and mix thoroughly.

Ideal Nutrient Levels for Cannabis

Here are the ideal nutrient levels for your plants, in teaspoons per gallon, using the General Hydroponics Flora series. Lower levels in proportion with the plants' intake needs.

TRICHOME TECHNOLOGIES' RECOMMENDED NUTRIENT CHART
For Use With General Hydroponics Flora Series Nutrients

Stage		Micro	Grow	Bloom
Stage 1 clones and seedlings	Early	1/4	1/4	1/4
Stage 2 vegetative stage	Early	3/4	3/4	3/4
		1	1	1
	Middle	1 1/4	1 1/4	1
	Late	1 1/2	1 1/2	1
Stage 3 flowering stage	Early	1 1/4	3/4	1 1/4
		1 1/2	1	1 1/2
		1 3/4	3/4	1 3/4
	Middle	1 1/2	1/2	1 1/2
		1 3/4	1/2	1 3/4
	Late	2	1/2	2
		2	1/2	3
	Later	2 1/2	1/2	2 1/2
	Last (if needed)	2 1/2	1/2	3

PPM depends on the levels and quality of the starting H2O.

At this stage we add a ¹/₂ teaspoon of hydrogen peroxide per 45 gallons of water to keep the water pathogen-free and oxygenated (see the section below on Pythium and Pathogens). Dissolved oxygen is essential to root formation and root growth. Do NOT add hydrogen peroxide to organic soils or nutrients.

Tea

Organic fertilizers and teas can also be used. By tea, we mean a mix of organic fertilizers—of bat guano, seabird guano, or earthworm castings—diluted in water. These teas are applied to the underside of leaves via foliar feeding and medium / soil drench.

Trichome Tech Foliar Feed Mix and Schedule

Using: General Hydroponics Flora series in teaspoons per gallon:

Flora Grow	Flora Micro	Flora Bloom
1	1	1

Spray-N-Grow

2 – Tablespoons

(one ounce) per 1 gallon agent / surfactant / spreader / sticker (they are all the same thing but just a different name)

6.2 pH

Apply this foliar feed every 4 days in the vegetative stage

Apply every 4 days for the first half of the flowering stage

Apply once a week for the next ¼ of the flowering cycle after that

Discontinue application of foliar feed for the last ¼ of the flowering stage

Nutrient Schedule and Mixing Chart

Teaspoons per gallon, water starts at 100 PPM and 6.9 pH

	Flora Micro	Flora Grow	Flora Bloom	pH	PPM	Notes
Stage 1 Clones and Seedlings						
	1/4	1/4	1/4	6.7	300	adjust pH to 6.2
Stage 2 Vegetative						
early:	1/2	1/2	1/2	6.5	500	adjust pH to 6.2
	3/4	3/4	3/4	6.5	700	
middle:	1	1	1	6.4	880	
	1 1/4	1 1/4	1	6.4	1030	
late:	1 1/2	1 1/2	1	6.4	1170	↓
Stage 3 Flowering						
early:	1 1/2	1	1 1/2	6.3	1150	adjust pH
	1 1/2	3/4	1 1/2	6.3	1090	between
	1 3/4	1/2	1 3/4	6.3	1040	5.8 – 6.8
middle:	2	1/2	2	6.2	1270	depending
	2 1/4	1/4	2 1/4	6.1	1360	on method,
late:	2 1/2	1/4	2 1/2	6.1	1650	media and
	2 1/2	1/4	2 3/4	6.0	1680	varietal
last:	2 1/2	1/4	3	6.4	1710	
	2 3/4	0	3	6.1	1730	↓

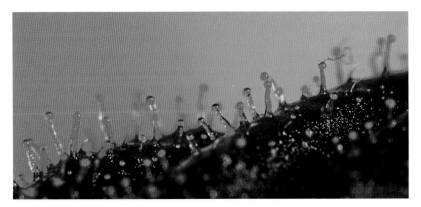

Trichomes stand tall like trees in a forest.

Foliar Feeding

The value of foliar feeding is well established. Plants can feed through the underside of their leaves. Foliar feeding is effective in correcting and preventing nutrient deficiencies. This method also increases yields and quality by overcoming limitations of the soil / media and its ability to transfer nutrients into the plants. The best time to foliar feed is mid-morning, one hour after the lights come on. This is the time when the stomata, the small openings on the underside of the leaves, are open. Also, this allows plants to completely dry before the lights go out for the night cycle. Excessive moisture can cause mildew and mold, so plants must be completely dry by the time the lights go out. If the temperature is 80°F or above, do not spray the plants, as it will have little effect. The best temperature for foliar feeding is around 72°F, and the pH of a foliar spray should be between 6.2 and 7.0.

If foliar feeding is done effectively, you should see noticable results in 48 hours. Always use a spreader, sticker, surfactant, or wetting agent. Always mix foliar feed nutrient solution thoroughly, and apply the spray in as fine a mist as possible. The best misters and sprayers apply a fine mist across a large area. Be careful of burning the leaves. Never foliar feed an outdoor crop in full sun, after 10am, since large beads of solution can magnify the sunlight and burn. It is best to spray small amounts of nutrients more frequently than to spray large amounts all at once. At Trichome Technologies we use General Hydroponics Flora series and organic teas. You can use any mild form of nutrients you choose, but they must be used in proper portions; for example, never spray high-nitrate fertilizers on flowering plants. Organic teas are also excellent.

Photo: K

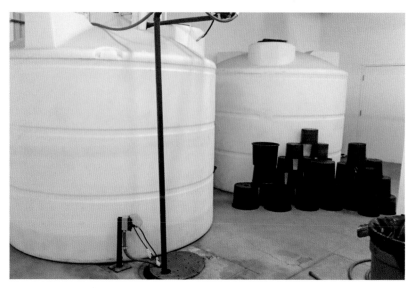

Large reservoirs for a grow. Keep the temperature at 72°F to get the most oxygen in your nutrient solution.

Never spray HID lights, because they could explode or cause serious harm. Besides, it's just a fucking stupid thing to do, don't you think?

The spray should be applied to the underside of the foliage until it's fully wet. In the vegetative stage, apply every 4 days. During the first half of the flowering stage, apply every 4 days. In the next quarter of the flowering cycle, apply once a week. In the last quarter of the flowering stage, discontinue use entirely to prevent the possibility of mold.

Temperature Control, Sterilization, and Oxygenation of Reservoirs

These are the methods and equipment recommended to keep nutrient reservoir solutions in perfect condition:

■ The optimum hydroponic reservoir solution temperature is 72°F.

■ To maintain this temperature we have titanium drop in probe water chillers and titanium core water chillers.

■ The titanium drop in probe water chiller is simply a titanium probe that is placed into the reservoir and cools the nutrient solution to exact temperatures with a digital thermostat.

■ The titanium core chiller simply cools the water that is circulated through

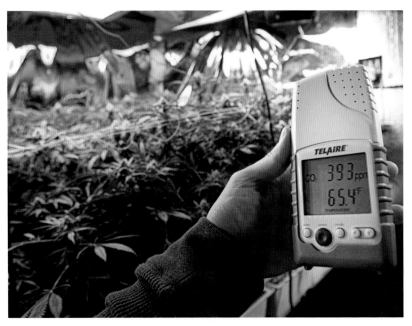

Temperature and PPM monitor for nutrient solutions.

the titanium core (titanium does not react to nutrients, unlike other metals – never use metal in proximity to nutrient solutions).

■ The core cools the nutrient solution to the desired temperature. Small / large water chillers are available that can cool any amount of nutrients.

■ For maintaining / heating nutrient solutions at 72°F, we use large / small (depending on size requirements) titanium aquarium heaters. These are also thermostat controlled.

■ To maintain oxygen levels in the nutrient solution in the reservoirs, we use aerators from www.O2grow.com. These aerators deliver 50% more dissolved oxygen than traditional bubbles or air diffusers.

■ Ultimately, we want large amounts of fine / oxygen rich air bubbles throughout the reservoir.

■ The pump itself should be kept out of the grow chamber for the atmosphere in the grow chamber is high in CO_2.

■ Place any air pump in an area that ensures fresh, uncontaminated environmental air.

■ After following all these procedures the nutrient solution is now ready to be given to the plants if it is at the proper temperature.

Photo: Freebie

Temperature and Watering

If using hydroponics or systems that utilize a reservoir, consider that the perfect temperature for the nutrient solution is 72°F. Water at average room temperature can only hold approximately 8% dissolved oxygen. Water at 86°F holds just 5% dissolved oxygen. Roots grow best at 75°F, so nutrients need to be well oxygenated or the plants will not grow well. The optimal conditions for your roots are 8% dissolved oxygen in the water / nutrients and reservoirs; the roots need as much oxygen as they can get. Aerated water will accept 5–8% oxygen and hold it for 24 hours.

A simple way to oxygenate your water and provide disease control is to add hydrogen peroxide once a week into reservoirs. When it breaks down, the resulting byproduct is oxygen. For 45 gallons of nutrients, add $^3/_4$ teaspoon of 27% food grade hydrogen peroxide. Never apply hydrogen peroxide to organic soils or nutrients.

To Recirculate or Not to Recirculate

Whether or not to recirculate water is an important question. At Trichome Technologies we run to waste, and do not recirculate our water. One of the theoretical hazards in a recirculating irrigation system is the possibility that pathogens may spread throughout the recirculating solution. The most effective approach to preventing disease is knowing where a pathogen comes from, whether it's the soil, the substrate, the walls, underneath tables, from cuttings brought into the environment, or from the water source. Plant pathogens can cause serious losses in a recirculating irrigation system. Pathogens spread quickly, and in most cases where crops have been lost, it can be traced to pathogens, either bacterial or fungal, which have gotten into the nutrient solution. Pythium, which causes root rot, is the most common plant pathogen spread by irrigation systems. It can get into a recirculating irrigation system from incoming water. See the section on pythium below for more information.

In outdoor and soilless mix situations, never under- or over-water the plants. Soil must be wet but never soggy. The soil must be allowed to dry out slightly between waterings, in order to draw oxygen into the root structure. Allow the top 1 to 1½ inches to dry out, then water again. Observe the plants and understand their water and nutrient needs. As the plants' growth rates accelerate, so do their water and nutrient requirements. Over- or under-watering causes low yields, poor health, or eventual death.

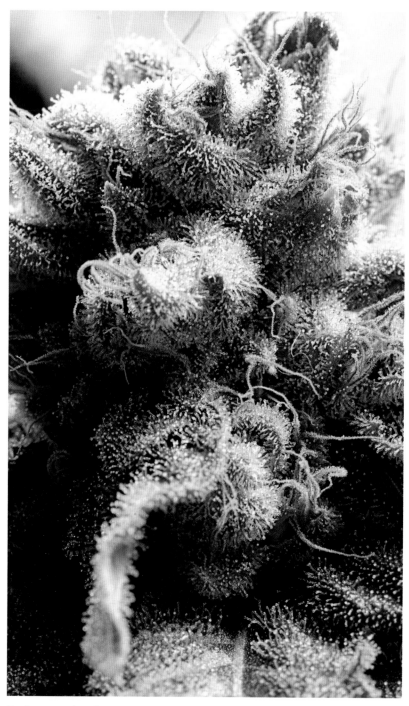

Resin-coated and ripening.

Photo: Samson Daniels

Humidity

A main cause of mildew and mold is the night-time "dew point," which is basically the same phenomenon as when evening dew forms suddenly on leaves on trees outside in spring or fall and saturates them with moisture, making them completely wet. A plant's leaves can accumulate moisture in a rapidly falling temperature when day turns to night and there is excessive humidity in a greenhouse or growroom. Once your environment is contaminated with mildew or mold, it can be difficult to eliminate. Always maintain a clean, debris-free grow environment. To minimize the risk of fungus development, limit the temperature drop and potential condensation onto the leaves of the plants. Using large exhaust fans to evacuate the air from the room, particularly if cool night air is replacing the exhausted air, makes the situation worse. You should use smaller fans controlled to match the climate. They make slow, even changes to the room's climate, which lowers both the humidity and temperature at the same time so that the dew point situation cannot occur.

Dew Point Explained

■ A main cause of mold is night-time "dew point," which is basically the same as when the spring and fall evening dew forms suddenly on clothes on a clothesline, and saturates them with moisture making them completely wet.

■ A plant's leaves can accumulate the moisture from a rapidly falling temperature when day turns to night and there is excessive humidity in a grow room.

■ Once your environment is contaminated with mold / fungus, it can be difficult to eliminate.

■ Always maintain a clean, debris free environment.

■ The best way to minimize the risk / potential of fungus / mold development is to limit the temperature drop and potential condensation onto the leaves of the plants.

■ By using large exhaust fans to evacuate the air from the room, particularly if the cool night air is replacing the exhausted air, and cool night air is being drawn in. This makes the situation worse.

■ The utilization of smaller fans, or fans controlled to match the climate, they make slow, even changes to the room's climate, which lowers both the humidity and the temperature at the same time so that dew point does not occur.

■ We recommend using quality climate controllers, available at hydroponic supply stores, that will aid in limiting the temperature drop into the night

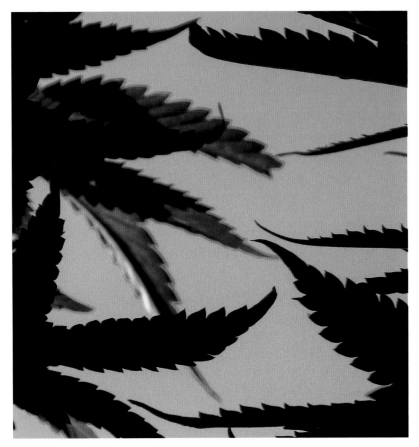

Blue skies and fresh air.

cycle. They monitor, manage, and control the environment / conditions to prevent dew point.

■ This reduces plant stress, and maximizes plant health, leading to bigger yield.

■ Plants photosynthesize more in less time at higher temperatures.

■ Maintaining the balance of temperature, humidity, and light, along with other aspects of climate control, is key.

■ Plant metabolism rises with temperature.

■ Wide open stomata are required to allow a higher CO_2 transfer rate to accommodate the increased plant metabolism. Therefore humidity levels should be kept higher to limit / slow transpiration and a nutrient / elemental facilitation, uptake, and assimilation.

Photo: K

■ CO_2 is one of the most important components of plant growth.

■ Rapidly growing, healthy, and vigorous plants require high (1400-1500 PPM) CO_2 levels. Then you can add nutrient levels to match accelerated growth produced.

■ Humidity and temperature go hand in hand, and both climate variables are very important to the growth of all plants. This explanation relates primarily to indoor growing.

■ Climate plays an important, vital role in the production of plants in an indoor environment. Controlling climatic conditions indoors can be expensive.

We recommend using a good climate controller from a hydroponic supply store. They will aid in limiting the temperature drop into the night cycle as they monitor, manage, and control the environmental conditions to prevent dew point, which reduces plant stress and maximizes plant health, vigor, and yield. Plants photosynthesize more in less time at higher temperatures. Maintaining the balance of temperature, humidity, and light, along with other aspects of climate control, is key to maximizing plant growth. Climate controllers manage the temperature, humidity, light cycles, and CO_2 of an enclosed growing environment. Good climate controllers produce fast, high-yielding crop rotations with minimal maintenance and management.

Basic Facts

Plant metabolism rises with temperature

Wide-open stomata are required to allow a higher CO_2 transfer rate to accommodate the increased plant metabolism. Therefore, humidity levels should be kept slightly higher to limit / slow transpiration and aid nutrient facilitation uptake and assimilation.

CO_2 is one of the most important components of plant growth. Rapidly growing, healthy, vigorous plants require high CO_2 levels, around 1,400–1,500 PPM, depending on the situation and environment. Then you can add nutrient levels to match the accelerated growth produced.

Humidity and temperature go hand in hand, and both climate variables are very important to the growth of all plants. This explanation relates primarily to indoor or greenhouse growing. Climate plays a vital role in the production of plants in an indoor environment. Controlling climatic conditions indoors can be expensive. The environment needs to be completely sealed with both filtered intake and exhaust fans, climate controller, lights, etc. The

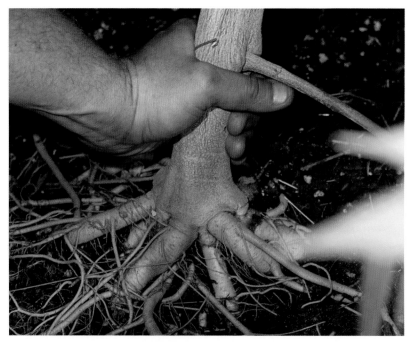

Large root system on a cannabis plant. Transpiration begins at the roots of the cannabis plant.

three main factors of indoor climate to consider are temperature, humidity, and light, as these are the factors that you have the greatest control over. If you can precisely control these three factors, you'll notice definite increases in growth, health, and yield. Indoor grow lights affect environmental temperature, and the temperature in turn influences the humidity. In hydroponic cultivation, there are usually large quantities of water present, which act as a natural environment humidifier through plant transpiration and evaporation of the water in the reservoir and medium. However, there is a point at which water in a growroom can become excessive, and will cause elevated levels of humidity. In this case, you will need to remove some of the moisture in the air by using a de-humidifier.

It is important to understand that all plants need elevated humidity during the propagation, germination, and vegetative stages of growth for healthy, strong, vigorous growth without deficiencies or other problems. However, you do not want too high a level of heat and humidity in the room either. A balance must be achieved—not too dry and not too humid.

Photo: Freebie

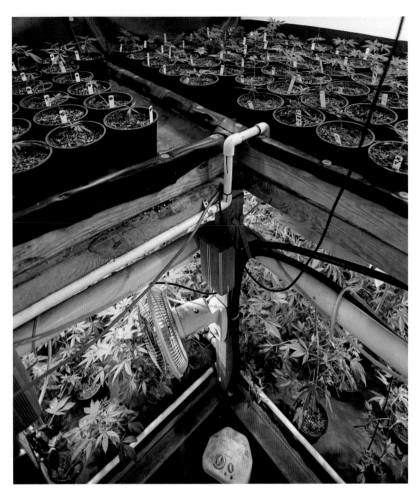

Tiered cannabis garden with tubes for runoff water.

Photo: Freebie

Extra Background

Plants are similar to humans in some respects: when they become hot, they perspire and lose water. If you do not replace the lost fluids when you sweat, you risk the chance of becoming dehydrated; therefore, you must drink more water. Plants require relatively high humidity for vegetative growth and lower for flowering. When the air surrounding your plants is too dry, plants will transpire more in an attempt to elevate the amount of humidity in the air, which in turn stresses the plants. They will become lethargic and tired, leaves will turn a pale green color, and eventually leaves will curl up, turn a rust brown color, and dry out. Cannabis plants grown indoors in soil must

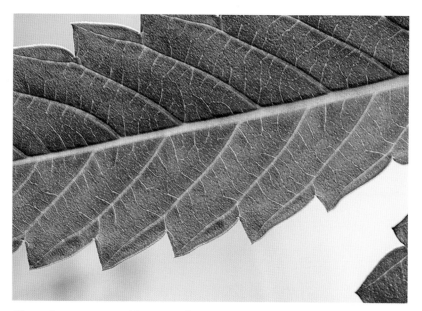

Always inspect top and bottom of leaves for any pest or disease.

absorb more water in low humidity environments because they are transpiring at an accelerated rate, yet may be unable to do so because of the lack of moisture in the growing environment, causing major stress. Therefore, a humidifier is necessary to elevate the humidity in the room, and will lessen the amount of water that must be applied to the soil. This will slow down the rate of transpiration, resulting in plants that are less stressed and have darker, healthier, lush green leaves with a waxy look to them.

Indoor growers should consider humidity and temperature control a top priority. Excessively low humidity is unacceptable and will cause many problems. It is more preferable to have a high humidity level than a low one. There are problems that materialize in high humidity environments, but not as many as when the humidity is lower than 40%. High humidity becomes a real problem when the plants are in the flowering cycle. The perfect temperature and humidity for the vegetative growth stage of cannabis is 74% relative humidity and 75°F temperature, although these should be higher when using CO_2. Warm air is capable of carrying more moisture than cool air can before it turns to mist, which means that an environment with a 75°F temperature and a relative humidity of 74% holds more moisture than an environment with a 68°F temperature and the same humidity level.

Photo: Samson Daniels

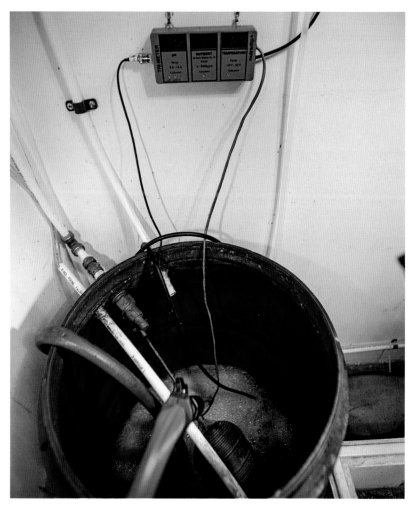

Water and nutrient mixing station with PPM monitor visible to ensure a proper mixture and temperature.

Temperature and humidity are the two main factors that contribute to overall healthy, vigorous plant growth. Humidifiers are not only beneficial for soil-grown plants; hydroponics growers can also utilize a humidifier in their vegetative growth stages, primarily in winter months, when multiple lights are confined in a small space, or when reservoirs are completely sealed or the reservoir is in a different room, preventing available moisture from evaporating into the environment. A quality humidifier is available from your local garden supply center or hydroponics store.

Photo: Freebie

Manipulating the Light Cycle to Conserve Electricity

The cost of electricity is high and is expected to rise in the future. If electricity usage in your growroom is a concern, you may consider manipulating your light cycle to save electricity and money. Simple, basic steps can be taken to conserve energy and continue to reap incredible harvests. For smaller gardens, we recommend using a good quality climate controller from a hydroponics supply store. The climate controller should feature an "any length" day / night light timer and should have a timer that allows a "fast flowering" cycle of 18 hours per day. This allows for a six-hour daylight period, followed by 12 hours of dark, to make sure the plants stay in the flowering cycle. Every day, you gain six hours for your plants to begin a new day. In three days, the plants will have had four days' worth of light. In three weeks, the plants will have seen four weeks. Basically, every month the lights, AC units, intake / exhaust, and dehumidifiers, etc., will be on for only about 240 hours in a "fast flowering cycle" as opposed to the usual 360 hours in a 12/12 regular flowering cycle. This simple process will save you approximately 34% on electrical consumption.

A good quality climate controller will help growers using smaller rooms or larger rooms if one controller is being used for each separate room. These climate controllers produce more growth in less time, with less power usage.

PPM (Parts Per Million)

PPM meters are extremely useful. They enable you to apply precise amounts of nutrients and to maintain desired PPM levels. They are easy to use and maintain. The insurance they afford and the precise info they provide make them a must-have item for any serious grower. To find out the concentration of water or any nutrient solution, you must measure the PPM. Pure water is not conductive, but it is conductive as soon as salt-based nutrients or acid is added. Municipal water usually contains many impurities and dissolved minerals, and it's not unusual to see municipal water with a PPM of 50–100. Adding nutrients will increase this level. PPM meters measure the total quantity of dissolved solids in the water. They work by determining the amount of current passing between two electrodes, either in the cup that you pour the nutrient sample into, or on the tip of a pen-type meter. The meter you choose must measure from 0–3,500 PPM. A reading of 100 means that for one million solution molecules, 100 molecules are total dissolved solids and 999,900 are water molecules.

Transpiration

Transpiration begins at the root. Super fine roots take up any water, nutrients, and oxygen available in the growing medium and transport them through the stems to the leaves. The transportation and flow of water and nutrients from the medium throughout the plant is referred to as the "transpiration stream." Some of the water is retained and utilized for photosynthesis. Unused water, nutrients, and waste products are evaporated into the air through the stomata on the underside of the plants' leaves. Some of the water that is retained transports manufactured sugars and starches back to the roots via the stems and main stalk. The fluids are transported throughout the veins or "vascular bundles" of the plant. The internal fluids transport nutrients and aid waste product disposal, as well as providing internal pressure that keeps the plant erect and standing tall.

Inspecting Runoff Water

As the PPM increases, the ability of the plant roots to take up water and nutrients decreases. Soil and hydroponic growers are advised to monitor the runoff water from the soil or medium of the solution in the reservoirs for its pH and PPM and to flush and replace nutrients when it exceeds the desired levels for that stage. An increasing pH and PPM indicates that the elemental concentration buildup of the nutrient solution is too high. You must flush soil and replace reservoir nutrients every week. Flush using pure, pH adjusted, room temperature water.

Stomata

Stomata can be defined as small openings or "pores" on the undersides of leaves, similar to the microscopic pores on human skin, except the stomata's purpose is to regulate and enable the plant to intake carbon dioxide and release water and oxygen through the leaves. The larger the leaf, the more stomata it has on the leaf. The larger the plant, the more leaves the plant has, and therefore more stomata it has to help with transpiration. The more plants you have and the larger they get, the greater amounts of available CO_2 you will need. It's quite simple: large numbers of plants or big plants require lots of fresh air and CO_2 for optimum health and growth. The stomata on your plants can become clogged by dirty, unfiltered air as well as nutrient residue left behind after foliar feed applications or other sprays. Clogged stomata can inhibit transpiration /

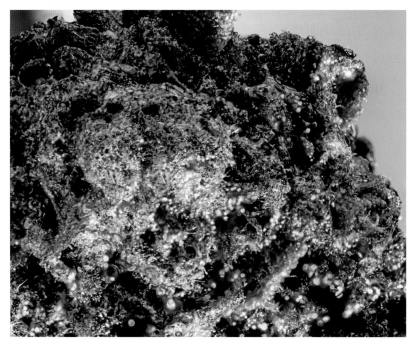

Honey oil-coated bud.

respiration and healthy growth. Twenty-four hours after foliar feeding or any other chemical spray application, you must wash off any chemical residuals from the leaves. To prevent stomata clogging, wash the undersides of the leaves with a spray applicator, using pure, pH-adjusted, room temperature water.

Water Preparation, Step-by-Step

If you follow these simple steps, the result will be perfect quality water in the exact form that your plants want it. This will promote superior growth characteristics, resulting in the most healthy, vigorous, productive plants, roots, and buds possible.

1. Analyze the water you intend to use. Check the water's PPM. If it is 50 or lower, the water is good and may be used. If it is 100 or higher, the water must be purified using RO or charcoal filtration. There are many water quality testing services available. They should offer water and soil testing services as well as retail pH and PPM testing equipment. Fill a 45-gallon container with this water, mixed 50/50 RO and charcoal-filtered.

Photo: Samson Daniels

181

2. Place large air stones or air curtains at the bottom of the container. The air stones should be attached to a large aquarium pump. When you turn on the pump, the water is aerated. Leave the water to aerate for 24 hours.

3. Sterilize water: UV sterilizers are used to sanitize and disinfect the water. UV sterilizers kill pathogens and bacteria that may be present in the water. They are available from most aquarium supply stores. They circulate water past a UV sterilization light bulb, and the UV exposure kills all of the unwanted waterborne pests. Do not use on organic based nutrient mixes, as it will kill any beneficial bacteria and microbial life forms.

4. Try to keep water temperature between 72°F and 75°F. At 72°F, water will retain the most oxygen. Water that is too hot should be cooled, and vice versa. You can use water chillers, refrigerators, or titanium aquarium heaters for this purpose. Both can be purchased from your local hydroponics store.

5. Because air has been bubbled through the water, there is the possibility of bacteria and pathogen contamination. For this reason we add $3/4$ teaspoon of 27% food grade hydrogen peroxide to the 45 gallons of filtered, aerated, temperature-adjusted water.

6. Apply the nutrients and then the amendments you have already chosen in proper proportions to the water. Know exactly what you are feeding your plants and understand what you are giving them in relation to their stage of growth. Stir the water thoroughly after nutrient applications; water must be completely mixed!

> **Important:** When using organic fertilizer or tea, or any other organic-based amendment, you must skip this step. Use no hydrogen peroxide, as it will kill all beneficial bacteria and desired life forms in addition to pathogens.

7. Using a pH test kit or pH meter, adjust the pH. Note that if using a meter you must inspect and recalibrate it prior to every use to prevent inaccurate readings. Depending on your cultivar, your pH should be between 5.8 and 7.0: never below 5.8; rarely above 7.0. We prefer 6.2. For hydroponic use, we

employ General Hydroponics pH up and pH down for adjustments; for organic use, see the section on organic amendments for more options.

Note: True organic soil does not typically require the pH to be meticulously maintained. Organic media usually self-regulate their pH levels with the aid of beneficial bacteria and living organisms in the soil.

8. After water has been deemed pure (filtered, decontaminated, aerated, dechlorinated, temperature-adjusted, pH-adjusted), it is time to check the PPM of the water. If the PPM is below your desired level, simply add more nutrients; if it is above, slightly dilute your water using more purified water. When diluting high-PPM water, it is best to completely mix it, then check the levels again; repeat this step until you have the ideal PPM.

9. As covered in step two, always prep twice the amount of water that you need. The first half is used for nutrient application and watering, and the second half is used to dilute high-PPM water if needed, or to pre-water or flush out your medium and any unused fertilizers, salts, or undesirable nutrients it holds. Another reason for pre-watering is that delicate root tips can burn when put in contact with full strength fertilizers. Pre-watering ensures that the roots are aerated, moist, and ready to take up available nutrients.

pH

pH stands for potential hydrates. pH is the inverse measurement of the concentration of hydrogen ions. Low levels of hydrogen ions correspond with a high pH reading; high levels of hydrogen ions correspond with a low pH meter reading. If your pH levels climb too high or fall too low, some nutrients become available to your plants at toxic levels while others become completely unavailable. Ranging from 0 (acid) to 14 (base), the pH scale is used to determine the acidity or alkalinity of a substance. pH is best kept approximately in the middle of the range. 7.0 pH is considered neutral; under 7.0 is considered acidic; above 7.0 is considered alkaline. Vitamin C / citric acid and common vinegar, both mild acids, are perfect organic forms of pH down. Alkaline substances are referred to as "bases": ammonia is an example of a mild base; potassium hydroxide is an example of a strong base. Cannabis prefers a pH range of 5.8 to 6.8 for healthy production, with 6.2 being perfect.

Evaporation, temperature, and light intensity can all effect pH levels, so constant monitoring of nutrient solutions is critical. If growing hydroponically, check your nutrient reservoir at least twice daily, once in the morning and once in the evening, with a handheld pH meter.

Blending the Ultimate Organic Soil Mix

Start with 100% organic soil such as Fox Farms' Ocean Forest or Light Warrior. Mix with equal parts organic soil and mushroom compost or top quality potting soil—not topsoil. The mushroom compost or topsoil should have a minimal nutrient content, but the consistency should contain chunks of broken up bark, mulch, oyster shells, or other medium-sized organic matter to aid in beneficial bacteria and microbial digestion.

The evenly mixed Ocean Forest blend and mushroom compost is then mixed with 30% of an additional mix, which is half medium / small vermiculite and half medium / small perlite. With a well-blended organic soil mix you will not need to fertilize the plants for the first three weeks; your soil should contain ample amounts of available nutrients for the plants' early stage of growth. After three or four weeks you can start using compost tea organic fertilizer amendment or Fox Farms' Big Bloom, if flowering the plants.

Nutrient Timing and Burn Periods

It's important when growing cannabis to understand the basics of the primary, secondary, and trace elements you intend to use. How long do they remain active? How strong are they? What is their exact elemental content? For instance, blood meal will release high levels of nitrogen for 70–120 days and then slowly begin to taper off and burn out for another 50–75 days. Therefore, it should not be used as an amendment in early-finishing cultivars—plants that have only eight weeks until they are finished flowering. Blood meal would release an excessive amount of nitrogen for an eight-week cultivar. Instead, you should use bat guano, which is also high in nitrogen, but only for about 45 days. Basically, you want some elements to become depleted earlier than others, but you want all elements to remain present at proper levels throughout growth, burning out only two weeks prior to harvest.

Seaweed / Kelp Meal

Seaweed meal contains a multitude of primary, secondary, and trace minerals in an excellent organic source full of beneficial hormones and enzymes that aid in pest and disease resistance and overall productive growth. Seaweed also promotes healthy, beneficial bacteria and microbe levels, and works in conjunction with organic fish emulsion.

Potassium Sources

Green sand, blackstrap molasses, seaweed, and kelp meal all contain available potassium. These sources release potassium slowly, over a long period of time in dry fertilizers. If your plants are deficient in potassium (which should not occur if you have amended your soil properly) they can be quickly corrected using a high-potassium content compost tea or Botanicare's Liquid Karma.

Phosphorous Sources

Phosphorous is a primary element that contributes heavily to the flowering process. Powdered soft rock phosphate is a perfect source of phosphorous and sulfur and is immediately available to the soil's beneficial bacteria and your plants' roots. It is best to combine more than one organic source of phosphorous in conjunction with other amendments such as steamed bone meal or bat guano.

Sulfur Sources

Caution: Never apply pure sulfur to your media. Straight sulfur will kill beneficial living microorganisms in the soil. Instead, use gypsum, soft rock phosphate, fish emulsion, or fertilizers such as Alaskan Fish Fertilizer or Down to Earth's Bio-Fish.

Dolomite Lime

Pelletized dolomite lime is a good source of magnesium, which is of major importance in the flowering stage. Dolomite lime is a perfect buffer and keeps other amendments that can drop pH to undesirable levels, such as guano and blood meal, in check.

Reusing / Recycling Your Soil

There is almost no reason to ever dispose of your organic soil, unless it is contaminated with an undesirable microorganism, such as pythium or some undesirable composition, or an unhealthy trait. Recycling your organic soil will dramatically increase its qualities and balance, as well as contributing

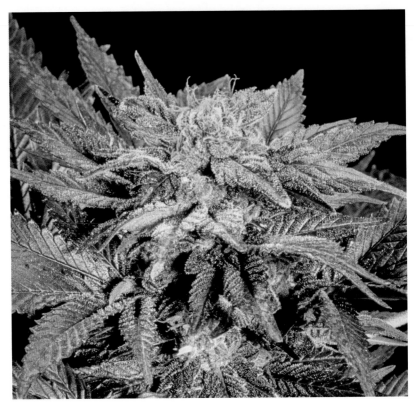

Two days from harvest.

to increased vigor, yields, and resistance to pests and disease. Many elements used in organic soils are broken down and available over a long period of time, normally longer than the life cycle of the plant. Many elements are just beginning to become available when your plants are finished, therefore if you replace the soil every crop you will never reap the full potential of the nutrients that are slow to break down.

Method

To reuse your organic soil you will need two compost containers or barrels if you have many plants or small containers if you have few. There must be holes in the tops of the containers to allow bad air out and good air in. One container is used for raw decomposing matter—fruit and vegetables, leftovers, egg shells, etc. No meat-based products should be present. Continually add matter to this container. The contents are imbalanced and pH-unstable in the initial

Photo: Andre Grossman

stages of decomposition, so they can't be used as fertilizer for plants.

The second container contains the amended soil you intend on using for your next crop. This allows you to continually add organic matter to the first container while allowing the second container to become balanced, pH-stable, cured, and ready to use for your next crop.

Earthworms

Live earthworms are an essential component in any organic soil. Earthworms (redworms) are nature's soil aerators. Keep them present at all times in both containers. Earthworms aerate and improve the condition of the soil as they burrow in search of food. Earthworms are available from live bait stores. Use two or three worms per square foot of matter.

Earthworm Castings

One of the most beneficial ingredients you can add to your compost is earthworm castings. Earthworm castings contain approximately five times the available nitrogen, seven times the available phosphorous, three times the exchangeable magnesium, 11 times the available potash, and $1^1/_2$ times the calcium found in six inches of top soil. It's an excellent amendment.

Amending the Depleted Soil

You must replace nutrients that have been depleted: nitrogen, phosphorous, potassium, etc. These elements are available in the organic form of guano, dolomite lime, and seaweed and kelp meal, to name a few. Guano is an excellent source of micronutrients and trace elements, but you must be careful in using it. Guano is "hot" when not fully decomposed and will burn roots and kill your plants by dramatically lowering soil pH.

This explains the role of the first container: it constantly decomposes the organic matter, balancing the elements and stabilizing the pH gradually. This, together with curing the compost after it has been amended, avoids burning, shocking of the plants that may be caused by unstable pH levels, and other compositional imbalances.

Important: Both containers must be periodically mixed and completely turned over to allow oxygen to permeate the soil and aid decomposition.

Straightforward Hydroponic and Soil Garden

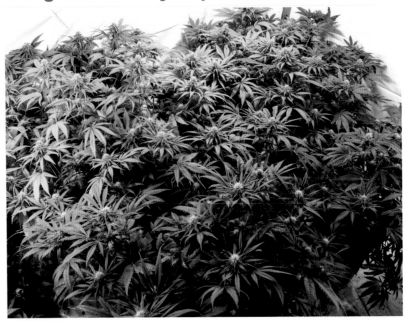

Canopy in a small grow. Plants are just starting to flower.

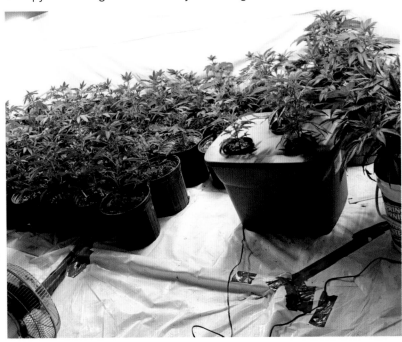

Photos: David Strange

Soil plants on the left and hydroponic bucket systems on the right.

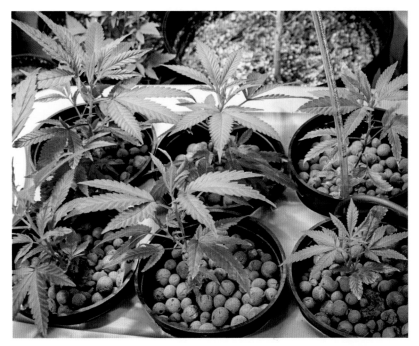

Homemade aerocloner system with hydroton pellets and fresh clones.

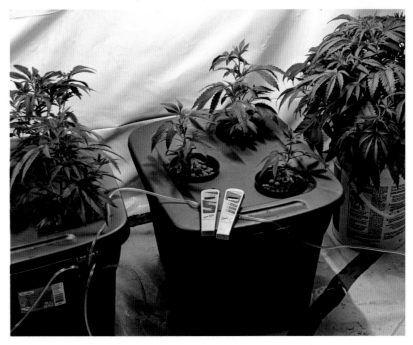

Hydroponic systems with plants in vegetative growth.

Straightforward Hydroponic and Soil Garden

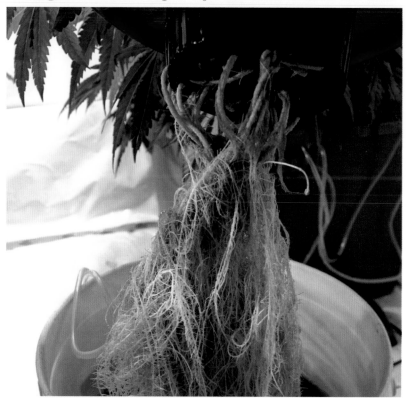

Roots in hydro system.

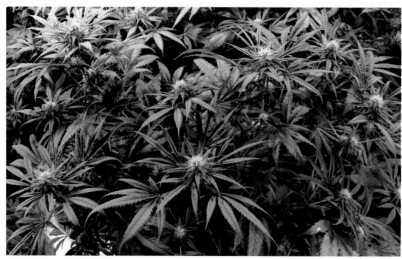

Photos: David Strange

Canopy of a small hydro tub grow after 22 days of flowering.

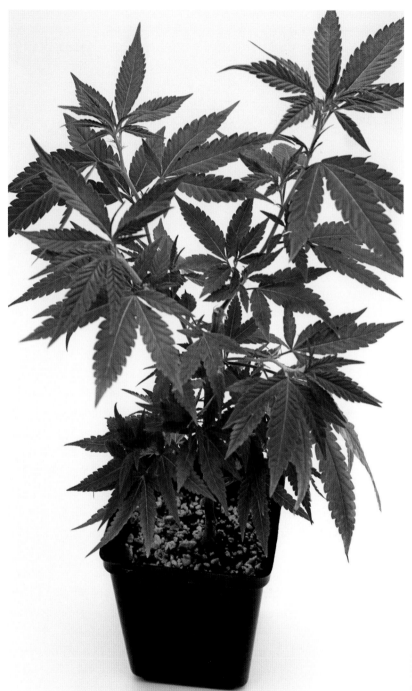

Small and healthy vegetative plant in soil.

Photo: Weado

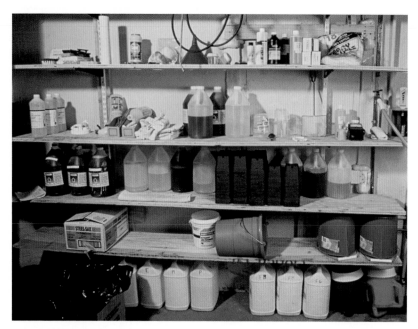

Many fertilizing options.

What Not to Do

Never use mineral salt-based synthetic, inorganic, powdered, or liquid fertilizer. Never apply chlorinated water to organic soil. All of the above are toxic to microorganisms and will kill all beneficial life forms in your organic soil. Never use non-organic soils or potting mix, redwood pine bark, walnut leaves, or pet waste in your organic compost.

Never allow the compost to become excessively dry. It must remain slightly moist at all times. If it becomes dry, the compost will decompose slowly and the beneficial microorganisms will be greatly reduced. This applies to both containers.

Before you add fruit or vegetables, place them on a window or door screen and allow them to completely dry out—this requires good air circulation. After it is dry, place it in a food processor or grinder and chop it up as finely as possible before adding it to the first decomposing container.

If you are using inorganic fruit or vegetable matter that contain trace amounts of synthetic herbicide, pesticides, or fertilizers, you must apply Biozome, an organic product that breaks down and neutralizes inorganic carbon-based elements. Follow the manufacturer's instructions for this.

Soil Amendment Options

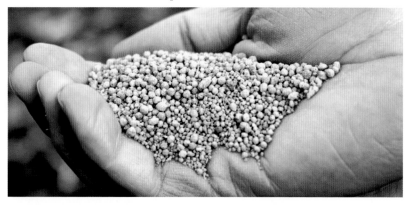

Bone meal is an excellent buffer for guano or blood meal. It raises pH.

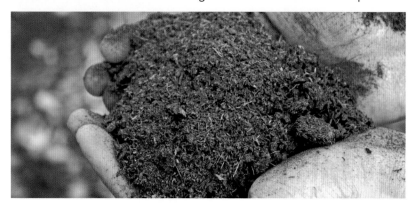

Peat moss can increase clay soil aeration and improves water retention in sandy soil.

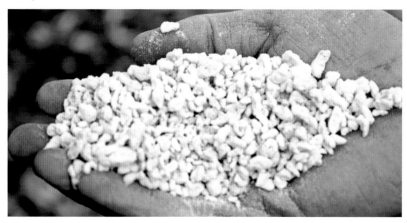

Perlite aerates soil and improves drainage without any effect on pH.

Photos: Sativa Steph

Soil Amendment Options

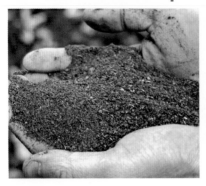

Blood meal lowers pH.

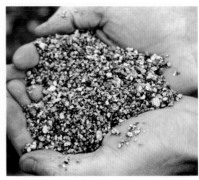

Vermiculite is a great soil amendment.

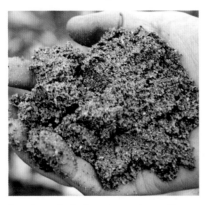

Sand can help break up clay soil.

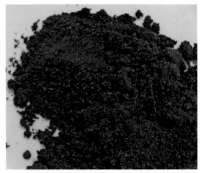

Topsoil is a great amendment for plants grown in the ground.

Unsulfured Blackstrap Molasses

Once you have added all of your chosen amendments to the soil in the second container, mix one teaspoon per gallon of unsulfured blackstrap molasses with pure, unchlorinated water. This provides sugars for microorganisms and accelerates the decomposition process, balances the soil and stabilizes the pH, and promotes healthy microorganism colonies in the soil. One application of molasses is all that is necessary. Do not over-apply. A healthy plant with a high Brix (the scale upon which we measure sugar content), will rarely be attacked by pests. They will not suck, chew, or perforate a healthy plant because they cannot expel the gasses associated with plant tissue that contains high sugar levels. Therefore, it is a good idea to apply molasses a few times during an outdoor cycle and a couple of times during an indoor cycle. Be conservative; follow manufacturer's instructions.

Photos: Sativa Steph

Curing Soil

Once the soil is completely amended and blended well, it must sit and cure for approximately 30–60 days. At the early stages the soil does not have to be perfectly balanced or have perfect consistency; as long as you allow it to sit and cure, it will become balanced. Even if you inadvertently over fertilize or over-apply any given element, the curing process will balance it out naturally. A large, healthy microorganism population and earthworms allow this balance to occur via decomposition and aeration.

The containers should be kept between 70 and 80°F at all times, in a dark, shaded, well-ventilated area. As noted previously, you should never allow soil to completely dry out—keep it moist but not soggy. Always allow soil to completely decompose; not doing so will cause a dramatic drop in the soil's pH level, which in turn will cause a myriad of problems such as nutrient excesses and deficiencies. Recycled, composted soil is the absolute best soil you can use; the more it is used and amended, the better it gets. For instance, amendments like green sand, bone meal, and soft rock phosphate decompose and break down slowly.

Recycled Soil Structure and Composition

Soil structure is the basic physical composition and make-up of your soil. Although you may have an excellent nutrient balance, you could still lack a perfect structure. The best method of correcting your soil structure is to use a 50/50 mix of vermiculite and perlite. Both are inert elements. Take this mixture and mix it with soil at a ratio of $1/3$ vermiculite / perlite and $2/3$ amended compost. This soil blend will fix any structural problems before they occur. The addition of small amounts of crushed oyster shells or mulched wood or bark (except redwood or pine) will add some chunky texture to the soil. Besides acting as a structure enhancement, the vermiculite / perlite blend will aid in soil aeration and drainage, helping beneficial organisms as well as nutrient breakdown and availability. Compacted soil with poor aeration or drainage will only produce unhealthy plants and poor yields.

Using Your Harvest Leftovers

The following applies only to your leftovers *after* you've made hash, of course. When you have finished harvesting, put your used soil and dried fan leaves through a $1/4$-inch hole size screen. Be sure to use goggles, particulate dust masks, and gloves during this whole process. Break up the medium as finely as possible prior to placing it into a container, and mix it thoroughly. Grind and chop all stems and branches in a food processor, as well as any other material to be decomposed, prior to adding it to the container.

Your reused soil should contain enough minerals and nutrients to get the plants all the way through their life cycle. If any deficiencies occur, they can be quickly corrected using Fox Farm's Big Bloom organic nutrient supplements, or by using an organic fertilizer tea. Never forget that the soil already contains available nutrients, so don't over-fertilize and burn the plants' roots. Be slightly conservative—let "slightly less fertilizer is better" be your somewhat odd motto!

Keep the tea / nutrient PPM at approximately 400–600 in the early stages of growth, progressively rising to roughly 700–900 in the later stages of flowering growth. When augmenting with organic fertilizers you must flush the soil, explained in the Flowering chapter. You can repeat this soil recycling process forever!

Beneficial Nematodes

Beneficial nematodes are microscopic, non-segmented roundworms that occur naturally in soil throughout the world. Inside the nematodes' gut is the real weapon—symbiotic bacteria that, when released inside a harmful insect, kill it within 24–48 hours. They are excellent for insect infestation protection. Nematodes come in an easily dissolved clay formation that you mix with water. The solution can be applied to the soil by hand-watering or with a hand sprayer. Apply every three or four days. Follow manufacturer's instructions.

Preferred Soil Amendments and Plant Spray Checklist

- Crushed oyster shells (small amounts)
- Mulched / composted wood bark (not redwood or pine)
- Vermiculite
- Perlite
- Water-retaining crystals
- Biozome
- Earthworm castings
- Earthworms (redworms)
- Crushed eggshells
- Unsulfured blackstrap molasses or Floranectar (from General Hydro)
- Mushroom compost

■ Seaweed or kelp meal

■ Bone meal, fish or animal

■ Blood meal

■ Guano—bat, bird, or herbivore animal

■ Green sand

■ Soft rock phosphate

■ Vegetable plant waste—leaves, stems, roots

■ Fruit waste—watermelon, cantaloupe, honeydew rinds, apple, orange, grapefruit, lemons, limes, banana peels, etc.

■ Beneficial nematodes

Organic Fertilizers

■ Fox Farm's Big Bloom

■ Age Old Bloom

■ Rare Earth

■ Diamond Black

■ Fulvic Acid 4%

■ Superthrive

■ Spray-n-Grow

■ Nitrozyme

■ Cornucopia Plus

■ Chitosan—Chi Foliar Spray (by General Hydroponics)

Recommended Organic and Non-Organic Soil Amendments

■ Banana Peels

Elements / Effect: Potassium. Good organic amendment.

Comments: Dry out, then chop and grind in a food processor before adding.

pH Influence: None.

■ Beneficial Nematodes

Elements / Effect: Microscopic roundworms that kill harmful insects.

Comments: Occur naturally in soils throughout the world. Apply to soil every three or four days to prevent harmful insect infestation. Nematodes can be dissolved into clean, pure, non-chlorinated, pH-adjusted water and used as a foliar spray and soil drench.

■ Blood Meal
Elements / Effect: Nitrogen and many trace elements and nutrients
Comments: Caution: very strong. It must be decomposed first for at least 30 days prior to application. Never apply directly to plants or roots.
pH Influence: Lowers.

■ Bone Meal (Steamed)
Elements / Effect: Phosphorous (high), nitrate, nitrogen, calcium and trace nutrients.
Comments: Excellent buffer for "hot" elements such as guano or blood meal.
pH Influence: Raises.

■ Chitosan—Chifoliar Spray (by General Hydroponics)
Elements: Contains chitosan salts, a naturally occurring polymer found in shells of crustaceans, insects, and many fungi.
Comments: Enhances resistance to disease and environmental stress. Improves plant vigor. Activates genes that stimulate protease inhibitors.

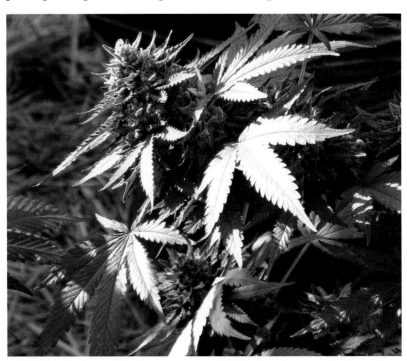

Photo: K

Outdoor plants should receive maximum sunlight.

■ Cornucopia Plus

Elements: A bio-engineered plant fertilizer.

Comments: Assists the biogenetic pathways of primary and secondary metabolic plant processes, enhancing the plant's development.

■ Cottonseed Meal

Elements / Effect: Perfect for long-term source of nitrogen (well into flowering); use sparingly.

Comments: Good for microlife and worms alike; long-term nitrogen release. Excellent for vegetative and flowering growth.

pH Influence: Lowers

■ Diamond Black (by General Hydroponics)

Elements: Pure mined mineral consisting of rich organic plant active humates.

Comments: Humates regulate the flow and enhance the transport of nutrients.

■ Dolomite Lime, Prilled and Pelletized

Elements / Effect: Magnesium and calcium are used in large quantities in the flowering cycle.

Comments: Excellent as a buffer for "hot" nutrients such as blood meal or guano.

pH Influence: Raises.

■ Earthworm Castings

Elements / Effect: Perfect organic amendment. Contains many micronutrients and humic acids.

Comments: Excellent source of micronutrients, enzymes, and trace elements.

pH Influence: Lowers (slightly).

■ Fish Bone Meal

Elements / Effect: Nitrogen (weak), phosphorous (medium), potassium (weak), trace elements and sulfur.

Comments: Superior form of bone meal. Use as a replacement for steamed bone meal.

pH Influence: Raises.

■ Fulvic Acid—4%
Elements: Accentuates the production of nucleic acids and photosynthesis.
Comments: Fulvic acid will supercharge the entire plant from the roots to the growing tips.

■ Grapefruit, Orange, Lemon, or Lime Peels
Elements / Effect: Good source of molds and an excellent vitamin C amendment. Again, the source matters.
Comments: Dry out first and then chop and grind in a food processor prior to addition.
pH Influence: None.

■ Green Sand
Elements / Effect: Potassium, approximately 32 essential minerals, plus trace elements.
Comments: Perfect source of trace elements and potassium. Breaks down slowly.
pH Influence: None.

■ Guano(s)
Elements / Effect: Sources vary, but it usually provides high and low levels of every required nutrient.
Comments: Excellent foundation for amending soil, good food source for microorganisms, and beneficial bacteria.
pH Influence: Lowers.

■ Lawn Trimmings
Elements / Effect: Nitrogen, phosphorous, potassium.
Comments: Use only if chemical and pesticide-free.
pH Influence: Raises slightly.

■ Liquid Fish Emulsion Fertilizer (Alaskan 5-1-1)
Elements / Effect: Nitrogen, phosphorous, potassium, sulfur, and trace elements.
Comments: Excellent organic source of nitrogen and sulfur. Beneficial to desirable bacteria, fungus, and microbes.
pH Influence: Raises.

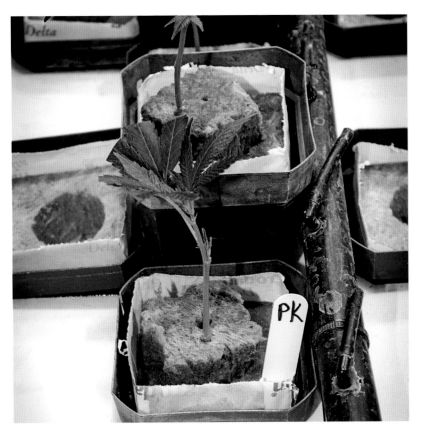

Drip system.

■ Mushroom Compost

Elements / Effect: Perfect source of beneficial soil fungus, some primary, secondary, and trace nutrients. Must be organic.

Comments: Large, porous consistency. Perfect soil structure amendment. Good for microorganisms in soil.

pH Influence: Lowers slightly.

■ Nitrozyme

Elements / Effect: An all-natural organic marine algae extract that contains many nutrients and growth hormones.

Comments: Promotes vigorous and healthy growth, earlier flowering, increased yields with heavier and denser buds. Foliar spray must be applied with surfactant (spreader).

Photo: Freebie

201

■ Perlite

Elements / Effect: Aerates soil and improves drainage.

Comments: Perfect for excessively moist and clay-dominant soils; very visible from the sky and the trail. Tends to rise to the top of soil and must be thoroughly covered with natural soil and vegetation or dyed ahead of time using wet soil or coffee grounds (to camouflage it and make it less visible).

pH Influence: None

■ Pine Needles

Elements / Effect: Slow release, long-term, low-level nitrogen source. Lots of microlife and worm-conducive.

Comments: Perfect amendment for promotion and enhancement of drainage and soil aeration.

pH Influence: Raises.

■ Rare Earth (by General Hydroponics)

Elements / Effect: Derived from ancient seabed deposits of pyrophyllitic clay.

Comments: Protects plants from environmental stress and nutrient extremes. Reduces susceptibility to insect damage and disease.

pH Influence: None.

■ Seaweed or Kelp Meal

Elements / Effect: Many trace elements and nutrients, micro and macro (except phosphorous), plus enzymes and hormones.

Comments: Seaweed or kelp meal add almost every element you need. Excellent source of trace elements.

pH Influence: None.

■ Soft Rock Phosphate (Powdered)

Elements / Effect: Phosphorous, magnesium, and sulfur.

Comments: Commonly referred to as colloidal phosphate. Excellent source of trace elements.

pH Influence: Lowers.

■ Spray-n-Grow

Elements / Effect: A micronutrient complex that uses soil nutrients and

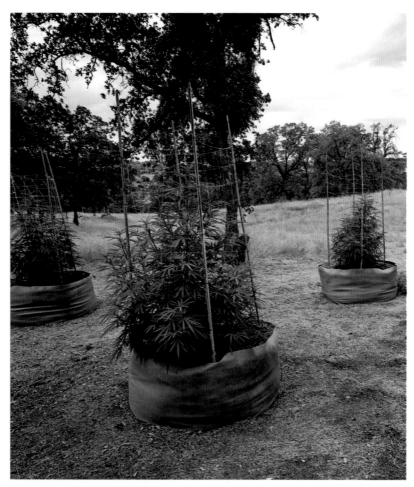

These medium-sized containers are used to allow plants grown outdoors to have specific soil mixes used, rather than the natural soil at the location.

natural plant qualities to the optimum.

Comments: Increases overall health of plants. Promotes larger, heavier, denser buds.

■ Superthrive

Elements: 50 vitamins and hormones.

Comments: Increases overall health of plants. Excellent for transplant shock and stressed plants. A good product is OrganiBliss, an organic plant growth enhancer available from www.organibliss.com

Photo: Freebie

203

■ Unsulfured Blackstrap Molasses
Elements / Effect: Nitrogen (weak), Potassium, trace elements, simple sugars.
Comments: Organic source of potassium and simple sugars which are beneficial to desirable bacteria, fungus, and microbes.
pH Influence: None.

Note
When using organic or synthetic / non-organic liquid fertilizers, you must pre-water the soil or media with pure, clean, non-chlorinated, pH-adjusted water. Delicate roots can be damaged by direct application of full-strength fertilizers. Simply water as you normally would until water begins to drain out of the media. After one hour you can apply your pH-adjusted fertilizers. When watering with (or without) fertilizers, you must allow 25% of the water nutrients to drain out of the media. This practice will wash out any salts or unused fertilizers, preventing buildups that can cause salt or fertilizer excesses or deficiencies and their accompanying symptoms and problems.

Preventing Soil Drainage Problems
Adequate drainage for your media is very important, although media that drains quickly and does not retain moisture will require extra effort and maintenance to keep it properly hydrated and fertilized. But compacted media with inadequate drainage will severely stunt and most often kill some plants, because the roots become oxygen deprived due to their constant immersion in stagnant water. In such a case, desired aerobic bacteria levels will be retarded, while undesirable bacteria flourish, causing overall poor health and diseases. And even if the roots are not damaged by inadequate drainage, healthy, vigorous root growth will be diminished, resulting in a shallow root development that will be unable to use deeper water sources in drought conditions (if you are growing outside).

Evaluate Your Soil
There are many and varying causes of draining problems. Most can be corrected without much effort and with a few simple materials.

   Method of Evaluation: This basic test will enable you to determine whether or not your soil has proper drainage and is conducive to healthy, productive growth. Prior to planting, you will need to get a growing con-

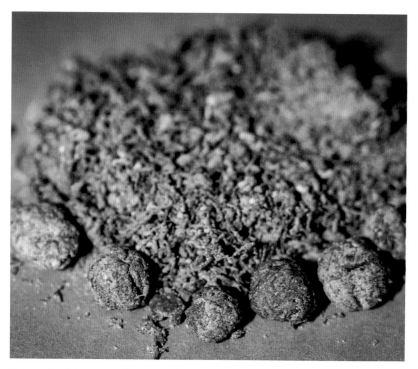

Scissor hash tastes unlike any other.

tainer with $\frac{1}{4}$-inch drill holes and fill it with the soil mix you intend on using, or dig a hole in the soil that you intend on planting in. Pack the soil into the container approximately $\frac{2}{3}$ of the way full or in a hole 2 x 2 feet deep in the ground. Dig the holes deeper than you think you need, which will ensure that even if the lower layers of dirt are not ideal, you will have good water retention and drainage. In the container, fill the remaining $\frac{1}{3}$ with water; the same applies to the earth.

If there is no water on top of the soil in the container after 10 seconds, or no water on top of the soil within one minute, the soil's composition is excessively porous and drains too fast. It will require amending to aid moisture retention. The application of water-retaining crystals, mulch, and amended compost will rectify the condition of the soil. Completely blend and mix in the amendments and retest.

If there is still some water in the container after 30 seconds or in the hole after one minute, the drainage composition is good and there is no need for any amendments.

Photo: Samson Daniels

If water remains in the container for one or more minutes or in the hole after two minutes, then the drainage composition is poor and drains too slowly. In the container you will need to amend soil with 50/50 blends of vermiculite and perlite, crushed oyster shells and mulched bark (albeit not Redwood or Pine), sand and gravel, or other aerating amendments. As for the hole, you must dig it twice as deep. Small plants will need holes three feet deep; medium plants will need holes 4 feet deep and 3 feet wide. Large plants will need holes 6 feet deep and 6 feet wide. The extra soil you extract from the hole will usually be undesirable in composition and will need to be amended with the same amendments listed above, or compost and earthworm castings.

Minimizing Water Loss / Evaporation

Whenever possible outdoors, place hay, straw or coarse mulch on top of the soil surrounding the plant's base. This will minimize evaporation and extend the periods between watering, saving water and time.

Examine Your Outdoor Soil

Clay-dominant soil, or soil with a red, blue-gray, rusty brown, or yellow coloration, possibly accompanied by a foul, stagnant odor, indicates inadequate drainage that will require amending. In poor drainage situations the addition of organic matter to the soil will rectify situations where drainage is not too severely restricted. The addition of generous portions of coarse sand or medium-sized gravel will also improve drainage, as will perlite.

Likewise, drainage will be severely impeded if the soil composition has a close-to-the-surface, non-porous rocky structure or a high water table or soil pan. In such instances the chosen location may be undesirable or not conducive to healthy growth. There is little to nothing you can do if the water table is too high, except to place containers in the soil and grow in them. If the soil pan is too high and the soil is shallow you must dig through the rock layer and replace lost soil. A jackhammer might come in handy.

Caution: snakes like to curl up in the shade around the moist base of outdoor plants in summertime; check with a stick before you dig around with your hands.

Your goal is to have a soil that drains fast—but not too fast!—and retains the desired amounts of water and fertilizer. Test and retest your soil prior to planting and augment it as the soil composition dictates.

Organic Tea

Organic amendments do not necessarily have to be mixed in to your media. Organic compost teas are an excellent method of nutrient delivery. Plants use essential elements such as nitrogen, phosphorous, potassium, and numerous other micronutrients. If these elements are not present, deficient, or not available in proper proportions in your soil, you will experience problems. A properly mixed organic compost tea can supplement all of a plant's nutrient needs. Organic compost is an aerobic mixture of decomposed vegetation and animal waste that contains soluble organic nutrients and beneficial microlife, as well as other healthy bacteria that assist in the breakdown and delivery of available nutrients and aid in pest resistance.

Use of organic compost tea amplifies the health, vigor, and yield of plants grown both organically and hydroponically. Basically, they use water to extract the beneficial elements and nutrients from compost and use the strained water to fertilize your plants. The key to healthy organic plants is to give them what they want in exact amounts, at the right time. With a little extra space and a few months for decomposition you can brew your own compost tea customized for any cultivar you choose to grow.

A good compost is comprised of extremely decomposed fruit, vegetable, and animal waste matter. See the section on Composts for more information. Worm castings make an excellent foundation for compost. They can be obtained at any gardening store, and pre-made composts are available there as well, but your choice between these will depend on the methodology and media you are using. It is thus best to manufacture your own compost to make sure it contains the exact elements you desire and in the proper proportions. Research the compost process, do your homework, and understand what exactly you are feeding your plants and why!

Note that fresh manures must be extremely composted and exposed to high temperatures, something that occurs naturally in the compost, for a minimum of 40 days to kill all harmful pathogens, diseases, or stray seeds that may be present. In addition, they should never be meat-based. Your compost must be stirred and turned over periodically to ensure proper decomposition and aeration.

When your new compost is completely decomposed and ready, and you are ready to brew your tea, you will need a few materials:
■ Rubber gloves

Making Organic Tea

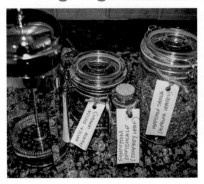

Vegetative matter (herbs) for use in organic tea.

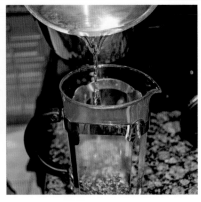

Add boiling water.

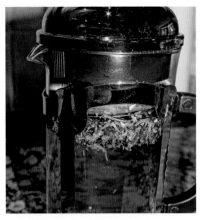

Steep for about 10 minutes.

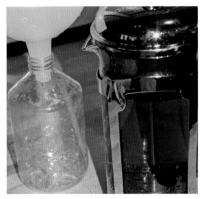

Let it steep until it is about lukewarm.

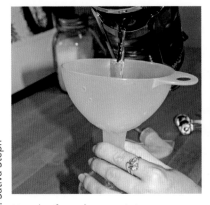

Use the funnel to put it in a spray bottle.

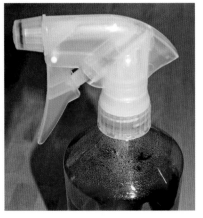

Spray leaves or add to soil.

Photo: Sativa Steph

- Dust masks
- Screens for sifting
- 5-gallon bucket with lid
- 50-gallon drum (if making large quantities) with lid
- Large aquarium pump
- $1/4$-inch air tubing with anti-siphon and regulation valves
- Large air stones or air curtain (last three items available at aquarium supply stores)
- Floor drop covering
- Strainer or stockings stretched around a rounded wire coat hanger or a paint filter funnel
- Purified, clean, non-chlorinated water

You must understand what you are doing, why you are doing it, which ingredients you are using, and what they contain. It's fairly easy to manufacture and use compost, but brewing compost tea demands dedication, care, and proper planning before you start to grow.

How to Brew Organic Compost Tea

Mix clean water and compost at a ratio of 4:1. This means that in a five-gallon bucket you would mix one gallon of compost to four gallons of water; in a 55-gallon drum mix ten gallons of compost and forty gallons of water. Stir and mix contents until all of the compost is completely saturated with water. Place air stones or an air curtain into your tea solution at the bottom of the container and turn on the air pump. This will integrate the necessary oxygen, which is an aid in the extraction of available beneficial microbes and essential elements from the compost. Periodically stir the mix and allow it to stand at approximately 80°F for at least five days, or a maximum of seven days. If the brew starts to smell rotten then inadequate oxygenation is causing proliferation of anaerobic (undesirable) bacteria; increased oxygenation and fresh water will be required to promote and reestablish the desired levels of aerobic bacteria. You can increase oxygenation by using more or larger air pumps or air stones.

Compost should be run through a fine metal screen before using it for tea. Again, always use a dust mask and wear rubber gloves during this process; the inhalation of compost dust is extremely unhealthy for animals and humans with compromised immune systems. Then, the tea should be thoroughly

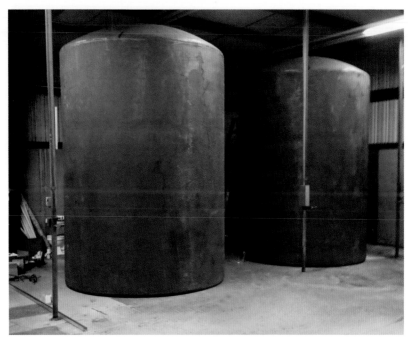

A sterilized water-source is essential, and must be utilized in all stages of growth as well as used for decontamination of all equipment.

filtered after brewing to ensure that larger particulates do not clog pumps, drippers, sprayers, foggers, or drains.

After filtration, your organic compost tea is ready for application. First, stir it very well and check the PPM of the tea; if the PPM is higher than you desire, dilute it using clean water as necessary. Next, check the pH to make sure it is within acceptable levels—5.8 to 7, depending on the cultivar of the plant. If it is not within acceptable levels, adjust using organic methods such as potassium hydroxide, for raising the pH, or lemon juice or vinegar for lowering the pH.

After PPM and pH are at desired levels your organic, nutrient-rich compost tea is ready for application as a foliar feed or soil drench. Use as needed depending on your plants' needs and cultivation method. When growing organically, the proper method of avoiding deficiencies is to apply compost tea to both the soil and the underside of the leaves, which is where nutrient uptake begins, through a foliar feed. Blending organic compost into media will aid in continual decomposition and allow the availability of necessary essential elements.

Photo: K

Basic Foundation Tea Recipe (for Vegetative and Flowering Growth)

- 3 parts seabird guano (high nitrogen)
- 4 parts bat guano (high nitrogen and phosphorous)
- 6 parts earthworm castings (high nitrogen and many other essential elements)

This recipe is meant as the base foundation of your tea; it must be composted with other elements, depending on your growth stage, as explained previously.

Introduction to General Hydroponics' Flora Series Liquid Concentrated Nutrient

For more than 30 years, General Hydroponics has been a leading innovator in the field of hydroponics. With factories in North America and Europe, their products are at the cutting edge of the industry. NASA uses their products in preparation for hydroponics on the international space station; laboratories and universities use them for teaching and research; and their products are used extensively for commercial crop production as well as high-tech cannabis crops.

Their Flora Series Liquid Concentrated Nutrient is the original building block nutrient system—often imitated but never duplicated. The Flora series contains complete primary, secondary, and micronutrients for enhanced yields and better crop quality. Users can adjust mixtures to suit specific plant needs. The Flora series enhances flavor, nutrition, aroma, potency, and essential oils in both hydroponic and soil-cultivated plants. It contains highly purified concentrates for maximum solubility and it is pH balanced for ease of use.

Products and Nutrients

Flora Micro: 5-0-1

Color: Red, purple

The foundation of the "building block" system; provides nitrogen, potassium, calcium, and trace elements.

Flora Gro: 2-1-6

Color: Green

Stimulates structural and vegetative growth. Builds strong roots. Provides nitrogen, phosphorous, potassium, and secondary nutrients.

Flora Bloom: 0-5-4

Color: Pink

Stimulates bud development. Enhances flavor, aroma, and essential oils. Provides high phosphorous, potassium, magnesium, and sulfur.

Caution

Never use Flora series nutrients in organic, "living" soil. Mineral salts will kill most beneficial microorganisms in the organic soil. For organic growing, General Hydroponics offer organic-based supplements, which are perfect for organic cultivation.

Water-Retaining Crystals

These crystals absorb up to 400 times their weight in water, and so increase the water-holding capacity of the soil or media they are in by 50% or more, depending on the type of media, the quality of the water, and the amount of applied fertilizers. During sunny, rainless days, they release their accumulated water. In so doing, they expand and contract, loosening the soil and keeping plants healthy and aerated. They prefer "soft" water, are non-toxic, and work for years. Plus, they are neutral in pH and non-toxic! You can find them at most garden and hydroponic supply stores.

Note: Because water-retaining crystals reduce the amount of fertilizer lost through drainage, you must sometimes reduce the amount of applied fertilizer to avoid potential fertilizer "burn." If nutrient excesses do occur you must flush the medium.

For outdoor or soil use, mix one teaspoon of dry water-retaining crystals for every two liters of soil. Use this mixture in the bottom half of your containers or holes, then add regular soil to top it off. Water lightly at first to hydrate the crystals.

Watering Interval

Since water crystals store water much longer than soil, you'll probably find that your soil will dry out before your plant does. The tried-and-true "finger test" for soil moisture will no longer be a reliable measure of plant moisture needs. Watch your plants for signs of moisture loss or stress, such as a lightening of plant color, leaf droop, or abnormal stretching. Each plant is different and each will have different watering needs. Be vigilant: check your plants

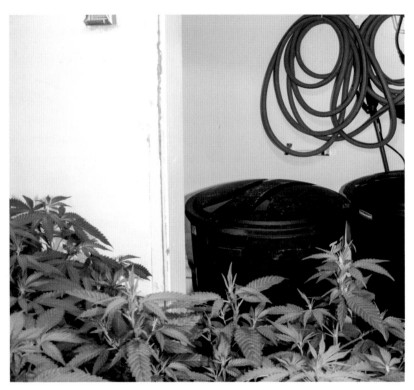

A good growroom always has a hose.

at least once a day! If they are in containers, lift them; if they feel light and the top two inches of soil feel dry, then they probably need water.

Outdoor Soil Augmentation

Augmenting existing soil in outdoor situations is relatively easy so long as the soil or terrain you begin with is not completely unacceptable. Outdoor cultivation is completely different from indoor growing; the methods, techniques, and susceptibility to problems are determined by the surrounding environment, over which you have little control. Your chosen climate and its relative humidity, rainfall, altitude, longitude, latitude, available sunlight, and soil composition will contribute to the overall health and vigor of your plants as well as the quality of the finished product. To grow superior quality organic cannabis outdoors, you need to examine your chosen climate and environment. If all parameters are acceptable, you must then find a cannabis cultivar that will thrive in your chosen situation.

Photo: Samson Daniels

Soil-Mix Augmentation

When cultivating cannabis outdoors, your major issues are soil content, structure, and pH level. pH levels can dictate which cultivars will do best in your chosen area; some cultivars are very temperamental in regards to excessively high or low pH. Consult seed companies and the Internet to make sure your cultivar is suitable for your chosen environment. Extremely soggy, sandy, or clay-dominant soils are unacceptable and you must either find another grow location or augment the soil to render it more conducive to healthy growth.

Your first step is to purchase a soil pH testing kit or soil pH meter for precise analysis. Samples can also be sent to a soil-testing laboratory, which will give you exact pH and mineral content information. Addresses of these may be found on the Internet.

Augmenting existing soil is basically the process of replacing all or part of the existing soil with a composite media that has a stabilized pH and high-nutrient consistency. How you augment your soil depends on the initial pH. Is it fairly low, i.e. 5.7, or extremely high, i.e. 7.6? Each will require a completely different preparation and soil amendment to set the pH to the desired levels.

If at all possible, always use some of the available natural soil; this will ensure the inclusion of many beneficial microbes and bacteria that promote vigorous, healthy growth.

Clay-Dominant Soil Augmentation

If your soil has high clay content, you must amend it with generous amounts of gypsum, compost, and green sand about six months prior to planting. These amendments will aid in pH stabilization and nutrient availability, and allow clay soil to homogenize into a more desirable form. At this time you can also mix in hay, perlite, water-retaining crystals, pine needles, kelp, seaweed-based fertilizer, earthworm castings, blood meal, and fish meal. Top it off with more compost and native soil.

Correction for Elevated pH Levels in Soil

Soil with pH levels higher than 7.0 will require amendments to lower and stabilize the pH to acceptable levels: between 5.8 and 6.8, depending on the cultivar. Organic fertilizers that are high in potassium, nitrogen, and phosphorous are excellent for correcting high pH soil conditions. Fox Farm's Peace of Mind, a fertilizer for acid-loving plants, is a perfect choice.

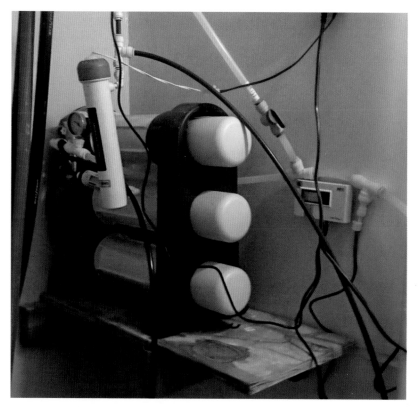

RO systems like this are perfect for small gardens.

Gypsum is the ultimate amendment for outdoor soil conditions, except in cases of soil pH levels of 5.6 or lower, in which case it must be applied in conjunction with bone meal and dolomite lime. Gypsum is an excellent source of sulfur and calcium, which are both important components of bud production, and it is good for elevated pH levels and clay-dominant soils, as well. Bear in mind that gypsum can take as long as ten months to decompose and become available to the plants. For application, combine gypsum with green sand (one part green sand to three parts gypsum) and mix it into the top layer of soil. Apply every six months if you intend on using the same location.

Correction for Lower pH Levels in Soil

Adding elevated levels of dolomite lime and bone meal to the soil provides buffering for other amendments that may contribute to a drop in the soil's pH such as bird and bat guano, cottonseed meal, fish emulsion, blood meal, etc.

Photo: K

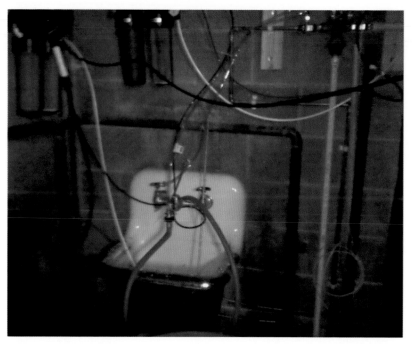

This is a mess. Never allow your equipment to become an entangled mess.

Replacing Soil

If you want to simply replace the existing soil because you deem it unacceptable for plant growth, you can use Fox Farm Ocean Forest or Light Warrior
potting soil as your foundation and then custom blend the aforementioned
amendments as your environment dictates. Amended soil and most potting
mixes usually do not need added fertilizers for the first few weeks of use, as
they should contain ample amounts of the required nutrients for healthy
early-stage growth. After approximately three to four weeks, you can begin
feeding with organic foliar spray, compost tea or Fox Farms' Big Bloom or
General Hydroponics' organic based nutrient supplements. This is very important as plants will use and deplete available elements rapidly—usually
within three weeks. Never over-fertilize; be conservative. You can always
apply more if needed, but too much fertilizer can burn plant roots.

Introduction to Fertilizers and Organic Amendments

Cannabis requires nutrients, be they synthetic or organic, in proper proportions throughout the lifecycle in order to keep vigorous and healthy and give amazing yields of fantastic buds. Nitrogen, phosphorous, and potassium (a.k.a. N-P-K) are the primary essential elements and, combined with trace elements, comprise the ingredients of all fertilizers designed for cannabis cultivation.

Plants sometimes deplete essential elements available in soil more rapidly than they can be made available, therefore nutrients must be applied to the plants when they need it, and in precise amounts.

N: Nitogen

Both nitrate and ammonium are responsible for overall health and vigorous growth of foliage and cellular division.

P: Phosphorous

Primarily responsible for root production.

K: Potassium

Responsible for pest and disease resistance; essential for high yielding, potent buds.

The required amounts of nutrients will vary depending on your growing methodology, chosen cultivar, environment, and soil composition or growing system.

Organic Fertilizers

These are basically decomposed matter derived from plant matter and animal waste. They are slow to release their elements and less prone to burn root and foliage than synthetics. However, caution must be used, as too much of one or another amendment can cause imbalance, resulting in nutrient lockout.

Inorganic and Synthetic Fertilizers

Synthetic / inorganic fertilizers, such as those in the General Hydroponics Flora series, are often salt-based and mixed with essential elements from natural sources, therefore they are not usually completely "inorganic" or "unnatural." Synthetic fertilizers, meanwhile, are derived primarily from man-made or mined-mineral sources. Both come in concentrated form and are diluted with water and pH-adjusted prior to application. Inorganic and synthetic fertilizers are designed for hydroponics; aeroponics; and mist, drip,

NFT, and fog systems. They are also perfect for soilless, rockwool media and for foliar feed applications. Both are rapidly absorbed by plants and therefore great care and precaution must be taken to prevent over-fertilization or buildups, but when used correctly as a foliar feed these fertilizers are ideal for correcting nutrient deficiencies and ensuring that plants maintain balanced nutrient availability.

Soil Amendments

Animal waste, fruit and vegetable composts, soft rock phosphate, and green sand, to name a few, all add essential elements to soils and tea fertilizers, but all must be given at proper levels at the appropriate time. Organic soil amendments also contribute to healthy, beneficial life forms and bacteria levels, proper oxygen absorption, and water drainage in organic soil environments. Soil amendments slowly and predictably decompose and provide essential macro and micro nutrients to plants in a form that is easily metabolized.

There are many pseudo-organic fertilizers available for sale. Make an educated purchase; do your homework and understand the contents and sources of your chosen fertilizers and amendments. Again, your method of cultivation and environment will usually dictate which fertilizers you ultimately choose. For example, fish-based fertilizers are very aromatic and may not be the best fertilizer choice in an apartment grow.

Powdered Fertilizers

These come in one-, two-, and three-part formulas, sometimes more! The fertilizer is dissolved in water, pH-adjusted, and applied to your media or as a foliar feed. It is critical that these (and all) fertilizers are mixed in proper proportions to avoid nutrient over- or under-fertilization. Follow manufacturers' recommendations and adjust accordingly.

Liquid Fertilizers

These are the most prevalent fertilizers on the market. As with dry fertilizers, they are available in one-, two-, three-, or even five-part nutrient formulas. The liquid nutrients are mixed to specific PPM levels, pH-adjusted, and placed into the reservoir, applied to the soil, or foliar fed to ensure a complete nutrient availability.

Application Timing

Organic matter fertilizers are mixed into soil prior to use and allowed to naturally break down and provide essential elements over an extended period of time. Should deficiencies appear, they are quickly corrected using compost tea or organic fertilizer. Hydroponic fertilizer applications are usually done via the reservoir. Nutrients are mixed and pH-adjusted prior to filling the reservoir. Depending on your media, system, and methodology, the watering schedule will be dictated by the plants and how rapidly they utilize their water and nutrients.

Animal Waste

Composted manures are excellent amendments for cannabis cultivation, though they should not be from meat-eating animals. Never use fresh manure, as it will burn and kill plants. It must be composted first, allowed to sit at 70°F to 80°F for 90 to 120 days. Animal waste provides the essential micronutrients required for vigorous, healthy plant growth and development. Not all manures are the same, and consistency varies from one type to another as far as nutrients are concerned, so you must augment any deficiencies with compost tea, foliar feeding, or amendment top dressing.

Pythium and Pathogens

Pythium, a.k.a. root rot, is a basic and prevalent waterborne disease that can have disastrous effects on indoor and outdoor crops. Pythium is a term used for many different root- and stem-rotting fungal species, commonly referred to as "damping off." Pythium will kill plants if left untreated, and it can infect plants at any stage—seedling, clone, vegetative, and flowering. Indicators of early pythium damage are:

■ rotting, discolored roots
■ yellowing or curling leaves
■ acidic pH
■ poor health
■ low yields

Eventually, it will result in crop failure.

Pythium can rapidly become a serious problem in both large and small hydroponic systems. Recirculating systems with interconnected reservoirs, irrigation—drippers, NFT, aeroponics, etc.—all create perfect environments for accelerating growth and spreading pythium spores. In recirculating systems, one pythium-infected plant will spread the disease to all plants in the system. Pythium proliferates best in anaerobic, warm environments and stagnant, unaerated nutrient solutions and reservoirs. Clay-dominant soil with inadequate drainage also creates perfect conditions for pythium.

Preventative hygiene is an absolute must! Unfiltered water, infected root material, roots from prior crops, decomposing plant matter, and unsterilized systems, tools, and surfaces can spread pythium. Growroom temperature and oxygen starvation both relate to pythium infection. As explained previously, oxygenation and temperature are interrelated in hydroponic systems. High growroom and reservoir temperatures cause oxygen starvation situations that will cause plant stress, increasing susceptibility to pythium and other opportunistic pathogens.

Advanced symptoms of pythium include dead, decaying, or slimy roots and sulfurous, decaying smells from reservoirs. Ultimately, the plant will die as the roots rot. Root death is irreparable, and there is no single product that can cure a pythium-infected plant. The only thing you can do once plants are infected is to manage the infection: eliminate and properly dispose of any and all infected roots and dead vegetation; cut off all dead roots and eliminate any loose root material in the system, including drains, drippers, containers, etc.; clean / decontaminate reservoirs and replace nutrients twice a week. As there is no cure for pythium, your focus must be on prevention.

To clean your system, sterilize it with ONA Bleech (hydroponics cleaner) or hydrogen peroxide (but caution! Never mix bleach and peroxide together), mixed at one part bleach / peroxide (27%) to ten parts water. You must clean everything thoroughly, period. A product called Pythoff, manufactured by Flairform, is used as a hydroponic nutrient conditioner for maintaining nutrient system sterility. It is available at most hydroponic supply stores.

Prevention is the only cure for pythium! Remember:
- Constantly inspect roots for discoloration
- Weak and stressed plants are infected by pythium first
- Eliminate all weak plants
- Only use healthy, uninfected clones from a known origin
- Monitor pH and keep it between 5.8 and 6.8
- Use sterilized soil and soilless media and purified water

Nutrient Delivery System

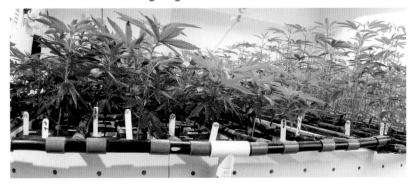

Vegetative plants with nutrient delivery tubes visible in foreground.

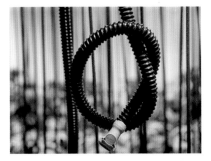

Unconnected delivery tube looped for tidiness.

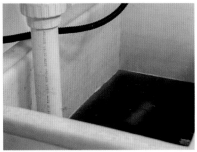

Reservoir seen here with nutrient solution.

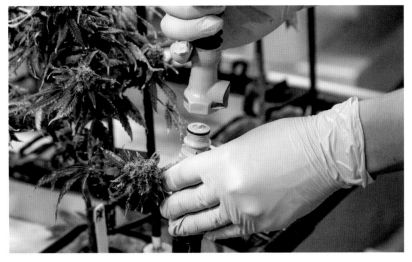

Male and female connectors on the nutrient delivery tubes make cleaning and set up / take down easy.

Photos: Freebie

Nutrient Delivery System

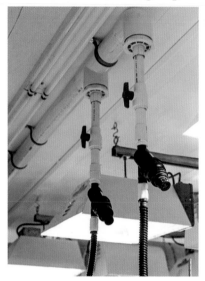

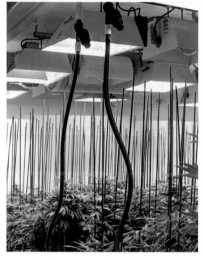

Plumbing is well organized with easily accessible connection points and valves.

In this system the reservoir is across the room and the nutrient delivery system travels across the ceiling and down to the grow system.

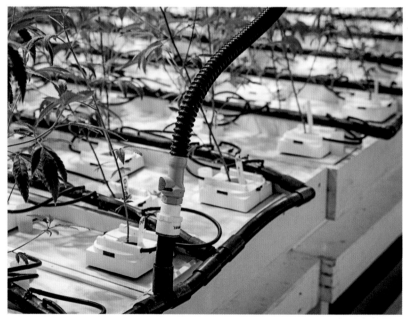

Here we have a closer look at where the nutrient delivery system links to the grow system.

Photos: Freebie

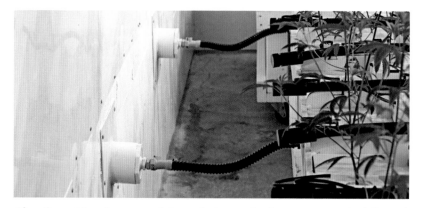

After the nutrient has passed through the media the wastewater is delivered via quick disconnects to a plumbing system in the wall.

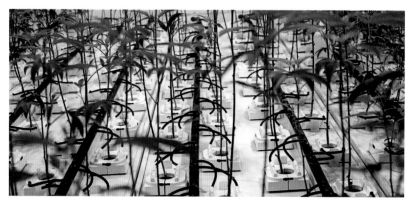

This grow system and the attached drip caps is the most efficient, eco-friendly, and is at the height of water conservation.

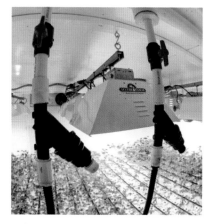

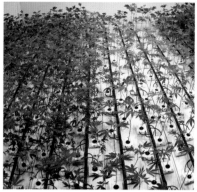

Valves and filters visible.

A good nutrient delivery system can keep all these plants thriving.

Nutrient Delivery System

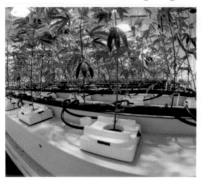

Cube caps on the rockwool cube keep algae from growing.

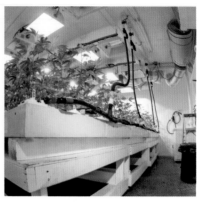

Nutrient delivery from above.

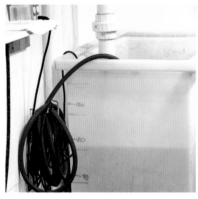

Reservoir with gallon measurements on the side.

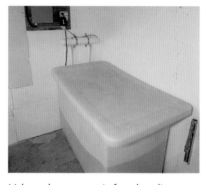

Lid on the reservoir for cleanliness and to minimize humidity by limiting water evaporation.

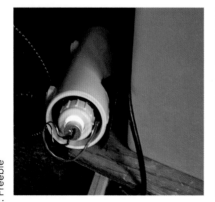

Small scale ultra violet water sterilizer.

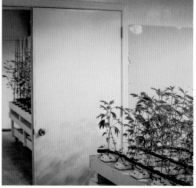

Partitions between growth chambers.

Photos: Freebie

■ Use Pythoff or other additives

■ Monitor nutrient temperatures and keep them at approximately 72°F

■ Maintain excellent ventilation in the growroom

■ Maximize oxygenation and circulation within nutrient tanks and reservoirs by using water circulation pumps, air pumps, or air stones

■ Sterilize all equipment that will be used in several reservoirs

■ Always maintain proper drainage of soil

Urgent care for infection:

■ Remove all plants and disinfect entire system

■ Dunk roots in diluted, ten-to-one water / food grade hydrogen peroxide (27%) solution

■ Remove all rotted, diseased roots from the plant and dispose of properly. Rinse the remaining roots and place the plant back into the system. Note, in a large scale grow, it is advised to discard the plant entirely. However, a small home grow where every plant counts can get away with this procedure.

■ Add beneficial root growth boosters, vitamin B1, Superthrive, etc.

■ Replace nutrient in sterilized tank reservoir at half nutrient strength and maintain at 72°F

■ Reduce light levels and intensity; move lights three feet away from plants to reduce radiant heat

■ After one or two weeks, when new root growth slowly increases, increase nutrient levels and return lights to normal position

Nutrient Enhancers

What follows is a list of the nutrient enhancers and amendments we use at Trichome Technologies to ensure proper health throughout the grow cycle. While the General Hydroponics Flora series nutrients are the building blocks of Trichome Technologies' fertilizer program the following products are the mortar that holds them all together. Combined, they provide for every nutrient need of our plants.

Liquid KoolBloom Ripening Formula
Manufactured by General Hydroponics
Concentrated potash and phosphorous
N-P-K: 0-10-10

Promotes abundant flowering, facilitates ripening, and enhances production of essential oils and fragrances; produces larger buds. Use at onset of flowering to manufacturer's mixing specifications. For indoor and outdoor use. Available at hydroponic supply stores.

Diamond Nectar
Manufactured by General Hydroponics
Premium grade humic acid
N-P-K: 0-1-1

Humic acid accelerates nutrient absorption at the root boundary zone, where minerals enter the plant. Excellent for indoor and outdoor use. Available at hydroponic supply stores. (Also available and excellent is Diamond Black: dry, premium grade humic acid, for use in soil and soilless media.)

Chlorine, Contaminants, Aeration, and Their Importance

Chlorine (and chloramines, which will be implied by the term "chlorine" in this section) in municipal city water kill all beneficial bacteria and living organisms in your medium, be it soil or soilless. Chlorine is not conducive to healthy, productive plant growth and must be eliminated. There are two easy methods to eliminate chlorine. The first is charcoal filtration. Second is a chloramine filter that goes before the reverse osmosis system. Charcoal filtration is the less expensive of the two. In charcoal filtration, a charcoal filter is placed in your water line, supplying you with unchlorinated water; make sure that the filter is guaranteed to eliminate chlorine. The second option is to leave water standing in a container—uncovered, but not able to collect dust or other contaminants. A common aquarium water pump should be used to aerate the water. It should be connected via $\frac{1}{4}$-inch tubing to an air stone or air curtain. All of these items are available online or from your local grow supply store, or any ordinary aquarium supply stores. Aerating water for 24 hours dechlorinates it!

Notes:
- You cannot over-oxygenate your water; the more oxygen, the better.
- Place the air pump outside of a CO_2-enriched environment and run a $\frac{1}{4}$-inch hose to the water storage container that is to be oxygenated.

■ Never place an air pump in an unventilated area with decomposing roots and vegetables; pythium spores and other organisms can infect your water— and besides, what good would it do to use stale air?

Water

Many inexperienced growers apply too little water too often, which encourages shallow root growth. When watering, 25% of the water should "run off," i.e. drain out of the soil or container. The plant should not be watered again until the medium becomes slightly dry. Overwatering encourages root rot and disease. How much water plants require per day varies throughout the cycle / season. It's dictated by the conditions and climate you are growing in. Even a small garden will demand significant amounts of water in hot or dry weather. Water first thing in the morning, at sunrise, or, if indoors, when the lights come on.

Serious growers all use purified, "clean" water to ensure a productive harvest. Many other growers water their plants with straight tap water. This is a bad idea. These are the common components and properties found in municipal water: alkalinity, aluminum, ammonia, antimony, arsenic, barium, beryllium, bicarbonate, boron, bromate, cadmium, calcium, chloride, chlorine, chromium, cobalt, copper, cyanide, fluoride, iron, lead, magnesium, manganese, mercury, molybdenum, nickel, nitrate, phosphorous, potassium, selenium, silver, sodium, strontium, sulfate, thallium, vanadium, and zinc. All of these, though they may vary in percentage, make up the PPM of the tap water. A full list of all contents and contaminants found in water, and their maximum limits, may be found at http://www.epa.gov/safewater/contaminants/index.html.

Water Hardness

The number one indicator of water quality for plants is hardness. Hardness is measured by the amount of dissolved calcium and magnesium, elements that make up the majority of the PPM in most water. While it is true that both components – calcium and magnesium – are critical for plant growth, they are only needed in certain quantities. With higher levels of hardness, plants can experience nutrient lockout problems. High levels of other minerals can also impede optimum growth. High PPM levels of iron, manganese, lead, copper, or zinc, for instance, can result in deficiency and lockout problems.

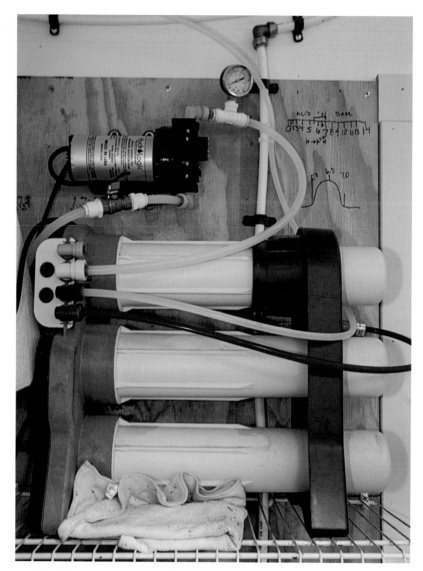

Small scale reverse osmosis filters are a must for obtaining purified water.

When is Water Too Dirty?

Here is a plausible scenario: after receiving the results from a water testing facility or a water quality report from your city, you learn that the PPM of your water sample is 300 PPM (high) and that the level of hardness (calcium and magnesium) is 150 PPM. The remaining 150 PPM will be made up of miscellaneous elements, including iron, copper, zinc, sulfur, and so on.

The water looks good and smells good. You decide it is acceptable water to grow with.

When it's time to transplant rooted clones into larger containers, you know that the new plants will require approximately 400 PPM in the water for the first week, and that new plants are sensitive to high PPM levels in their early stages.

Here's the dilemma: What do you do at this point? Add 400 PPM of nutrients to the water that is already 300 PPM? Or do you add 100 PPM of nutrients? In this situation, it would be impossible to accurately control the amount of nutrients necessary for optimum plant growth.

Beginning with pure water, which is as close to 0 PPM as possible, allows you to add every required element in precise, desired quantities, as needed for every stage of plant growth. Each part of the nutrient formula can be measured to exact amounts.

Precise control of the PPM makeup of your water is essential and will contribute to fantastic growth and amazing, consistent harvests, without the worry of nutrient deficiencies, lockout problems, or contaminants.

Well Water and City Water: Sources and Composition

Water from the tap can originate from a multitude of sources—municipal or city water, springs, wells, creeks, rivers, lakes, streams: all have potential water quality problems. Many believe that spring water is perfect for growing, yet the mineral content is usually way too high for optimum plant growth. Each water source presents a unique challenge when deciding how you are going to improve its quality. The filtration system required for well water treatment may differ from the requirements of municipal water. The majority of springs and wells require a water softener to filter out undesirable hardness and minerals.

Reverse Osmosis

A high quality reverse osmosis (RO) filtration system will remove all contaminants from water. Most small RO systems are affordable and do not require anything more than normal water pressure and periodic maintenance for them to operate properly. Understanding the pros and cons of RO will allow you to reap its benefits.

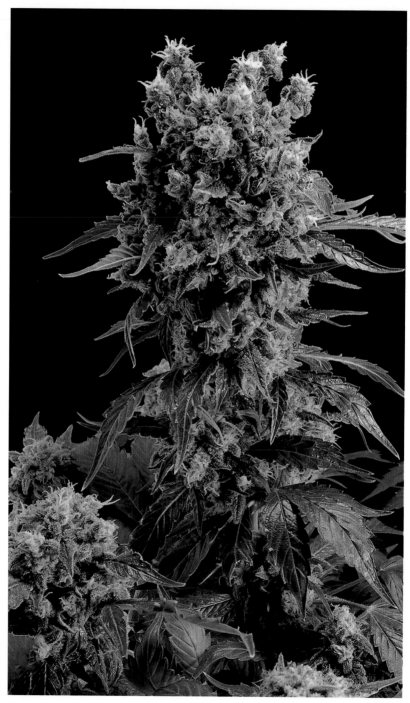

Photo: Dinafem

California Hash Plant.

Most RO systems offered perform very well, as long as you understand the quality of the water you are starting with (its PPM) and perform daily maintenance. Most systems can handle a maximum of 1,000 PPM (and 170 PPM of hardness) of incoming water to be filtered. If the source water is approaching the upper limits, or beyond what a typical RO system can filter efficiently, you must pretreat the filter using a water softener or charcoal filter.

In such a case, place the water softener or charcoal filtration system in the water line before the RO system to remove hardness. Pre-filtering allows the RO membranes to perform at maximum efficiency, resulting in very pure water with the least amount of maintenance costs, as RO filters and membranes will require less frequent replacement. Municipal water users dealing with chlorine and chloramines must use additional carbon and sediment stages to pretreat water before they reach the RO membranes as chloramine and chlorine will degrade the membrane of the RO filters.

As stated previously, intimate knowledge and understanding of your water quality is paramount in achieving quality results. Understanding water quality and filtration techniques will allow you to produce the purest water of a superior quality.

Reverse Osmosis vs. Charcoal

RO systems are extremely wasteful. For every gallon of purified water you get (at approximately 0 PPM), many gallons of unpure water are diverted. The gallons lost depend on the PPM of the source water you are starting with: the higher the PPM of the source water, the more water is diverted; the lower the PPM of the source water, the less water wasted. With this in mind, try charcoal filtration before RO. If RO is necessary, use its diverted water as "gray water" (which is safe but unfit for consumption) for watering your lawn or shrubs—but use it cautiously, and discontinue if the plants appear not to like it. Otherwise place the diverted water in the sewer to be reclaimed.

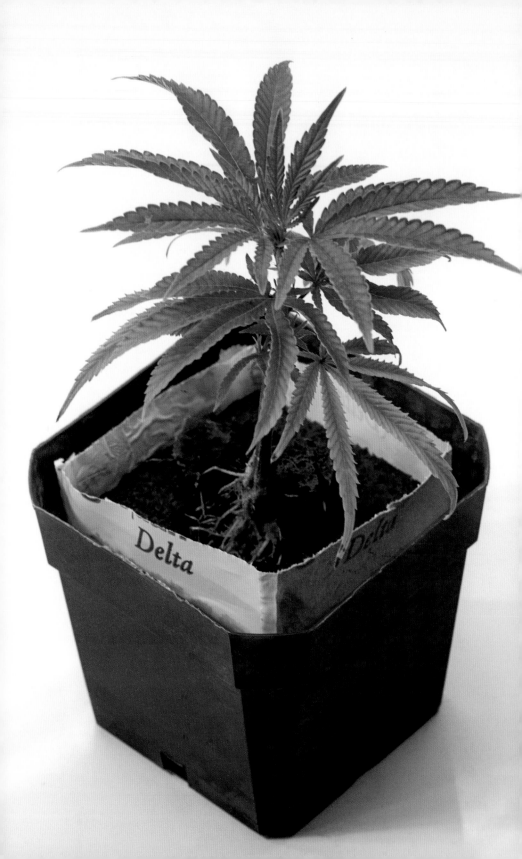

CHAPTER 12

Cloning

What is a Clone?

A clone is the exact replica of the plant from which it was taken: same sex, growth pattern, and harvest timing. Literally dozens of successive generations can be obtained with no particular degeneration. Some growers take cuttings from mother plants, others from vegetating plants before they enter the flowering cycle.

Materials Called for in this Chapter

- One razorblade or very sharp pointed scissors
- One alcohol Bunsen burner
- Two 2-cup measuring cups
- One small bucket for carrying cuttings
- One mini-greenhouse dome and one propagation tray
- Small potting containers / plastic drink cups with multiple holes in bottom for drainage
- Preferred medium (soil, rockwool)
- Fluorescent lights with cool white bulbs
- Rooting hormone (such as Wood's Rooting Compound or Olivia's Cloning Gel) that contains butyric and acetic acid
- Hand mister
- Clean, disinfected work area

◀ A small potting container. Note the green algae on top of the rockwool cube which inhibits nutrient uptake, oxygenation, and can contribute to the proliferation of fungus gnat larvae. You must always prevent light from reaching the top of your rockwool cubes.

Photo: Samson Daniels

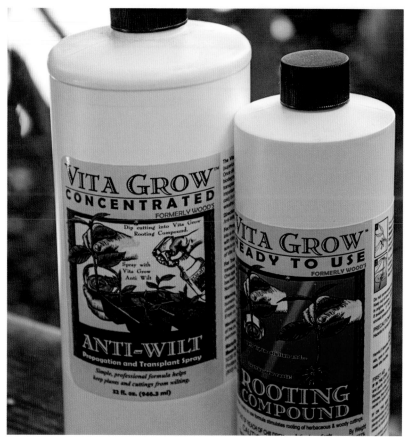

Vita Grow Rooting Compound (formerly Wood's Rooting Compound).

Clone How-To

Plants rooted from cuttings are the preferred method of propagation by many growers, particularly if they've experienced difficulties starting from seed, or if they want to be certain the offspring exhibit the identical traits of the donor plant. Cloning is easy provided only a sharp, sterile razor blade or scissors are used to make the final cut on the stem. Cloning solutions such as Wood's Rooting Compound, a ready-to-use rooting compound (available from hydroponics supply stores), are used to minimize susceptibility to embolism (an air bubble inside the stem) and transplant shock; it also delivers hormones and nutrients to encourage rapid root growth.

Aside from viable cuttings, you will need propagation containers with an insert tray and a translucent domed top, as well as a sterile, inert medium to

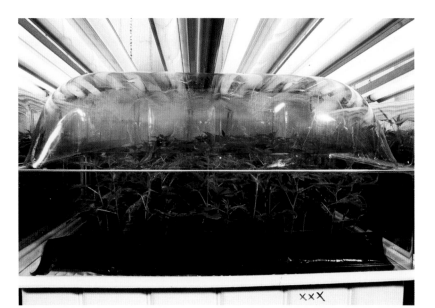

Propagation tray.

get started. There are many cloning machines and kits available on the market at your local hydroponics supply center. Fox Farms' Light Warrior soil—mixed equally with a mix of one part Light Warrior, one part perlite, and one part vermiculite—is a good organic cloning medium. So are Grodan rockwool cloning slabs.

Cuttings require warmth, moisture, oxygen, and light. Inside the dome, try to maintain a humidity of 74–80% and a temperature of 75–80°F. To maintain the temperature, use a heated propagation mat placed underneath the tray that holds the medium. Root zone temperature should be slightly higher (say 3–5°F higher) than the ambient temperature inside the dome. These mats help monitor and maintain correct temperatures, usually about 15°F above room temperature. As such, the growth of root rot or "damping off" disease is greatly inhibited.

Caution: to make sure your cuttings don't get too hot, avoid placing cloning trays directly on top of heat mats. Elevate the tray two or three inches above the heat mat and monitor the temperature with a digital Hi / Lo thermometer.

Bear in mind that the heat mat will increase evaporation, so you must keep your growing medium moist. Not too moist, though: plastic covers and humidity domes can get too much heat and moisture, which can lead to fungal

Photo: Andre Grossman

problems, such as pythium, so you should uncover them periodically, perhaps twice a day, or place a few small holes in the cover so that excess heat and moisture can escape. Once your cuttings form roots you can extend the period of time you keep the dome off of the plants, until ultimately the clones do not need to be covered at all, and are ready to be moved to the vegetative stage.

If you intend to transplant your clones outdoors, you must remember to acclimatize them in advance. As soon as the risk of frost diminishes, take your cuttings for a few hours at a time to an outdoor shady area protected from excessive wind, gradually increasing their exposure to the elements over a one or two week period.

Clone Considerations

Advantages:

Productivity; clones grow faster and accelerate the growth process more rapidly than plants started from seed; sex is usually pre-determined (female).

Homogeneity:

A batch of cuttings taken from the same plant will produce the same characteristics and yield uniform results.

Economical:

Clones typically cost between $5 and $10 each, depending on the source, and going to purchase and constantly transport new clones is costly and potentially risky. At the same time, you can take dozens, even hundreds of clones from just a few vegetative plants by taking cuttings over and over again.

Sources

There are three general sources for clones. The first is an outside source, such as a friend or a legal Cannabis buyers' club. The advantage of this is you save yourself time, space, and work. The disadvantage is the cost, unfamiliar genetics, and the possible introduction of pests and disease into the growroom. Using outside sources also allows other people to know what you're doing, which is never a wise move.

Keeping mother plants is another source. This enables you to perpetuate your genetics by taking cuttings from specific plants. In order to do this, keep a mother plant in a separate environment under an 18 on / 6 off light

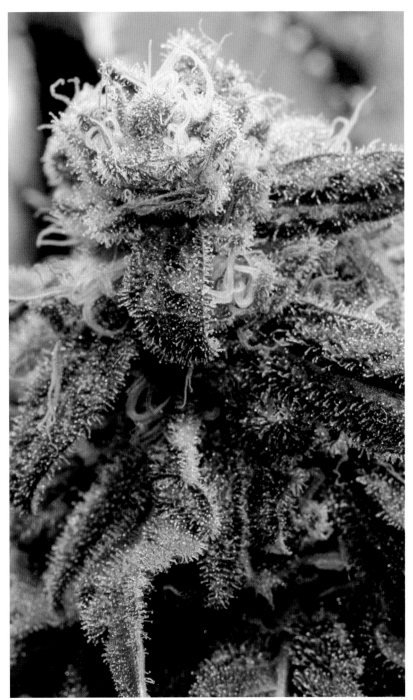

Sticky and stinky is the way I like 'em.

Photo: Samson Daniels

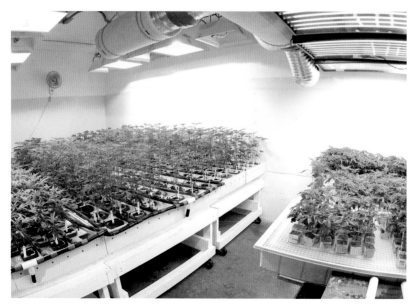

Vegetative and clone chamber with uniform canopies. Note the newly rooted clones in rockwool on the right.

cycle and never let it flower. Whether you're just keeping one mother or ninety-nine, the same rules apply. You give it the same light as any plant in the vegetative stage. I've heard that some people retain the mother for years. Myself, I like to create new ones when they get too gangly—usually every six months or so. Mother plants allow you to self-perpetuate your plants and dictate your own schedule. They also afford you the knowledge that your clone source is disease and pest-free. On the downside, they eat up time, money, and space.

The third source for clones is to take them straight off your vegetating plants. This works only in systems where you have achieved a solid rotation, when you have just harvested your finished flowers and are about to move your vegetating plants into flowering. The trick is to wait two days after they have been placed under a 12 / 12 light-cycle; this purges them of starches that can inhibit root growth. Then take your cuttings from any or all of the lower branches, always leaving at least the top two for flowering. Once you've taken the cuttings, they can sit under fluorescents for up to thirty days before it's time to transfer to your vegetating room. This completes the cycle and maximizes time and space.

Photos: Freebie

Traditional Cutting Methods

Below are two traditional methods for taking cuttings. Both use artificial lighting, but you can choose to use a soil-perlite-vermiculite organic medium, a hydroponic substrate (such as rockwool or Hydroton Clay Pebbles), or one of many others.

Mother / Donor Plants

You should choose bushy plants with many small, 4–6-inch branches to take cuttings from. Cuttings root more easily when they come from a plant in its vegetative stage rather than in its flowering stage. For small gardens the best solution is to maintain mother plants. A mother plant is kept in the vegetative cycle all year by maintaining an 18 hours on / 6 hours off photoperiod. The goal is to keep the donor plant in vegetative growth and not allow it to flower or produce buds. Then you can cut off the branches whenever you want clones.

Gardex Substrate

Gardex is a hydroponic substrate made up of a combination of mineral matter: vermiculite, perlite, and hydrophilic horticultural rockwool. Its water-retention capacity is 60% of its volume and the medium allows you to space out your watering intervals without fear of harming the plants. Gardex can be used for either automated watering systems or hand watering without fear of excess watering. Gardex is an excellent medium for rooting cuttings.

Advantages:

■ Maximum aeration of the root mass: 33% of the volume is made up of air
■ Higher water retention than soil
■ Neutral pH (7)
■ Accelerated growth and healthier foliage
■ Decreased watering frequency and easy rehumidification
■ Consistent volume with no compaction
■ Sterile because it is manufactured to contain no organic contaminants

Avoid Stagnant Water

Excessive water, especially stagnant water, increases the risk of rot, and the cutting will take longer to produce roots. Stagnant water is rapidly depleted of its oxygen by the plant and this prevents the growth of new root tissue.

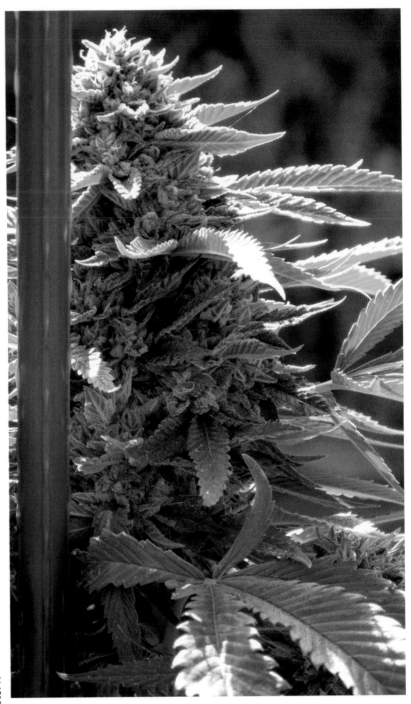

Photo: K

Stake support the buds to prevent them from bending over and breaking stalks.

On the other hand, aerated water promotes rapid root production and development.

Aeroponic Cloning Machines

Cloning machines (aeroponic propagation systems) such as the Rainforest by General Hydroponics, the EZ Clone, and the Clone Machine by American Agritech all work by directing a continuous spray of oxygen-rich mist onto the hydroponic substrate that holds the cuttings, which in turn encourages and promotes root growth. All of these propagation systems work very well and are available as both large and small models, producing just a small number of clones or as many as you need.

Rooting Hormones

Rooting hormones are manufactured, synthetic hormones similar to those naturally present in plant tissue that induce root growth. Placing hormones on a freshly cut branch enables it to produce roots faster and with more vigor and health. You will save time and have higher success rates when using rooting hormones. Many forms of rooting hormones are available in liquid, powder, and gel forms. Powders are impractical: the powder must cover the cut stem in a thin layer, yet it clumps up and sometimes seals the stem, preventing it from taking up water and clogging its pores. Gels are more practical in that they adhere to the cutting and are easy to use; Olivia's is a good gel brand. Wood's Rooting Compound is also a good product. Liquid is ideal, however, because it penetrates the stem wall and can't clump up or be wiped off as the cutting is placed in the media; here Vita Grow is a perfect option.

Types of Containers

Rockwool slabs are an excellent substrate and offer flexibility for the final method and system you decide to use. A rockwool slab, depending on the manufacturer, contains over 98 square $1^1/_2$ x $1^1/_2$-inch plugs; each square is its own grow cell that roots can develop in. The rockwool slabs can easily be cut in sections that fit your exact needs, but do not work with dry rockwool. Whole slabs fit perfectly into most propagation or mini greenhouse systems. Large plastic drink cups containing a media of equal parts of Fox Farm's Light Warrior, vermiculite, and perlite also works well when only propagating small numbers of cuttings.

Cloning

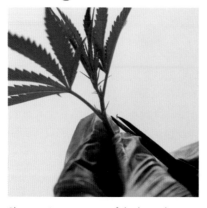

Sharp scissors are useful when cloning.

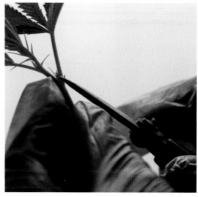

Removing excessive vegetation.

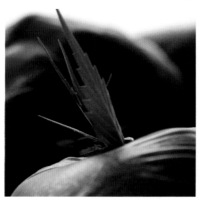

Carefully remove the tips of the leaves.

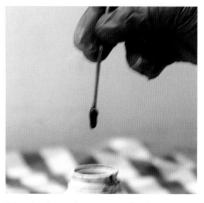

Dip the base into your cloning solution.

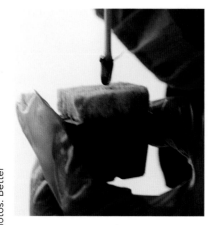

Insert into your media.

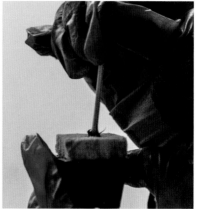

Make sure the clone is well inserted.

Photos: Better

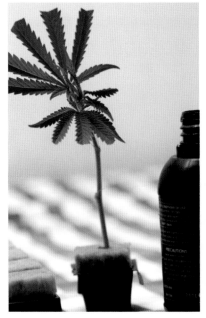

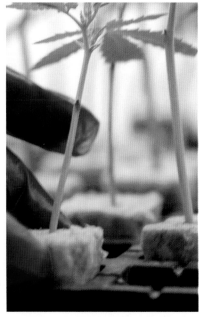

Finished clone.   Inserting clone in tray.

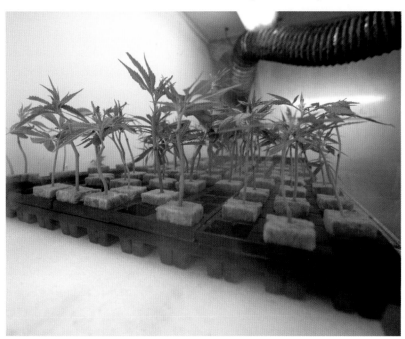

Mist plants with sterilized water before you place them into the humidity dome.

Water, pH, Nutrients

Use extremely low levels of nutrients in the rooting stage. Excessive salts found in fertilizers can block water absorption. General Hydroponics offer excellent pH-up and pH-down solutions; both are practical and work well, but use them sparingly and raise levels in small increments, thoroughly stirring the solution in between adding pH adjustment solutions. Do not use salt-based or synthetic pH-up or -down on organic soil or in organic nutrients. For organic pH preparation see the Water and Feeding chapter.

Plant Preparation

48 hours prior to taking the cuttings, you can prepare them on the donor plant for a higher rate of success. Choose the branches that will produce the best clones: nodes that are spaced every one or two inches; a succulent, green texture, not woody or hard. Lower branches are best for clones because they do not contain as much nitrogen and will root faster. All branches can root, some are just faster than others. On each prospective cutting, remove all of the lower leaves beginning at the lowest node, leaving only the top two to four youngest sets of leaves.

To cut off the lower leaves: hold the leaf and cut its petiole / stem with a razor blade, X-acto knife, or very sharp pointed scissors, one or two millimeters from the main stem. If you accidentally cut too close to the stem, it will cause unwanted damage. Using pointed scissors, cut off the tips of the two to four sets of remaining leaves to one half of their original size. This will stop the new clone from exerting too much energy on photosynthesis, respiration, or transpiration, and force it to produce roots.

Making these preparations 48 hours early enables the prospective clone to scab at places it has been cut and experience less stress when you take the cutting. Also, when using this method the risk of embolism is minimized to the final cut.

Taking Cuttings

To remove a cutting, simply use a razor blade, X-acto knife, or very sharp scissors and cut the stem diagonally, three to four inches below the lowest leaf-free node. Immediately place the clone into a measuring cup filled with pH-adjusted, room temperature, pure, clean, filtered water. The stem next to the fresh cut will release its sap and an air bubble can form when it is exposed to the air for too long a period of time. This air exchange must be avoided or the stem will dampen off and suffer necrosis and the clone will rot and die.

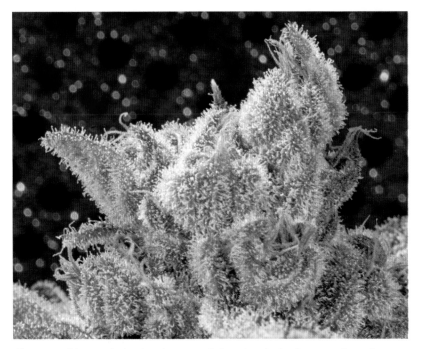

Choose cultivars wisely. Just because it has the desired name, doesn't mean it is a preferential copy of that cultivar.

Transporting Cuttings

Rooted clones may simply be placed in a container with a plastic bottom, or a bottom that won't leak or absorb water from the media – not cardboard. Place a plastic catch tray in the container to help cuttings stay upright and keep them from sliding around or from being root damaged. Get the cuttings to their final destination as soon as possible. Do not leave them in a hot car or any such environment for extended periods of time. Unrooted cuttings can be transported by cutting them longer than you want them and then placing the fresh cut stem directly into pure water in either a small measuring cup or cutting tube (a test tube with a rubber seal on the opening that has a small hole which allows the cutting to slip in but not lose any water). Place the cutting upright in a sealable plastic bag, mist the inside of the bag, and seal it. This will prevent the cutting from drying out before it's given its final cut and placed into its media. If possible, transport in cool, dark conditions.

As described in the Water and Feeding chapter's Water Preparation section, the water you use for feeding your plants, especially when rooting fragile

Photo: Freebie

clones, should be filtered, decontaminated, temperature-adjusted and pH-adjusted, in order for it to be considered pure and safe for your cuttings and plants. References to 'pure' water in this text mean water that has been through this process.

There are many other methods of transporting clones and some will allow you to stall them for two or three days, yet as time goes by chances of success will diminish. I know of someone, for instance, who placed rooted clones into a videotape, sealed it in plastic and sent it wherever in the world he needed.

Cloning Tips

Some growers make a few scrapes or superficial wounds on the base of the stem nodes' bark. This will create a few sites where the hormonal activity is more concentrated. Basically, the plant will attempt to heal the damaged tissue and add cells that will ultimately aid in the generation of rapid root development. Never cut through the stem's core; the goal is only to scrape through the stem's outer bark (approximately 0.1 millimeters).

When inserting the cutting into the medium / container, avoid excess pressure and do not bend the cutting or force the stem into the medium. Cuttings are very delicate.

Start Clean

Most failures in cloning occur because of disease. Unsanitary environmental conditions are the foremost contributor to this problem. All areas used to handle, clean, and trim cuttings should be sanitized before you begin. If you plan on producing your own cuttings, start with plants from a reputable grower or seed bank. Mother or clone source rooms should be closely monitored to prevent disease and the introduction of insects. Wash your hands, and rotate and sanitize tools between taking cuttings from different plants. This will minimize disease and contamination.

Regular pest and disease monitoring of the clone source / mother plants will reduce potential problems in the propagation trays. It's difficult to produce clones if mother plants are loaded with mildew or spider mites. Even clones from a reputable grower should be closely scrutinized! Be sure of the integrity of your source. You might be able to get a great deal on extra cuttings from another grower, but will you also be inheriting a disease or insect problem that will cost you more in the long run?

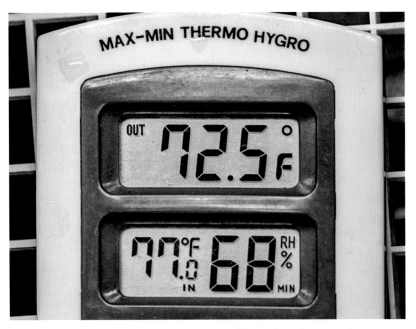

Always closely monitor the temperature and humidity of your environment.

The propagation environment should be managed to reduce fungal and bacterial disease. Sterile rooting media, benches, and tables eliminate a potential source of root-damaging diseases. Sanitize everything possible with a 10-to-1 water–bleach solution (or a 10-to-1 water-27% hydrogen peroxide solution) between crop cycles. Rinse everything afterwards. Bag and remove damaged and diseased plants and plant debris immediately. Inspect propagation trays each day. Continually removing infected, dying, and yellowing plant material reduces disease and dramatically reduces losses. Keep humidity levels at 74–80%. Irrigate and mist early in the day.

Reduce Stress

Stressed cuttings usually result from high light and low moisture levels. High light can be a problem during the early stages. Excessive light increases leaf temperatures, causing them to transpire and lose stored water. This contributes to cell collapse and dead tissue, making your clones easy targets for disease. Use cool white fluorescent lights, compact fluorescents, LEDs, or induction lights: they are more efficient, give off less heat than HIDs, and allow light and heat levels to be easily controlled by raising or lowering fixtures.

Photo: Samson Daniels

Step-by-Step Cloning

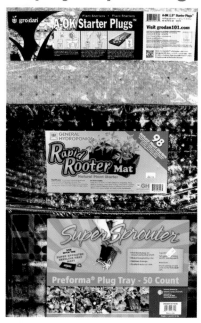

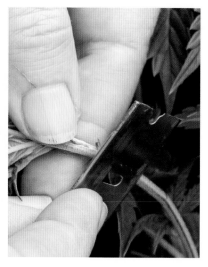

Use a razor to cut the clone (preferably a new, clean, un-rusted razor is to be utilized, unlike the one in this photo).

Cloning kits.

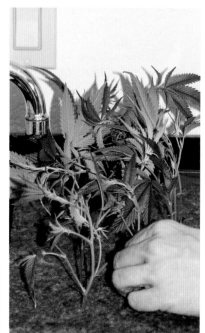

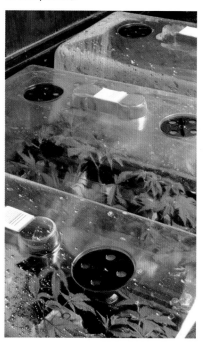

Placing clone into a media slab.

Put clones into humid environments.

Photos: Mel Frank

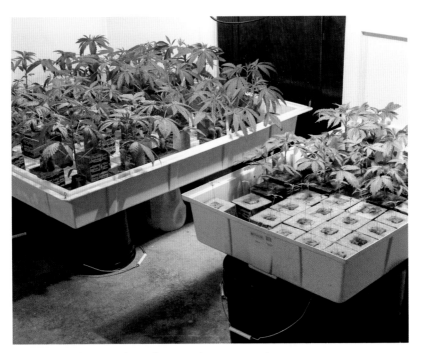

Vegetating plants and seedlings in the same environment.

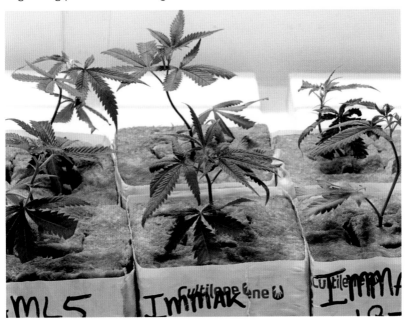

These clones have been placed into 1-inch rockwool cubes, and then after rooting, they were placed into 4-inch rockwool cubes.

Getting Clones From Budded Plants

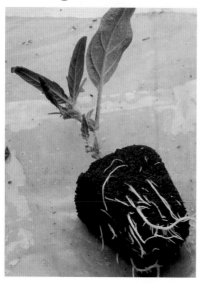

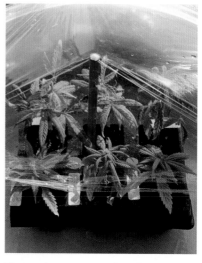

Healthy white roots on a clone that has been re-vegetated from a budding plant.

These clones were taken from a budded plant. Given 18 hours to 24 hours of light, they will root and revert back to vegetative growth.

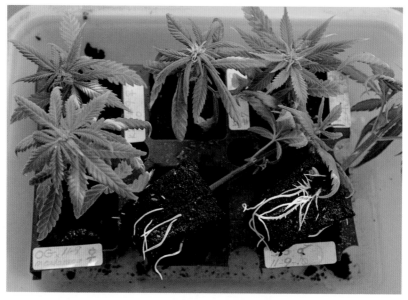

These clones have rooted and will soon begin to produce vegetative growth. This is a way to save your favorite plant if you were unable to take clones during the vegetative stage.

Photos: Mel Frank

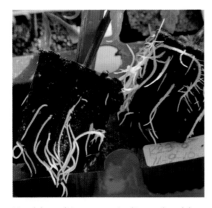

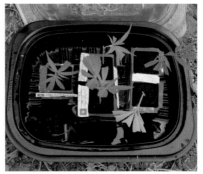

Healthy white roots indicate healthy clones.

Grower using a small, improvised cloning chamber from a roasted poultry container.

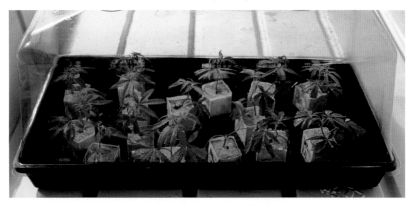

Clones in rockwool inside a covered cloning chamber.

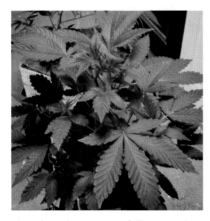

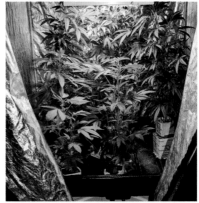

This clone has successfully rooted and is now in the vegetative stage.

Mother plants kept on 18 hours of light for a perpetual supply of clones.

Conversely, never allow clones to get too cold either; low temperatures will stunt clones and delay or inhibit rooting.

Minimizing moisture loss is the key to propagation. Once a cutting is harvested from a stock plant, the clock starts ticking. Keep cuttings misted and cool before you stick them in the growing medium, to reduce dehydration and increase rooting success rates. Cuttings should be stuck in the medium immediately following their removal from the mother plant. Delays add up to lost cuttings. It's a good practice to apply a pure water mist once or twice a day for the first 24 hours. Cuttings should be placed in propagation trays with clear domed tops.

The Right Cuttings

Professional propagators go to great lengths to harvest the correct cuttings. Cuttings that are either too soft or too hard will present problems in the propagation trays. Also, cuttings that are too large will crowd neighboring cuttings, causing uneven rooting and promoting disease. Generally, soft cuttings taken from firm tissue will develop callus and roots quickly, and be relatively problem-free. Remember, the further from the growing tip the cutting is taken, the harder the tissue. This harder tissue roots slowly. Rooting hormones containing indolebutyric acid, Indole-3-butyric acid, or 1-Naphthalene acetic acid are a must for cloning; we use Wood's Rooting Compound. Avoid dipping cuttings into a common container. This practice can spread disease from one clone to an entire group. To avoid spreading possible disease through an entire garden, it's best to change your solution multiple times throughout the process when making many cuttings.

When cloning from mothers, take clones from wherever they're available on the plant. It's preferable to have at least two nodes above where you will be cutting. Your stage of growth and cultivar will ultimately dictate this, as an indica will have a shorter internodal length than a sativa. However, you want a cutting that is 4 to 6 inches long. Some people do a diagonal cut, some a cross cut; some use scissors, others a razor; it's up to you. After cutting, there are those who scrape the side of the cutting to promote faster rooting. We trim the ends off all the leaflets and minimize all unneeded foliage. Your goal should be perfect uniformity in height. It's best to take two or three times the number of cuttings you will need, so when the time comes, you will have a large stock to choose from and can select only the best specimens for your vegging system.

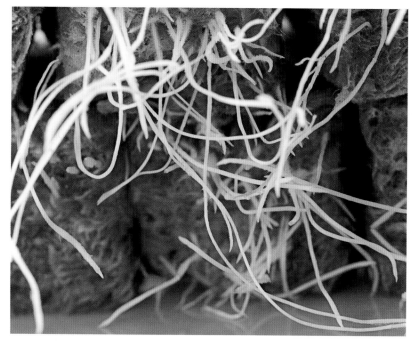

Healthy, white roots show no signs of degradation or infection.

Proper Media

The correct medium can make or break your crop. We use Grodan rockwool slabs or Fox Farms' Light Warrior soil with perlite / vermiculite amendments. Sterilized media are a must, and will help eliminate disease pathogens such as pythium. Media can sometimes dry out very quickly, causing root damage, so careful monitoring is required. The relationship of air and moisture separates a good medium from a bad one. A good medium is able to maintain a balance between the two variables. Too much aggregate can cause a medium to dry out too quickly and wilt cuttings. Too little aggregate creates soggy conditions that promote disease and fungal gnats.

Proper Temperature

Root-zone heating that maintains temperatures between 70–80°F is a good starting point. If your room does not already provide ideal temperatures, there are many thermostat-controlled heating mats available for purchase. Lower temperatures will slow plant metabolism and delay callus and root formation. A delay of even a few days can mean the difference between single-digit losses

Photo: Samson Daniels

and catastrophe. Be aware that excessively high temperatures become a hindrance, too. Heat stress varies depending on the cultivar. Some tolerate temperatures well over 80°F, but most prefer high 70s and low 80s.

Rooting Hormones

Tips:

- Wear rubber gloves to avoid contamination.
- Ventilate the room while working with it.
- Store the hormone in a dark, room temperature location.
- Avoid breathing it in or getting it in your eyes—wear goggles and a mask!
- Clean spills with water. Remember to triple rinse.

Sticking

Clones should be stuck 1 to 2 inches deep into the rooting medium (depending on your medium). Cuttings stuck too shallow are liable to be washed out of the medium or loosened to the point where rooting is delayed or inhibited. Cuttings stuck too deep may be in the part of the rooting medium cell that is constantly filled with water, depriving them of the air they need to callus. The base of cuttings stuck too deep will turn black and appear diseased. This means the tissue has died due to lack of oxygen. Once this happens, secondary infections can occur, killing the cuttings. Maintaining a proper sticking depth will produce uniform product.

Proper Density

Sticking cuttings at the correct density is an exact science. Crowded cuttings will stretch and be susceptible to botrytis. We use $1^1\!/_2$ x $1^1\!/_2$-inch rockwool cubes interconnected as a slab, and that dictates our spacing.

Fertilization and pH

We like to start our clones using $^1\!/_2$ a teaspoon per gallon of both General Hydroponics Flora series fertilizers and $^1\!/_2$ a teaspoon per gallon of liquid vitamin B1. Adjusted to a pH of 6.2, we use this mix to flush the medium. We only use the B1 on the first flushing / feeding, and then switch to the fertilizer alone. We water the medium every three days, but your environment will ultimately determine your schedule. With the first callus, cuttings begin to take up moisture from the medium.

The Rooting Process—Toning

Rooting cuttings is a multistage process. Stage 1 is where the cutting develops callus. Callus is basically where the fresh cut seals itself like a scab. This keeps it from losing moisture, enabling it to encapsulate and retain the moisture it already has. During stage 2, the first root initially develops. Stage 3 is when the shoot and root tissues develop. Stage 4 is for toning the cuttings prior to transplant. This step is often overlooked. This process should begin at least one week before planting and consists of increasing light levels and exposure to vegetative growth conditions. Clones that have been properly toned will respond to the environment shift that occurs in the finished containers with little or no wilting and subsequent leaf damage.

Determining Sex

Cloning is a simple method to determine the sex of plants. Take cuttings as described, except place the fluorescent lights on a 12 on / 12 off flowering light cycle. Cuttings will show signs of being male or female in approximately 14 days. This is the proper method of sexing plants. Inducing the whole plant to flower instead of a clone causes stress, plus you will have wasted two weeks of vegetative growth, unless you plan to flower at that time. Taking a clone and sexing it makes much more sense.

Root Development

Signs of visible roots produce a gratifying sense of satisfaction. After about seven days for faster cultivars and up to 14 for slower cultivars, the cuttings will develop roots. Allow the roots to develop and grow for approximately five to 10 more days until they are ready to re-pot or be installed in a hydroponic system.

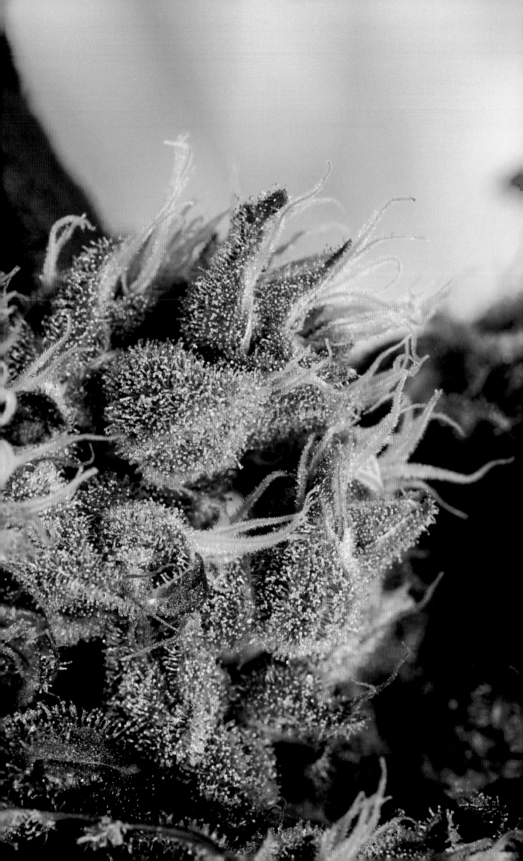

CHAPTER 13

Flowering

Males / Hermaphrodites / Sinsemilla

Male plants are only to be used for breeding and, before they are allowed to do so, they must be examined closely to determine whether or not they possess characteristics or traits that are desirable. For sinsemilla production, you want no male plants present in the flowering room. Male pollen will pollinate the buds and create seeds, so be sure to only expose flowering female plants to flowering male plants if you want seeds.

Hermaphrodites have both male and female characteristics. These are either determined by genetics or caused by plant stress. Improper breeding practices can produce an abundance of hermaphrodites, as can irregular light cycles, light leaks, chemical stress, nutrient problems, irregular watering, or excesses in temperature. Typically, a plant of either sex will start to show hermaphroditic traits in the later stages of flowering. They can cause pollination and should be separated or eliminated.

Sinsemilla's literal translation is "without seeds." To eliminate the possibility of seeding your plants, there must not be any male or hermaphrodite plants or pollen in the flowering room.

The Flowering Stage

The flowering stage of cannabis is fairly straightforward.

◀ The bract in the middle of this photo is just beginning to ripen and will reach peak potency in approximately two weeks.

Photo: Andre Grossman

The flowering cycle can be short or long, depending on the cultivar you choose to cultivate. Cannabis sativa, indica, and sativa-indica hybrids all mature at different rates. Indicas typically mature in approximately 50 to 60 days; pure sativas can take as many as 60 to 90 days; and sativa-indica hybrids take 55 to 65 days.

As stated previously, the flowering cycle begins as soon as the photoperiod is altered to induce flowering (cannabis leaves contain a light-sensitive hormone known phytochrome, which is responsible for triggering the flowering cycle to begin), duplicating conditions such as those in outdoor scenarios when days become shorter. Indoor HID lights are switched to a 12 on / 12 off light cycle. For me, the flowering stage is truly an amazing thing to witness, each and every time. This is the stage in which you will see the fruits of your labor rapidly begin to develop.

Nutrient Management

The nutritional requirements for flowering are completely different from those of the vegetative cycle. Ammonium nitrates are eliminated from the nutrient feed mix and nitrate nitrogen is dramatically decreased. Phosphorous, potassium, calcium, and macro- and micro- nutrient levels must be increased proportionately (see nutrient chart and soil amendment explanation in Chapter 11). Never over-fertilize with nutrients—this will cause leaf burn, root death, stunted growth, and poor development. Fertilizer buildup can be avoided with proper watering methods and periodic flushing: simply water with pure water (without nutrients applied) every 10 days. In combination

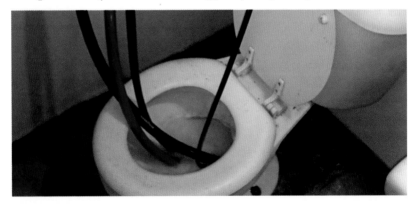

A-Mac chose to dispose of his wastewater like this, which is unacceptable. Always dispose of wastewater properly and professionally, to safeguard the environment.

Photos: K

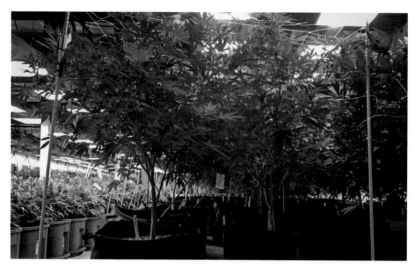

These plants are supported by a netting / trellis system which enables the grower to place multiple levels that provide total support, as the plant grows taller.

soil / soilless mix situations, 25% of all water given must run off.

Examine the runoff water. Any anomalies, such as excessive PPM or abnormal pH, must be examined and corrected. If the pH level is high or low, you must flush using water that is slightly higher or lower, depending on the pH of the runoff water. For example, if the runoff water exits the container at 6.8 and you prefer 6.2, then try giving the soil a flush using water that is adjusted to approximately 6.0. Likewise, if the runoff pH is 5.8 and you prefer 6.2, flush with water adjusted to 6.4. This will slowly and safely readjust the medium's pH to a more desirable level.

After plants are induced to flower, and after cloning, tie up the plants using plastic plant ties or a product called "vine clips." Vine clips offer great support throughout growth; use them to tie your plants to stakes, trellis, or whatever supports you use—even yo-yo plant supports. Clip them to the main stem and the support. Tying up your plants enables you to work on them before they have flowers and while they have less vegetation to get in the way or possibly break. It is best to place the stake in the soil as early as possible to prevent root damage—even as early as the beginning of the vegetation stage. Caution: Never drive a stake through a plant's root system, as it will damage roots. Place stakes before roots proliferate.

Flowering with Landrace Hindu Kush

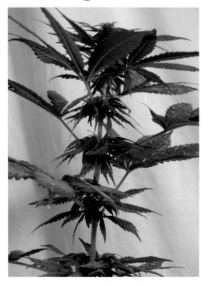

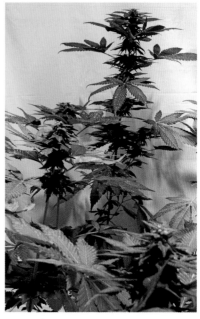

The Hindu Kush plants from the Vegetative chapter are now flowering, five days later.

One week later.

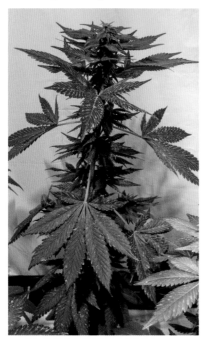

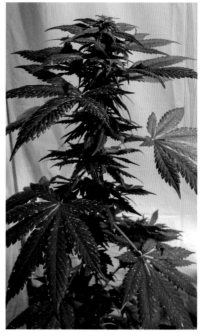

Five days later. Good growth.

After a further 10 days of growth.

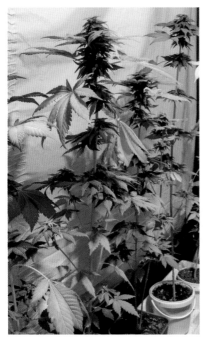

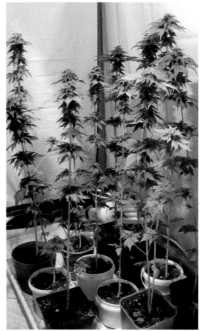

After another four days of growth.

Two days later.

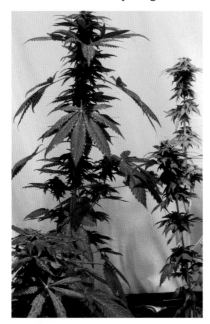

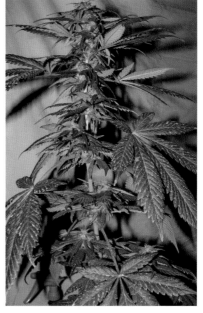

The next day. Fast growth at this stage.

The next day.

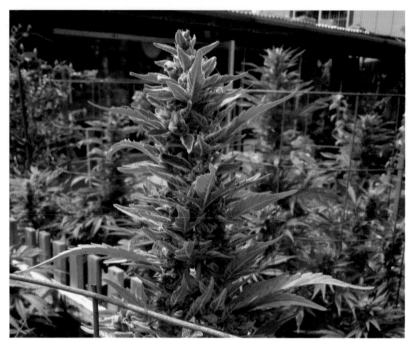

Heavy buds will always need support to prevent breaking of the stems, which can result in the total loss of the branch or an open wound which can lead to gray mold / stem rot and kill the whole plant.

Cleanup and Secondary Stripping

After induced flowering, cloning, and tying up, we allow the plants to grow undisturbed, except for watering and foliar feeding, for about 14 days. Then we once more clean up and strip off all unwanted vegetation. Any buds or branches that will not receive direct light will appear airy, light or pale green in color, and will never mature to their full potential and thus must be removed. After this material is removed, all the plant's energy is transferred to the remaining vegetation and bud / flower production. Do not over-strip (see following photos for a good example of cleanup and secondary stripping), and be sure not to strip off all the fan leaves. Large leaves can be trimmed by cutting off the tips (half of the leaf) to allow light to penetrate the dense canopy, which in turn allows the lower branches to produce quality product as well. Clean up and strip all dead or dying leaves—they do nothing but steal energy and increase risks of insects, disease, mold, and mildew.

Never strip or remove viable, healthy vegetation past day 14: it can result

Photos: K

262

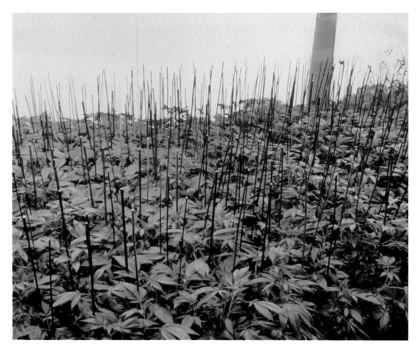

Staked plants that include eleven different cultivars, which accounts for the diversity in canopy height.

in stunted growth and reduced production, i.e. yield and quality. Stripping past day 14 also stresses the plant. The plant can perceive the late trimming as a threat and force itself to mature early, which will in turn reduce yield. If you accidentally break or split a branch or stem, you can fix some of them with a splint. Simply cut a drinking straw to the length that you need, slice it up one side, slip it around the injured, broken, or split stem, and tape the straw shut. Eventually, the stem inside will heal. Larger stems will require a length of $1/2$ or 1-inch tubing, split and applied as above and attached using plastic zip ties.

Accelerating Maturation

If you are using the symbiotic rotation cycle and are trying to slightly shorten the flowering stage, have chosen a cultivar that matures slowly, or have a sativa phenotype that takes an exceptionally long time to finish, consider these methods:

Shorten the light cycle to 11 hours on / 13 hours off in the later stages of

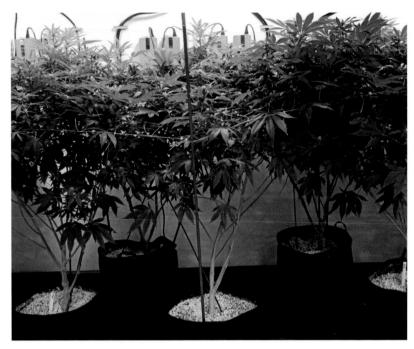

These plants have been cleaned-up perfectly, to allow for proper air circulation and to encourage healthier growth of the remaining vegetation.

the flowering cycle (about the last quarter of the cycle).

Slightly increase bloom nutrients and amendments like phosphorus, potassium, calcium, and other micronutrients. Fertilizer adjustments completely eliminate all sources of ammonium nitrate and nitrate nitrogen. (Perform these actions in the last quarter as well.)

Lower temperatures in the growth chambers by 10–15°F after 60 days of flowering cycle.

You can employ these methods singly or all together; they simply encourage earlier maturation in cultivars that are slow to mature.

Note: Maturation time is ultimately dictated by genetics. You can slightly encourage maturation times, but you will never be able to force a cultivar that naturally matures in 12 weeks to finish in eight. Experiment with your chosen cultivar and explore its limit; keep records pertaining to yield vs. shortened maturation time and quality, and you will discover exactly where the limits and requirements are. Each environment and cultivar is different; figure out what works for you.

Photos: K

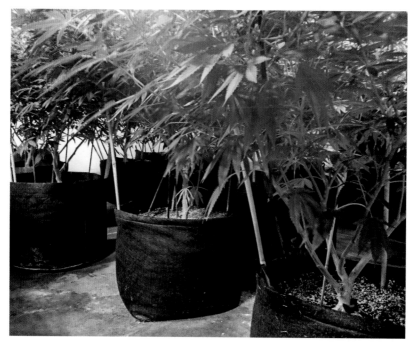

You must remove all lower vegetation that does not receive light. This allows for proper air circulation, and enables the remaining vegetation to utilize all available light without wasting energy on lower vegetation.

The Flowering Cycle Timeline

Day 1–14

Staminate flowers (see the section on Sexing your plants) on males; bracts and stigmas / stigmata begin formation on females. Bud production is slow at this stage. Internodal elongation and vertical growth continue. Plant structure strengthens in preparation for bud formation / growth. Roots uptake and the plant retains nutrients needed to begin bud production. Foliar feed to encourage rapid growth. Be extra vigilant for any nutrient deficiencies.

Day 14–28

Bud production starts to accelerate. Rapid bract, small leaf formation, and slight resin production begins. Stigmata elongate and buds begin to form. Internodal elongation and vertical growth continue, as does strengthening of the plant structure. Nutrient requirements escalate incrementally. Foliar feed with recommended amendments and fertilizers.

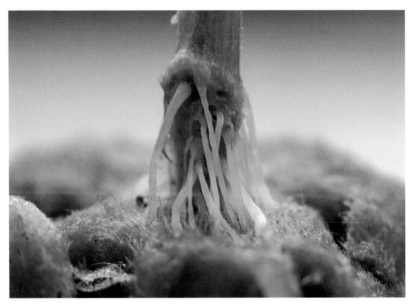

Roots emerging from the callus of the stem and into a one-inch rockwool cube.

Day 28–42

Internodal growth starts to slow. Bud formation continues to become denser and bud production is the plant's main priority. Nutrient requirements continue to escalate incrementally. Continue to foliar feed. Resin production begins to accelerate and essential oils (terpenes) develop and begin to give off a strong aroma.

Day 42–56

Nutrient uptake and retention levels are at their highest. Buds become heavy and dense. Resin production is rapid and aroma is strong. Stigmata start to dry out and turn brown / red. Internodal elongation and vertical growth cease. You must avoid over-fertilization of nutrients; be vigilant and flush when necessary. Plants may require a slight increase of calcium / magnesium (Cal Mag), phosphorous, and other macronutrients.

Day 56–Harvest

Buds are 90% mature, if pure indica or indica-sativa hybrids. Bud production slows. Stigmata continue to dry out and turn brown / red. Bracts swell to maximum size and resin production will soon peak. Discontinue foliar feeding

Photo: Samson Daniels

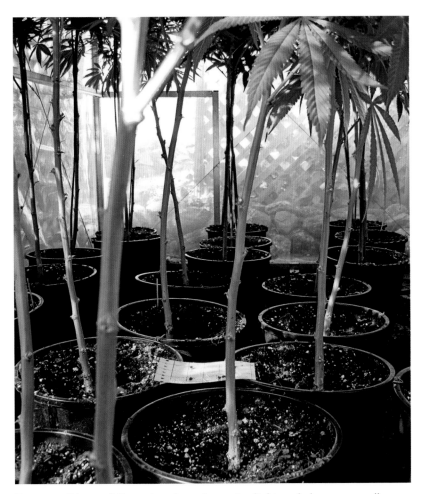

Remove all lower foliage that doesn't receive light and always use yellow sticky traps so that you know exactly what type of pests are present in the greenhouse.

when bud formation becomes dense to avoid problems with mildew and mold. At approximately 60 days, most indica and indica-sativa cultivars are fully matured and finished. Pure sativa cultivars mature at a slower rate, but are well worth the wait. Pure sativas can take 12 to 16 weeks to fully mature; even then they seem to do it reluctantly. It is best to grow pure sativas outdoors.

Outdoor and Greenhouse Flowering Methods

Outdoor and greenhouse plants can be forced to flower via light deprivation.

Photo: K

267

Greenhouses are covered with light-proof materials (black or white plastic or Visqueen), creating complete darkness at the same time every day, recreating a 12 hours on / 12 hours off light cycle, which allows plants to mature earlier. Outdoor plants can be covered with refrigerator-sized boxes or a tent with blackout (black plastic) covering the inside. Lift off the tent every morning and replace it every evening, again recreating the 12-on / 12-off photoperiod. Smaller plants can be covered with large plastic trash bins.

Flowering Tips

These tips are for the final weeks of flowering. They primarily affect flavor, and the purpose of these small adjustments are to enhance the taste. Simple, slight adjustments to temperature, sulfur levels, watering methods, drying / curing, or the distance of lights to plant canopy can make the difference between cannabis that smells and tastes very good or very bad. To realize the full genetic potential for both flavor and potency, just follow the tips listed below.

Excess Temperature

Excess temperature is the number one cause of resin and THC breakdown in cannabis buds. You must make sure that canopy and bud temperatures never exceed 85°F. Many cultivars are heat sensitive in the later stages of flowering and will respond to higher temperatures by producing hermaphroditic sexual mutations. 65°F to 70°F is the perfect temperature for the flowering room during the last couple of weeks of the flowering cycle.

Light Distance, from Bulb to Plant

Radiant heat given off by lights will also cause rapid trichome and THC deterioration. Excess light and heat are very detrimental to both flavor and potency. Be careful, be vigilant: never allow the plants to get too close to lights. Problems that may arise include burning—a yellow striping between the veins of the upper leaves—and "bolting": a sudden stem elongation within the bud structure, often referred to as a "fast super stretch" that grows straight up into the lights, resulting in burning.

Follow this chart to make sure you keep your lights the correct distance from your plants.

Light Source	Minimum Distance	Comments
Metal Halide (MH) 1,000-watt	18-24 inches from plant	If using light movers, 12–18 inches from plant is acceptable; 24 inches is best for the last 14 days of flowering
Metal Halide (MH) 600-watt	18-24 inches from plant	If using light movers, 12–18 inches from plant is acceptable; 24 inches is best for the last 14 days of flowering
Metal Halide (MH) 400-watt	18 inches from plant	If using light movers, 12–18 inches from plant is acceptable; 24 inches is best for the last 14 days of flowering
High Pressure Sodium (HPS) 1,000-watt	24–30 inches from plant	If using light movers, keep HPS 24 inches from canopy; 24 inches is best for the last 14 days of flowering
High Pressure Sodium (HPS) 600-watt	24 inches from plant	If using light movers, keep HPS two feet from canopy; 24 inches is best for the last 14 days of flowering
High Pressure Sodium (HPS) 400-watt	24 inches from plant	If using light movers, keep HPS two feet from canopy; 24 inches is best for the last 14 days of flowering

Sulfur

Sulfur is an essential element to aid plants in reaching their full genetic potential and flavor. Sulfur should be applied to soil during the last transplant prior to the flowering stage. Outdoors, it should be applied during the initial planting. Two good sources of sulfur are soft rock phosphate and K-mag, which is also distributed as Sul-Pro-Mag or Langbeinite; for outdoor use, gypsum is an excellent sulfur amendment. Never use Epsom salts on organic soil or substrate; although they are rich in magnesium and sulfur, they will kill all beneficial microorganisms in the soil. You can dissolve Epsom salts in water—one to two teaspoons per gallon—and use them as a foliar spray, but this is only a quick fix for magnesium and sulfur deficiency problems. Remember to rinse the leaves 48 hours after application.

Prewatering

It is very important to either water the plants slowly or prewater using pure,

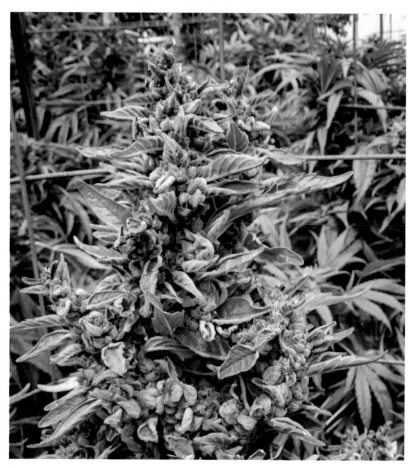

Sun-grown outdoor medicine, grown by Mom.

adjusted water. For indoor growing, allow 25% of all water to run out of the media / containers (inspect the pH and PPM) and wait one hour. After this time, thoroughly water with your normal nutrient application levels, taking into consideration the levels of the runoff you just sampled. The reason for this process is to allow water to break down and flush built-up salts or minerals that may be in the soil, avoiding any excess.

For soil growing, you must saturate the entire medium or areas will form that remain dry, allowing minerals to bond to insolubles that cannot be used by the plants. Calcium and phosphorous, for instance, commonly bond with other elements, such as iron, ultimately rendering them unavailable to the plant. This can in turn affect the flavor of buds and overall health of the plant roots.

Photo: K

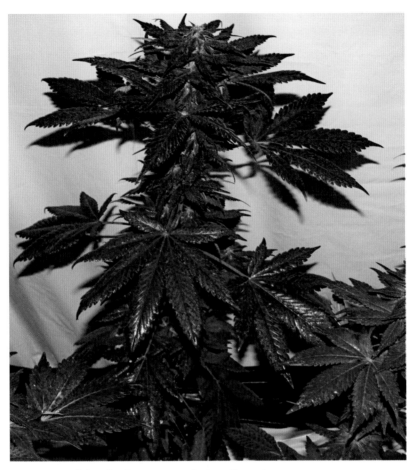

Discontinue foliar feeding two weeks into flowering.

Foliar Sprays

It is important that the plants' leaves and stomata are free of dust and debris so that they can properly transpire (breathe), which is critical to maintaining proper metabolism and overall health. To "wash off" plants and leaves use enough water that it will run off the leaves. The best time to wash plants is early in the morning, 24 hours after any foliar application and every seven days, under normal circumstances. Do not spray water into the buds themselves, only onto the big fan leaves. You must make sure the leaves are dry when the lights go out or the sun goes down, as residual water can encourage mildew and mold. Only wash plants if you have adequate ventilation and humidity levels are 50% or lower.

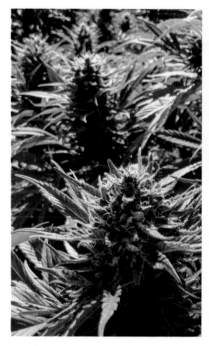
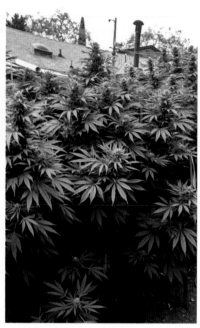

Outdoor sungrown cannabis in flower, grown by the author's mother and stepfather.

Flushing and Organics

If you are using true organic media you don't need to flush, unless you're excessively amending with liquid fertilizers. In such a case, there are no excessive elements to flush away, nor are elements in forms conducive to flushing. The main purpose of flushing is to remove any excess or synthetic nutrients or mineral salts that can cause nutrient excesses and reduce the quality and flavor of the final product. Basically, do not feed properly augmented organic plants any liquid fertilizers, organic or not, during the final stages of the flowering cycle, one to two weeks before harvest.

Note: Flushing will not compensate for poor cultivation practices! Follow the tips in this section.

Mineral Salt-Based Synthetic Fertilizers

Mineral salt-based synthetic fertilizers work fantastically. They are ideal for hydroponic, aeroponic, NFT, and ebb and flow systems. However, synthetic fertilizers can sometimes alter flavor and aroma when used in excess or im-

Photos: K

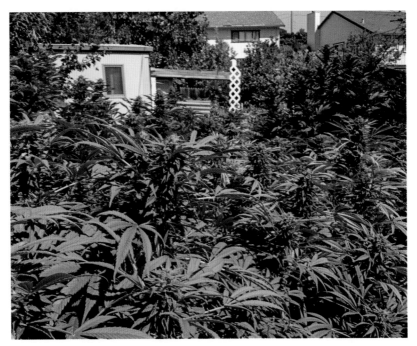

Cannabis grows and flowers like many other plants in one's garden. It thrives in well-lit conditions like this and grows like a weed.

properly, especially when you have not thoroughly flushed the medium through the plant's life cycle. This is also true of pseudo-organics—organics that contain even trace amounts of synthetic materials. You will never get the same quality using synthetics as you will using organics. Regardless of how much you flush, there will always be slight levels of residual salts and nutrients left in the plant that can alter the flavor no matter how low the levels are.

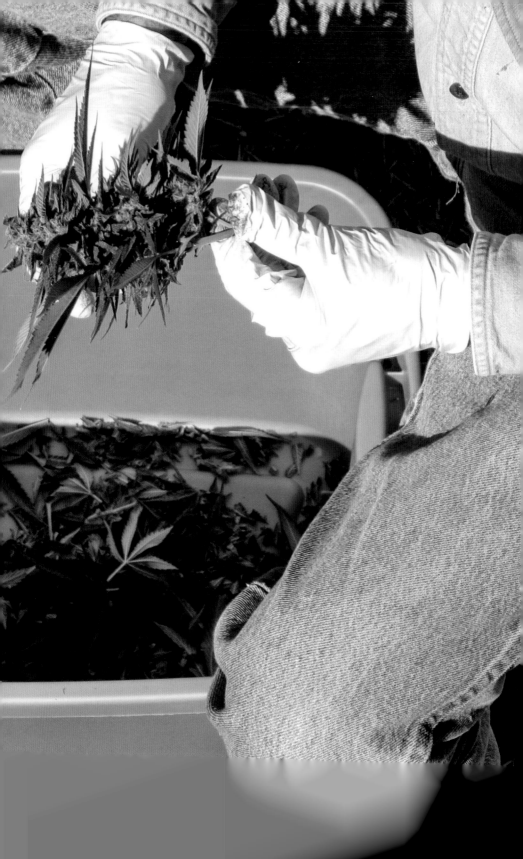

CHAPTER 14

Harvest

Harvesting and manicuring is an art, a science in itself. You must pay close attention to your every action. At this juncture you will have invested time and resources, so much so that if you do not maximize the full potential of what you have grown you will have rendered all this information pointless. You should strive to produce the best medical-grade marijuana possible. After all, the best marijuana in the world is the marijuana you have personally grown with loving care.

Harvesting

At Trichome Technologies we employ two different techniques when harvesting: one for our boutique or connoisseur cultivars, and one for commercial production. It would be nice to harvest, dry, and cure all of our crops with the same time and care we use for the boutique cultivars, but when you're talking about 99 or so plants, it's simply not practical or economical to do so. Large-scale harvesting will be covered in my next book, which will focus on advanced and industrial techniques.

Trichomes

Some misinformed people judge harvest time simply by the color of a plant's stigmas, and while that is a good pre-harvest indicator, we prefer using a 20x or 100x magnification loupe to look directly at the trichomes.

There are four distinct types of plant hairs, better

◀ Wet flowers being harvested in the sun.

Photo: K

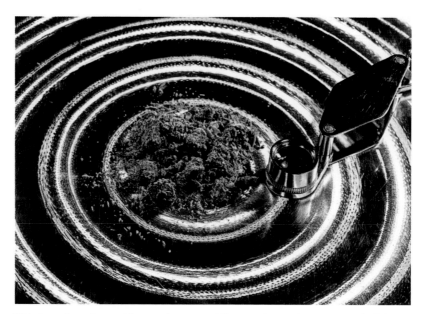

This is resin collected from scissors and fingers. It produces a wonderful flavor and smells incredible.

known as trichomes. There is a half-bubble, larger, egg-shaped resin gland that clings to the surface of the leaves and bud and contains only smell and taste terpenes (no THC): this is called a *bulbous trichome*. It is basically a plant hair without a stalk. There is also a *crystolith trichome*, that basically looks like a hair with a long, pointed tip; these trichomes appear primarily on the underside of leaves and their main purpose is to protect the plant from insects and spider mites. They are protective trichomes that discourage insects and mites from eating foliage. They also contain no THC.

The third trichome is called a *sessile stalked capitate trichome*. It is several times larger than the bulbous glandual trichome, but is still very small. It begins to develop in the plant's vegetative stage and stays very close to the plant's surface. It contains very low levels of terpenes and THC and is considered a contaminant to hash makers.

Stalked capitate glandular trichomes, the fourth, which under the microscope appear more or less like translucent mushrooms, are made up of a stalk or clear column with a resin head. They form on buds / bracts and smaller surrounding leaves. The resin head on top is psychoactive: this is the one that produces Delta 9 THC, so that's what we're looking for.

Photos: Andre Grossman

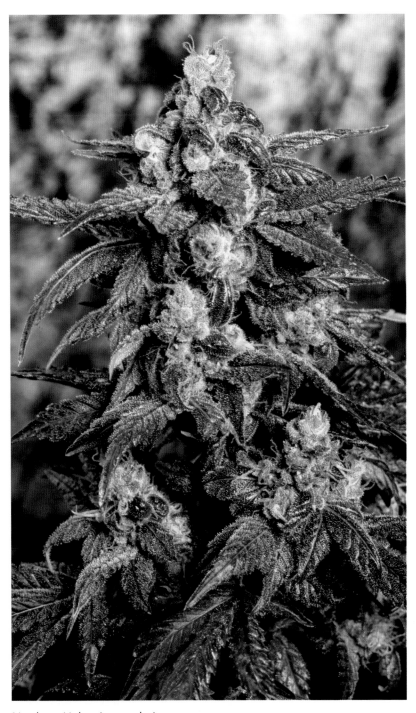

Northern Lights 6 at peak ripeness.

Trichome Guide for Harvesting

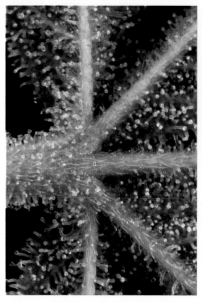

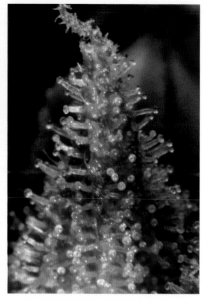

This cultivar is called Garlic. These trichomes are on the lower surface, viewed at X4 magnification.

Skunk #1 bract viewed at X5 magnification.

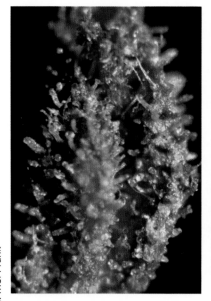

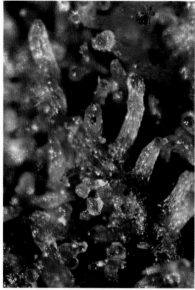

Photos: Mel Frank

This plant has been left very late. Trichomes viewed at X25.

The same plant was left too late. Note the trichome coloration.

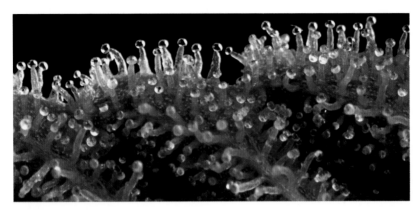

Sea of resin glands with only slight darkening indicating harvest should not happen yet.

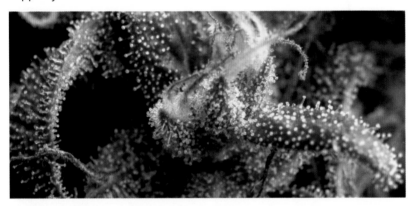

Stigma have turned orange and the trichomes look very full of cannabinoids.

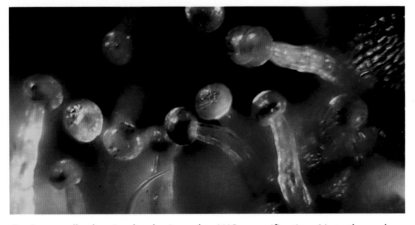

Capitate stalked resin glands viewed at X63 magnification. Note the amber heads: harvest time is soon.

Timing

We harvest when 70% of the glandular trichomes are ripe and 30% are just starting to get ripe, making sure that the majority of trichomes have turned slightly amber and that 30% are opaque white, or milky (this produces the strongest body high / euphoric effect). Once everything is properly dried, cured, and stored, those trichomes that hadn't fully ripened should be at their peak. If we don't harvest at the 70% point the majority of the trichomes would go past their peak while waiting for the other 30% to ripen, and at the end of the process we would have too high a percentage of overripe glands and the THC would have converted / degraded into other cannabinoids, such as CBN—not the peak Delta 9 THC we're aiming for.

We usually harvest after approximately 55 or 60 days of flowering growth cycle for pure Indicas, and about 60 to 70 days for others, including Indica–Sativa hybrids. We work with cultivars that have similar growth schedules; i.e., they all reach maturity in the same amount of time. Once the plants have reached what I would consider to be peak potency, it's time for the harvest!

Harvest Timing

When to harvest is a very controversial subject. Some prefer their cannabis harvested early, some prefer their cannabis harvested late.

In a nutshell, research at this time indicates that harvesting slightly early results in bud that has a more uplifting effect, and harvesting later than normal results in bud that has a more sedative effect.

Time of Day To Harvest

■ What time of day you harvest determines your final quality.

■ You must harvest, preferably in the dark, before the light has been scheduled to come on.

■ Whenever possible, do not allow the plants to see direct light while the roots are attached. Direct light on a plant will cause more starches and sugars to be drawn up from the root system.

■ During the night cycle, plants store food in their root system that they process during the daylight hours.

■ During the night cycle, starches and sugar produced by photosynthesis during the day cycle migrate downward to the root system.

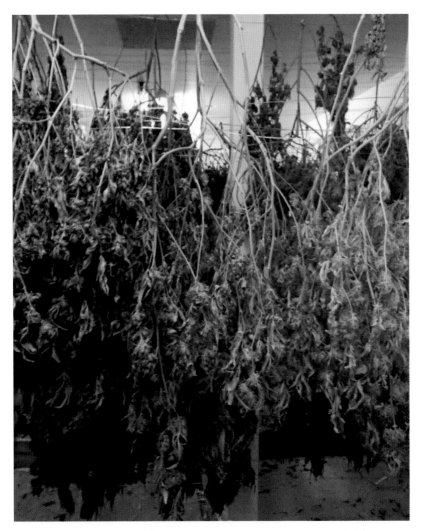

These plants have not been properly trimmed prior to hanging. The large fan leaves, leaves with no resin on them, and yellow leaves should be removed prior to hanging them on the line.

■ Understanding this, you can see that you want to cut the plants away from the root system before the lights come on which causes the starches or sugars to migrate back up into the buds.

■ Outdoor plants are often harvested during the daytime hours and the result can sometimes be a harsh tasting final product that is difficult to burn, and sometimes takes longer to cure.

Photo: K

Trichome Technologies Screen Drying

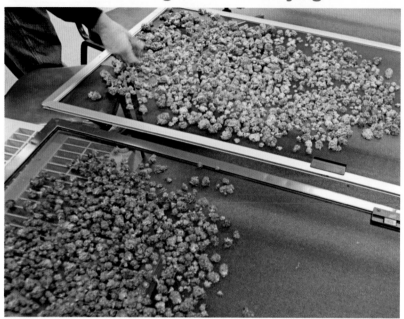

Screen drying.

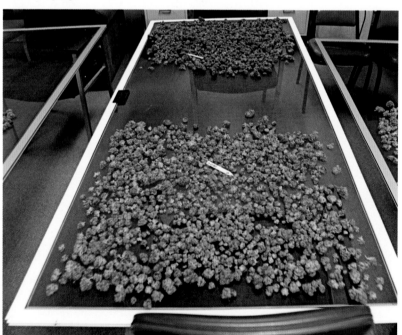

Photos: Freebie

Manicured buds drying.

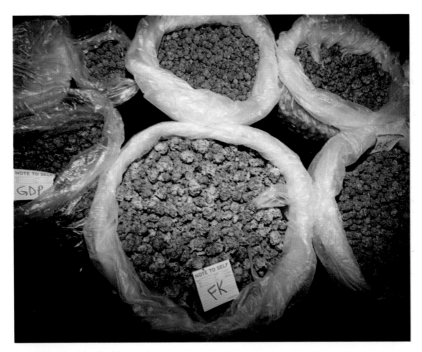

Dried buds labeled by cultivar.

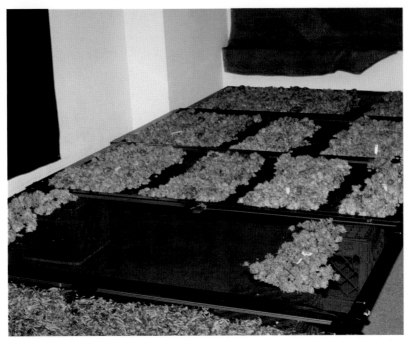

Old school Trichome Tech drying screens.

Top Photo: Freebie Bottom Photo: Mel Frank

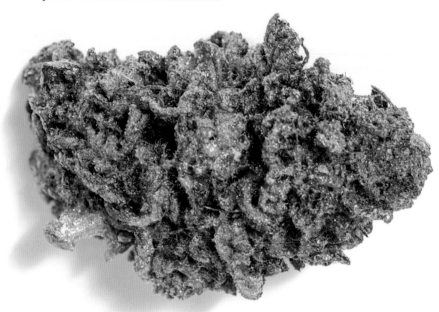

Bubba Kush dipped in honey oil.

....

■ The starches and sugars present in plants that were harvested at daytime can act like a type of fire retardant not allowing the plant material to completely burn.

■ The sugars and starch also change the composition of the chemicals you are ingesting, meaning the THC and CBD, as well as other cannabinoids, can't vaporize at optimum temperature because they were not able to properly convert to psychoactive forms.

Flushing

■ Flush media 7-14 days prior to harvest.

■ Discontinue nutrient application (in hydroponics or soilless mix medias / substrates) 7-14 days prior to harvest.

■ In soil media / substrates, discontinue watering 1-2 days prior to harvest (never allow soil to completely dry out or plants to wilt).

■ We like to remove all large fan leaves (unless they have trichomes / resin on them, if they have resin on them then we leave them on) 2-3 days prior to harvest. However, if you prefer, you can remove the leaves after you harvest the plant / branch. Note that removing the leaves earlier makes manicuring the harvested buds faster and easier.

Photo: Samson Daniels

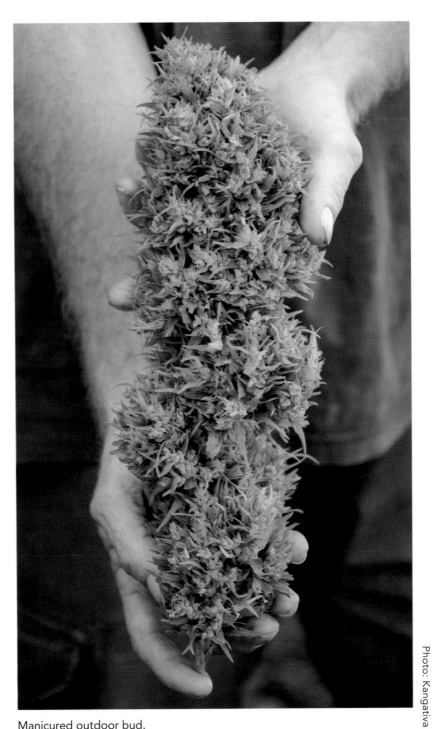

Manicured outdoor bud.

Photo: Kangativa

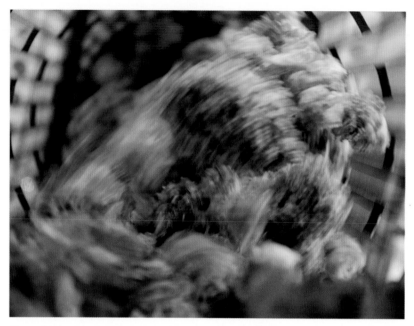

Cannabis inside the Twister power trimming machine.

Prepare for Harvest

7–10 days prior to harvest	discontinue primary and supplemental nutrient application in soil gardens
3–4 days prior to harvest	flush your medium
2–3 days prior to harvest	discontinue nutrient application in hydroponic or soilless gardens; flush medium, and remove all large fan leaves (unless they have trichomes on them, in which case leave them on)
48 hours prior to harvest	gently spray and wash off any residual dust or fertilizers on your plants; do this early in the morning and turn on all oscillating fans to make sure all of the plants are dry by the end of the day
24 hours prior to harvest	leave the plants in complete darkness
On harvest day	begin first thing in the morning, before the sun rises or the lights come on: this is when the THC is at its peak

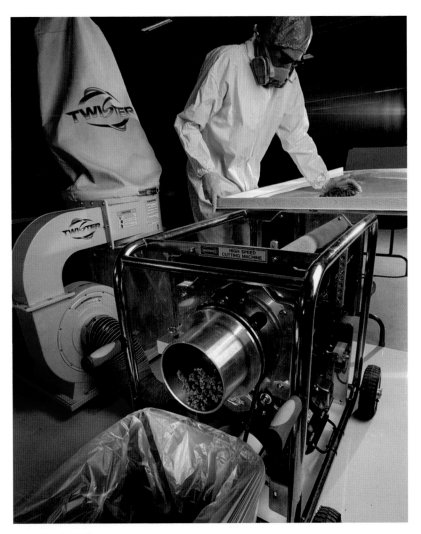

Trimmer in action.

Clothesline Method

If you're harvesting a small amount of plants, like ten or twenty, it's best to use the clothesline method. Cut the entire plant at the base or one branch at a time as they mature and ripen. Hang by putting one of the lower branches over the clothesline or by cutting the branches off and hanging the plant by the remaining 'V' in the branch. This way the flowers don't touch any surfaces where there's a possibility of losing the valuable THC-laden trichomes, which can fall off or be rubbed off quite easily.

Photo: Freebie

Clothesline Drying Method

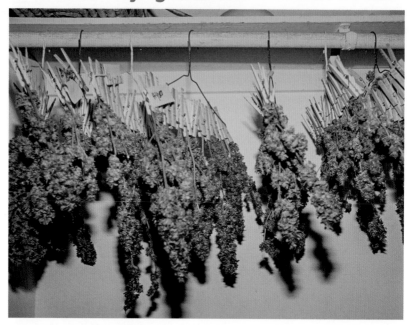

Drying with clothes pins.

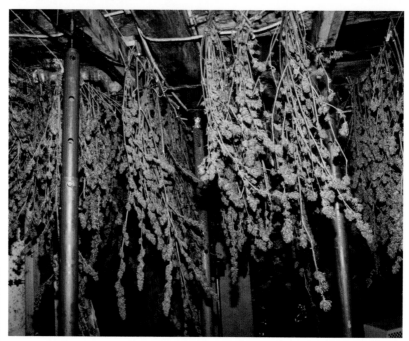

Photos: Mel Frank

Hang drying in a basement with fans and a space heater.

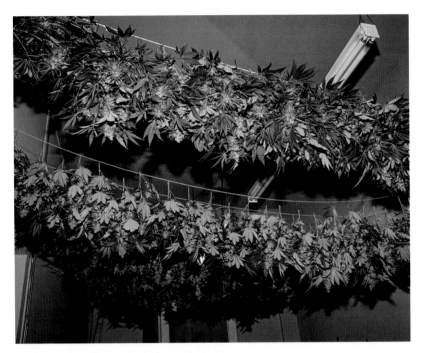

Old school Trichome Tech hang drying.

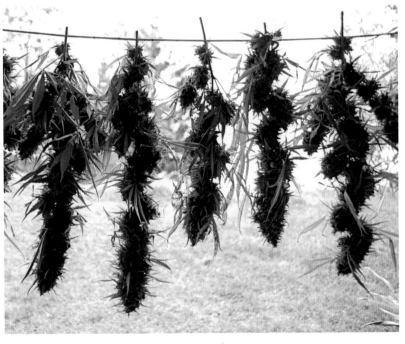

Clothesline method employed for an outdoor grow.

Top Photo: Mel Frank   Bottom Photo: Kangativa

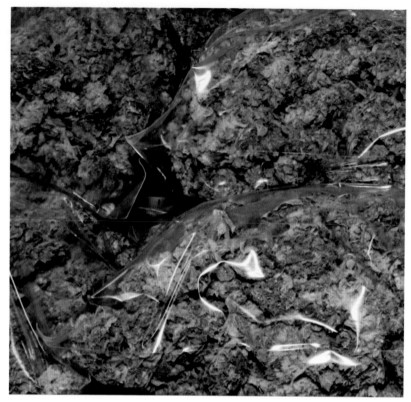

Buds in storage bags.

Manicuring

After all the plants are hung, clip off all of the remaining fan leaves. Leave the buds to dry for 48–72 hours, depending on environmental conditions, such as heat and humidity, until everything is just right for the second manicure. Next, go through them completely and cut off everything that is unwanted: leaf, stick, stem, etc. Do this over screens with Plexiglas underneath so that you can collect any resin that may fall off.

Cannabis buds are delicate, whether they're wet or dry, and should be treated as such. Rough treatment will cause resin glands to be knocked off or damaged. Never manhandle buds. Be gentle; don't just grab a handful. Every time you grab a bud you transfer resin glands from the bud to your skin or gloves, which is how finger hash is made. Grab the bud by the end of the stem and hold it like a popsicle. This way you can turn the bud any way you want it to trim off unwanted leaves with minimal trichome loss. In a nutshell, your goal when manicuring is to trim off and eliminate any material that has no trichomes on it.

When cutting off all medium and large leaves you must *always* cut off the entire leaf, including the leaf stem (petiole). You must cut the leaf stem off at the base, where it meets the main stem. If you do not cut it off, the petiole can retain moisture and begin to decompose, both of which can promote mold and bud rot. After removing all large and medium leaves, trim (using very sharp small pointed scissors) the non-resin-gland-covered leaf tips. Periodically scrape the resin off of the trimming utensils for "scissor hash."

I have seen many so-called manicuring machines, bud trimmers, and mechanized leaf cutters. For small gardens, I do not recommend any of them. Nonetheless, the "HarveStar" trimmer is a nice small trimmer that will help trim off all medium and small leaf tips, leaving you the task of removing all of the leaf's petiole. Be careful: trimming machines can also remove fingers—seriously. There is no substitute for hand manicuring; try to make the bud look like one you would want to buy. For large amounts, Trichome Technologies recommends the Twister Power Trimmer which will be featured in the large-scale second volume of this book. This is truly the finest trimmer on the market, and its quality and craftsmanship is literally unrivaled. Go to TwisterTrimmer.com to order..

Bagging and Moisture

Once the buds have been successfully manicured and are completely dry to the touch, but with a very slight amount of moisture still trapped in the inner core and some buds dryer than others, and with the stem still easily bending (we're trying to sweat them; homogenize and pull out moisture). Place the buds in sealed containers, glass jars, plastic containers, or what have you. Glass is preferred.

Put the containers into a drying room at 70–80°F for 24 hours, after which, remove the bud from the containers and replace them on drying screens. The moisture from the inner core will have been drawn into the previously dry outer bud and all the buds will be of the same consistency. Have the dehumidifier on at 0%, the temperature still set to 70–80°F, and check the buds every hour. When they are evenly dried and the inner stem cracks when bent (not breaks—if it breaks it has been overdried), the buds are now ready for glass containers.

Again, make sure the buds are dry. Wet buds will rapidly mold if stored in sealed containers.

That said, never overheat or over dry buds. It will destroy essential volatile oils that contribute to flavor and aroma, and will deteriorate the THC. To preserve essential oils and prevent molds, keep drying chambers between 70 and 80°F and at 40 to 50% humidity. Frequently inspect bud and leaf, and rotate both periodically to ensure even drying and eliminate the possibility of mold or mildew infection. Use charcoal filters on all exhausted air from the drying chambers to eliminate odor. Ultimately, the decision to produce top quality product is all yours.

Curing

I prefer to allow buds to cure for one to two months before consumption. In that period, the trichomes release more moisture and certain cannabinoids will convert to THC, resulting in a more potent end result. While they are stored, the buds are in a constant state of change.

If you try this curing process, you will need to inspect the bags every week. It's very important to take the stale air out of the containers and replace it with fresh air, as well as make sure that no moisture or mold is present.

Unfortunately, these days most growers aren't afforded the luxury of curing because they need reimbursement for the cost of their production, and the demand of the market.

For the boutique cultivars, and for my own personal use, it is always nice to put the manicured buds away for that extra month. The difference is astounding!

Harvest Tips

Cleaning Up

When manicuring or handling buds, wear surgical gloves and collect resin that builds up on them. When gloves are not available or are impractical, after scraping the hash off your fingers, you can clean your hands using olive oil—simply pour a little in your palm and rub your fingers and palms together, paying special attention to areas that are very sticky. Afterwards, wipe your hands off with paper towels and, if needed, repeat. Washing your hands with olive oil is much nicer than washing them with alcohol or just leaving them sticky—and smelly! Clean all scissors and utensils with 70% alcohol. It quickly dissolves cannabis resin.

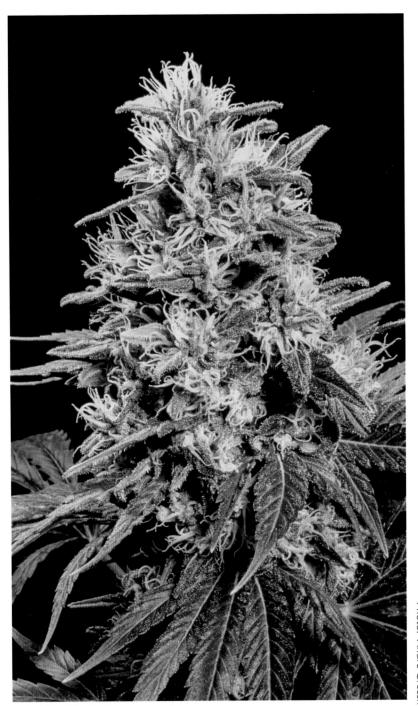

This bud still has two to three weeks until harvest.

Photo: Andre Grossman

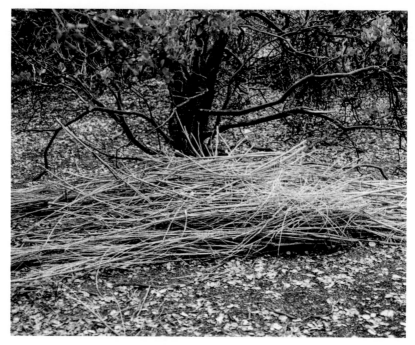

Harvested stalks from an outdoor grow.

Dry Air = Increased Resin

Resin production increases with a decrease in humidity. When the relative humidity in the growroom is slightly decreased, resin production will increase. This is a natural reaction that cannabis has to dry air. It is an attempt by the plant to protect itself from dry, hot environmental conditions. Decreasing the relative humidity in the flowering area 24 hours prior to harvest will contribute to increased resin production and swollen trichomes.

Harvest Tips

■ Bud should hang dry for 5-7 days at a temperature of approximately 70°F with 50% humidity.

■ The goal is to get most of the water out in the first 5 days without over-drying or sacrificing essential oils.

■ At this point you should be vigilant: you must monitor temperature and humidity in the drying room at all times.

■ To cure your cannabis properly, follow the guide to curing in the Curing chapter.

Photo: Mel Frank

■ Breaking up a mid-sized bud will give you a good indication of the moisture level. The bud should be smokeable and seem almost done.

■ Don't feel intimidated if this process confuses you. This process takes a bit of practice. If you are totally unfamiliar with this process, you may want to first experiment with a small amount of buds so that you do not risk your whole crop.

■ The next step is to slowly pull the moisture out of the buds, which is the ultimate goal.

■ Slowly pulling the moisture out will result in a superior product that burns properly and preserves all essential oils.

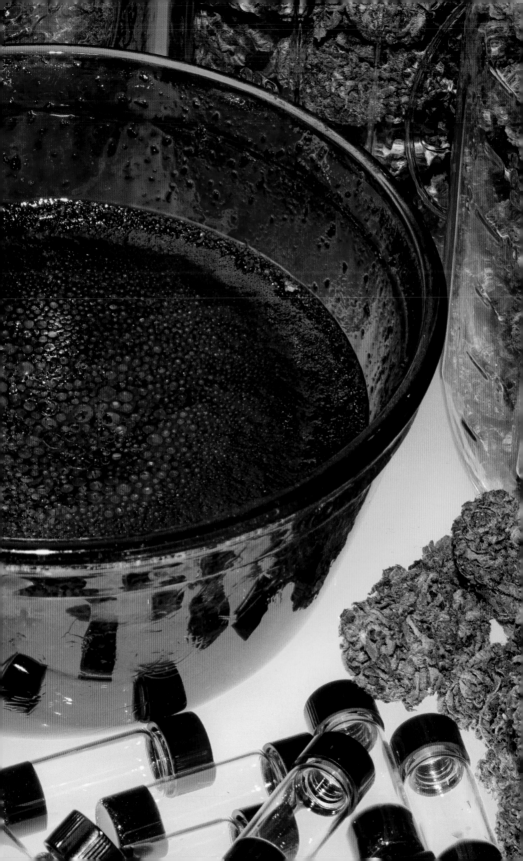

CHAPTER 15

Curing

Curing is the process of allowing buds to slow dry in the final stages of drying, which facilitates slow and even moisture release. The first stages of drying simply dissipate external and internal moisture. In the final stages of drying, the buds seem to be dry yet still contain internal moisture. How this moisture is eliminated will partially dictate the quality of the final product: the smell, flavor, and potency. Curing allows for the slow removal of remaining moisture, homogenizes the condition of all the buds so that they have consistent moisture content, and preserves and converts available cannabinoids.

At Trichome Technologies our situation is unique. Medical marijuana dispensaries want top quality medicine consistently and rapidly, without the product being too moist or too dry. Providing product that is too moist is dishonest and it can develop molds and decompose, causing ill health effects for consumers or patients. Too dry of a product will degrade and crumble during transportation, handling, and packaging; it will also be harsh to smoke. When we harvest large quantities of medicinal buds they are placed on drying racks (see the images in the harvesting chapter) after they have been completely manicured.

When all buds are completely dry to the touch, I use a dustpan to scoop them off the screen and place them into 30-gallon containers, $^3/_4$ of the way full. Seal them and place into a 70–80°F environment for 24 hours. After this

◀ Cured cannabis in glass jars and raw unrefined cannabis oil.

Photo: Freebie

Packaging for Transportation

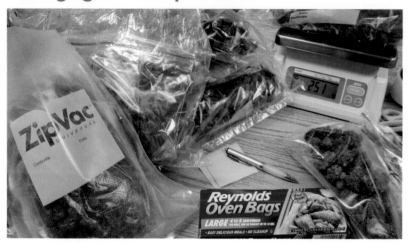

1 Materials needed.

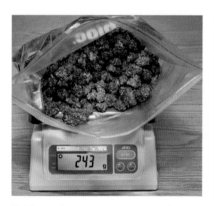

2 Always have an accurate scale.

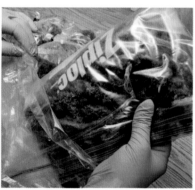

3 Bag sealed and into Turkey bag.

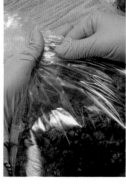

4 Leave some air.

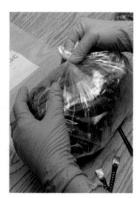

5 Tie a knot.

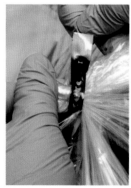

6 Seal bag tightly.

Photos: Samson Daniels

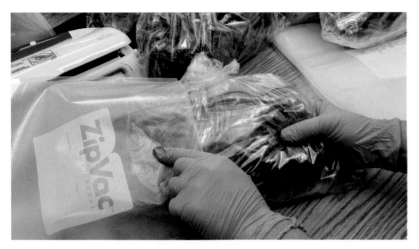

7 This will prevent unwanted odors from escaping.

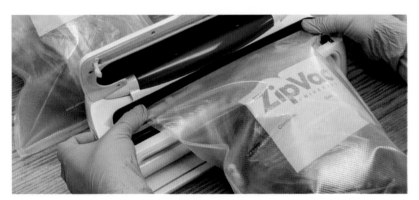

8 Buds then go into a vacuum sealed bag. The air in the Turkey bag prevents the vacuum-sealed bag from crushing the contents.

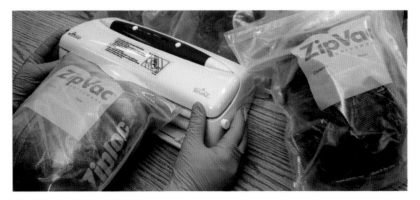

9 Make sure not to over vacuum so you don't crush the buds. *continues*

Packaging for transportation

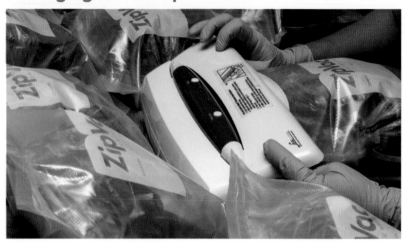

10 Air is then vacuumed out of the vacuum bag for double security.

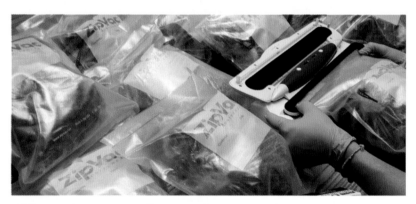

11 Repeat the process until you are done.

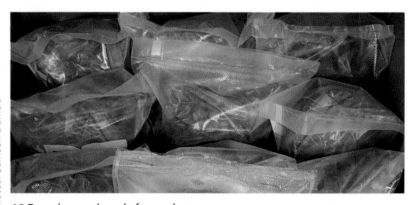

Photos: Samson Daniels

12 Boxed up and ready for market.

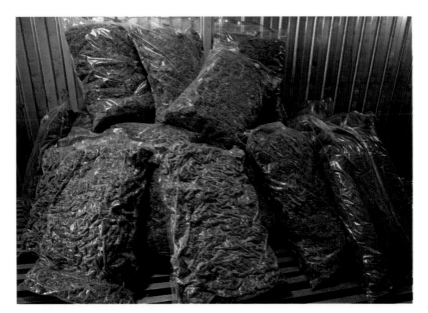

Cured cannabis vacuum packed.

period, the buds will have homogenized and their moisture content will equalize.

The buds are then placed back on the racks or screens. The environment is still 70–80°F and 40–60% humidity. The buds are inspected every hour for 4 to 6 hours, depending on temperature and humidity, and when they are 95% dry, they are placed back into the containers and into the 80°F environment again for 24 hours. After this 24-hour period, the containers are opened and any remaining residual moisture is evaporated into the environment. We periodically rotate the buds in the container and leave them open until the desired moisture content is achieved.

If you accidentally over-dry the product, you can place strips of water-moistened paper towels into the containers and seal them up again. Allow them to reconstitute and absorb moisture for 24 hours in a 70–80°F environment. Never over-dry or quick-dry cannabis, as it will destroy volatile oils responsible for flavor, smell, and potency.

Cannabis should be stored in cool, dark, dry environments in airtight containers. Ideally, we prefer to store the cannabis for two months until it is at its peak. All medical cannabis dispensaries package their medicine in different ways, so we do not utilize any fancy packaging. We place buds into large

Photo: Better

301

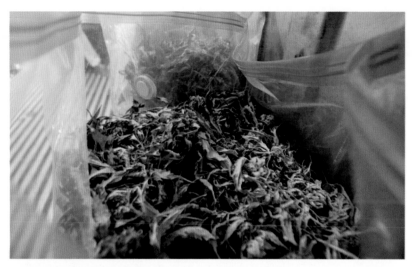

Loose cannabis leaves utilized later for an extraction.

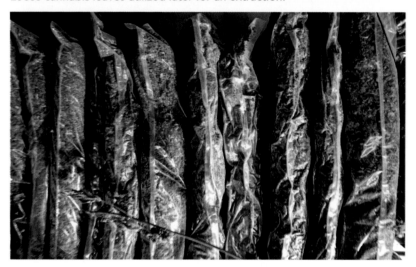

Cannabis packed in vacuum sealed bags for transport.

Ziploc bags, weigh them, and seal them. For smaller amounts we utilize large glass vacuum-sealed jars. These jars are placed into a cool, dark, dry environment, preserving essential oils, cannabinoids, aroma, flavor, and potency.

Do not place cannabis in a freezer. Freezing crystallizes any remaining moisture, destroying the composition of the bud. Refrigerators are acceptable but containers must be airtight. Refrigerators have high humidity and will reconstitute dry cannabis, requiring a second round of drying. Most

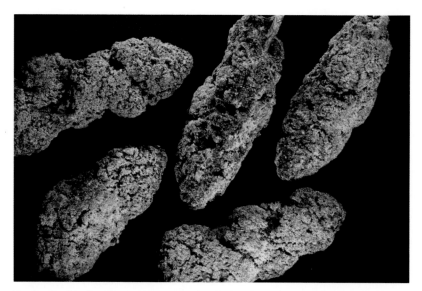

Perfectly dried and cured cannabis buds that have been dipped in cannabis oil and then coated with cannabis resin.

cannabis in a refrigerator will mold and decompose, if improperly stored.

When buds are perfectly dried, cured, packaged, and weighed, they are placed into clear plastic turkey baking bags. They allow no cannabis smell to escape or penetrate the plastic, thus eliminating the volatile aromas created by a large amount of cannabis. When delivering medical cannabis to a dispensary, or carrying cannabis on your person, safety is a huge issue. Cannabis aromas can cause unwanted attention. Use airtight containers when you possess cannabis and cannabis-related paraphernalia.

Curing Tip

Do not rush the curing process. It's delicate, kind of like aging wine prior to bottling: practice makes perfect. You may first choose to experiment with a small amount of buds to prevent the destruction of an entire crop. If mold does develop or if you over- or under-cure your crop the buds can smell like cat piss or lawn clippings. The goal is to dry the buds as evenly as possible and at an even, slow pace.

A good product is the BOVEDA Humidity Protectors. The purpose of this product is to maintain perfect humidity levels in your curing buds. Learn more at www.Bovedainc.com.

Photo: K

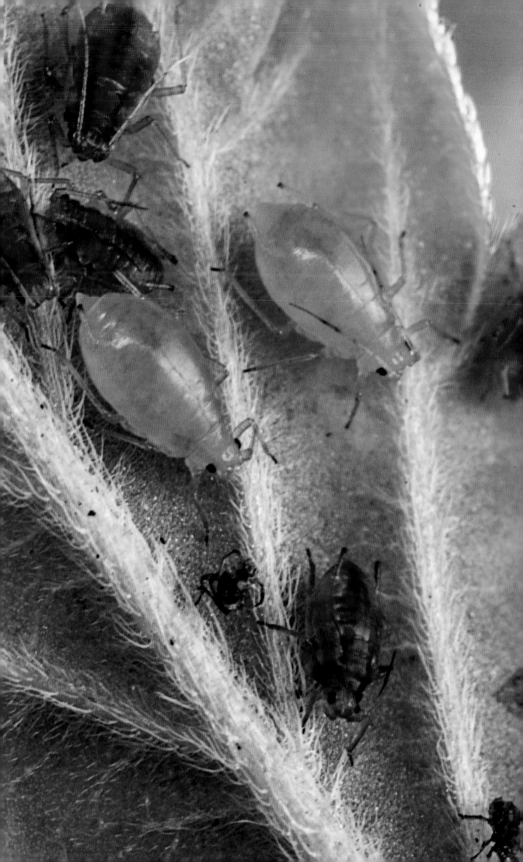

CHAPTER 16

Problems: Mold, Pests, Diseases, and Nutrient Deficiencies

What follows is just the tip of the iceberg as far as mold, pests, diseases, and nutrient deficiencies are concerned. There is much to learn, and there is an astounding amount of information available to you today in the form of published books, papers, and magazines, and especially on the Internet. Whole books have been written on each of these subjects, and one cannot possibly explain every single threat to your plants. Thus, the goal has been to describe the most common threats that growers experience. But don't stop here! Educate yourself: read everything you can concerning these subjects.

Typical Problems

There are many factors that can contribute to slow growth or poor health; so many that it is often difficult

◄ Aphids on an outdoor plant.

Photo: Mel Frank

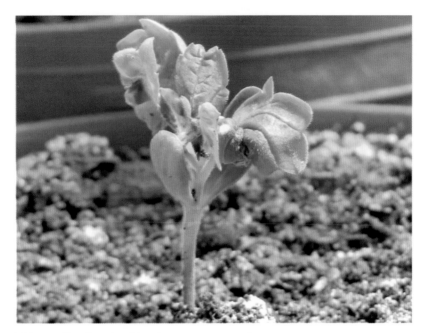

This seedling is unhealthy due to excess nutrients.

to interpret just what the problem might be. Similar symptoms can relate to different problems over the course of a plant's life. When you are diagnosing problems, many aspects of growing must be considered. In the following we list some of the possible causes for problems. Use the list as a basic troubleshooting guide and add to it as your knowledge and experience increases.

Seeds and Seedlings

Problem	Potential Causes
Poor seed emergence	Old seed
	Planted too deep
	Planted too shallow
	Fungus rotted seed
	Overwatering (saturated media)
	Medium too compact
Seed emergence good but growth poor	Insufficient nutrients
	Insufficient lighting
Seedlings dying at media line	Damping off due to fungi
Seedlings with leaf tip burn	Excessive nutrients

Established / Young Plants

Problem	Potential Causes
Yellowing leaves	Light too intense or insufficient
	High temperature
	Nutrient deficiency
Young leaves yellow	Low light intensity
	Excessive nutrients
	Iron or manganese deficiency
Old leaves yellow	Nutrient deficiency (see nitrogen, magnesium, and potassium)
	Overwatering or poor drainage
	Root rot or pythium infection
	Insufficient light intensity to lower leaves
Dead or yellow irregular spots or brown / white specks	Thrip infestation
	Spider mite infestation
	Pesticide damage
	Nutrient deficiency or excess
Yellow or brown spots on leaves	Overwatering
	Fluoride or chlorine toxicity (from water source)
	Pesticide damage
	Nutrient excess or deficiency
Camouflage pattern of light and dark on the same leaf	High temperature
	Pesticide damage
	Major elemental deficiency
	Viral infection (pythium in roots)
Leaves with abnormal color	Nutrient deficiency (especially with yellowing, reddening, or purpling)
	Viral infection

Flowering Plants

When plants are flowering, the potential for problems multiplies. Apart from nutrient deficiencies or excesses, which are covered below, there are a whole host of other potential problems to consider. A daily log will help you note the day's temperature, humidity, nutrients and additives, foliar spray feeding schedule, pH, PPM, and so on. A journal is an essential purchase for monitoring the status and health of your plants. Be on the alert for any unusual

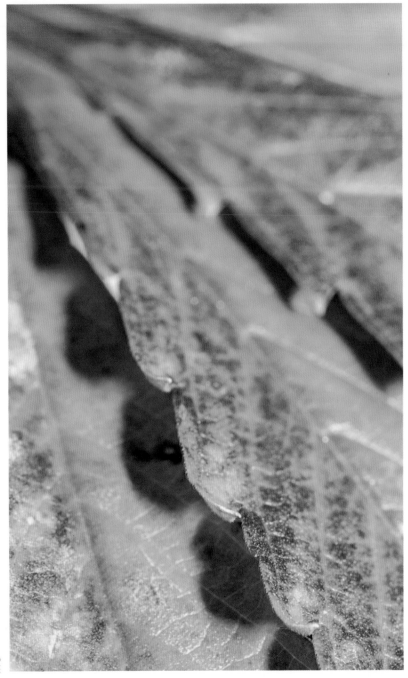

Photo: MG

Always inspect the top and undersides of leaves for any symptoms or signs of nutrient deficiency, pest, or disease.

behavior or erratic changes! Also note down the general condition of your plants. What color are they? How tall? What shape are the leaves? Do they have mold? Mildew? Insects? If you pay enough attention and get to know your plants, you can prevent costly errors and crop loss.

Compare the following parameters to your own measurements; if you notice any sudden erratic behavior, make alterations—but don't alter everything at once! Try one change and see how it works; if it doesn't fix the problem, try another change; and so on.

When the plant is in a VEGETATIVE state, it should be
- receiving light for 18 hours a day from a bulb between 400 and 1,000 watts
- at a humidity level between 65 and 75%. 74% is best
- at a nutrient reservoir temperature of 72°F, room temperature of approximately 75°F
- within pH levels of 5.8 and 6.8—we prefer 6.2
- maintaining CO_2 levels of 400 to 1,500 PPM, depending on stage of growth and cultivation method

When the plant is in a FLOWERING state, it should be
- receiving light for 12 hours a day from a bulb between 400 and 1,000 watts
- at a humidity level between 50 and 60% (this can increase a bit at night without concern)
- at a reservoir tank and room temperature of 70°F to 75°F
- within pH levels of 5.8 and 6.8; we prefer 6.2
- maintaining CO_2 levels between 400 and 1,500 PPM (depending on the stage of growth and cultivation method; discontinue CO_2 for the last $1/4$ of the flowering cycle)

Remembering and monitoring these levels will leave you prepared and ready to go!

Note: Trichome Technologies does not advocate the use of inorganic fungicides, insecticides (other than pyrethrums), or miticides on cannabis. Most organic control methods are perfectly acceptable forms of control, yet will not completely eliminate pests—they simply control the population until the crop is harvested and all rooms can be sterilized.

Identifying Bud Rot, Mold, and Fusarium

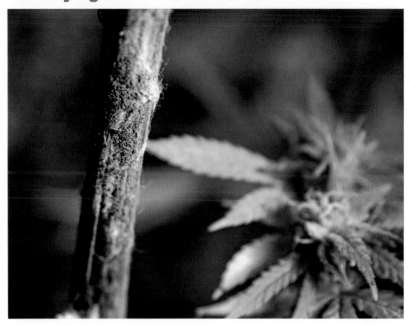

Mold on stem.

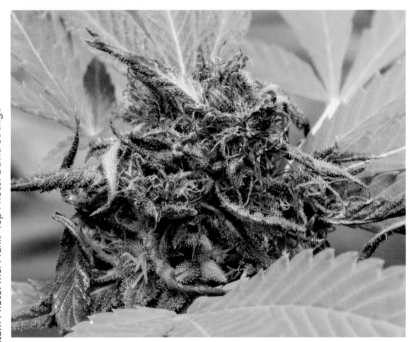

Bud rot.

Bottom Photo: Mel Frank Top Photo: David Strange

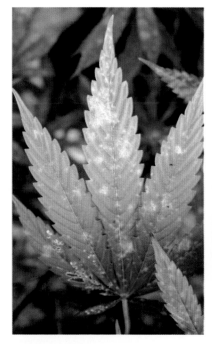

Powdery mildew.

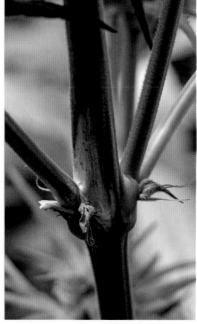

Fusarium on the stem of a plant.

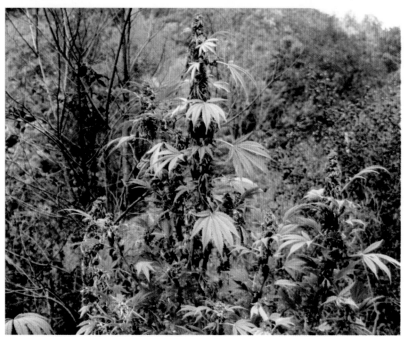

Botrytis fungus can devastate a plant in a few days.

Top Left Photo: David Strange Top Right Photo: Hanna Bliss Bottom Photo: Mel Frank

Grey Mold

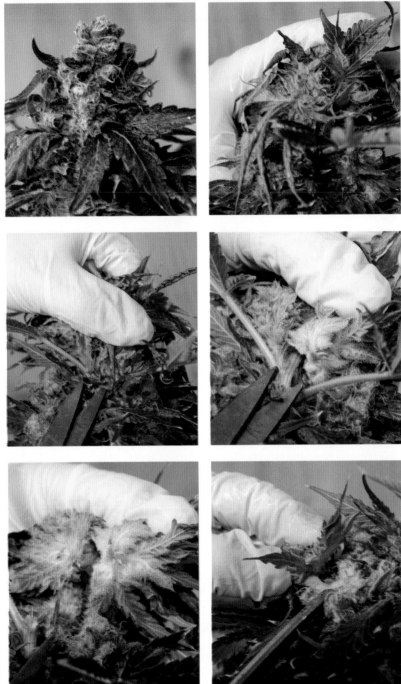

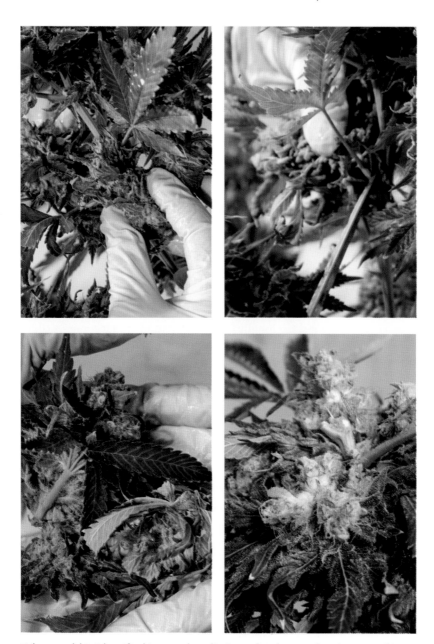

When mold is identified it must be eliminated to lessen the chances of it spreading. The infected material must be removed and immediately sealed and discarded in a garbage outside of the growing environment. All scissors / utensils need to then be sterilized using 90% isopropyl alcohol. Caution: never consume moldy or mildewy cannabis.

Fungi

Botrytis, Botrytis Blight, Gray (or "Grey") Mold, Bud Blight

All of these names describe the same problem. Botrytis affects the stems and inner core of buds. Eliminate all contaminated and moldy material with sterilized scissors. If buds are infected, keep humidity below 50% and increase air circulation. Narrow the temperature difference between night and day as this lowers the chance of dew formation. An ambient temperature of 77°F inhibits spore germination and also prevents condensation.

White, Powdery Mildew

A plant becomes infected with white, powdery mildew when an airborne spore named conidia lands on a leaf surface and germinates. It quickly grows a guide tube that anchors the spore to the leaf, and then penetrates the plant cell wall and membrane with a syringe-type hollow tube that is used to rob the plant of essential nutrients. After five to seven days, depending on environmental conditions, the fungus fully develops and produces microscopic mushroom stalks that distribute millions of new spores, which in turn infect even more of the leaf surface. At the same time, the fungus also produces a secondary spore, to ensure survival, which is dormant and can survive in the winter outdoors and in growrooms for many months after plants have been harvested.

Powdery mildew prefers to infect plants that are at least two or three weeks old and then spread to the whole plant; it can also infect clones if they are taken from infected mothers / donors. Two distinct fungus species are responsible for powdery mildew: Leveillula Taurica and Spaerotheca Macularis. The former prefers to attack warm and humid environments, while the latter prefers cooler spaces. That said, the aggressive strain of S. Macularis present in cannabis gardens has adapted to tolerate higher temperatures. Neither strain is harmed by contact with water; in fact, spores can be spread by water movement.

Powdery mildew in advanced stages looks like fine, gray-white powder that has been spread on the tops of plant leaves. In early stages it might appear on just a few big leaves as irregular circular spots, ranging from $1/8$–$1/2$-inch in circumference. It rapidly spreads to infect the surrounding vegetation, and eventually covers the whole leaf.

The infection causes stunting and death of leaves, buds, and growing tips. Yellowing of leaves and death of tissue can result in premature leaf drop. Be-

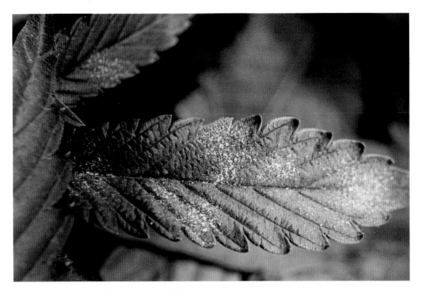

Early indication of powdery mildew.

cause of the removed nutrients from the plant by fungus, the plants will experience a general decline in health and vigor.

Management and Control

1. Use charcoal filters on all ventilation intake, discussed elsewhere in this chapter. This helps prevent contaminants from entering your grow space.

2. Isolate or eliminate all infected material and plants; this helps prevent spread of the fungi.

3. Use a UV sterilizing light inside your air intake ducting. UV lights kill airborne organisms like gray mold and powdery mildew spores.

4. Spray neem oil or potassium bicarbonate on the plant weekly. Neem oil acts as a physical barrier and a chemical deterrent and potassium bicarbonate changes the leaf surface pH and is detrimental to all mildew and mold. We recommend using Azamax, a neem oil derivative from General Hydroponics.

5. Foliar feed compost tea weekly. Beneficial microbes and fungi work as a natural deterrent.

Photo: Samson Daniels

Other Management Considerations Include the Following:

■ Avoid over-watering—which causes excess humidity—or under-watering, which causes drought stress, and in turn encourages susceptibility.

■ Reduce the garden density and provide good ventilation with a good quality environmental climate controller.

■ Water only at the beginning of the daylight cycle.

■ Control humidity so that it never exceeds 60%; use a dehumidifier if necessary.

■ Eliminate any standing water that may evaporate and contribute to elevated humidity; consider sealing reservoirs or moving them out of the growing environment completely.

Cultural Control

Pruning for Powdery Mildew

Trim any infected leaves, branches, or buds and eliminate any contaminated plants. If one or two leaves of a plant are infected with a few small white or gray spots, get a container or plastic bag big enough to hold the leaves and cut them off of the plant. Seal the bag and dispose of it. This prevents reinfection from spores. If infection persists and you see reinfection a short time later, chances are that your chosen cultivar is a good host to powdery mildew and examination of the source of the powdery mildew is in order.

After handling infected plants, you must always sanitize your scissors and other tools with alcohol, hydrogen peroxide, or bleach, and clean your hands with soap and water.

Recommended Organic Sprays for Powdery Mildew Control

These are a few organic sprays that you can use to prevent and control the proliferation and infestation of powdery mildew. All are safe, organic methods of prevention and control that can be washed off with water—foliar spray or rain.

Hydrogen Peroxide

Hydrogen peroxide (HP) works as a contact fungicide that leaves no harmful residues. When hydrogen peroxide makes contact with fungi, the fungi's spores' oxygen atoms attach themselves to molecules on the cell walls, "burning" or oxidizing them, thus killing them. Regular household HP contains 3% hydrogen peroxide; garden supply stores carry a 10% version; and Zerotol, available from organic food supply stores, has a concentration of 27%. Caution: this form of hydrogen peroxide is extremely hazardous and will cause severe burns if it contacts the skin—burns similar to those caused by exposure to concentrated caustic acids.

■ To treat plants using common household 3% HP, mix 4¹⁄₂ tablespoons HP with 1 pint of distilled water.

■ To use 10% HP, mix 4 teaspoons with 1 pint of distilled water.

■ If using Zerotol, mix 1 teaspoon to 1 pint of distilled water, or 2¹⁄₂ tablespoons Zerotol to 1 gallon of distilled water.

■ Dilute the 35% HP to approximate the other mixtures.

Neem Oil (Azamax from General Hydroponics)

Azamax in particular is fantastic for preventing and controlling the proliferation of white powdery mildew. At the first signs of infection spray neem oil onto the leaf surfaces. A neem oil extract acts as a natural barrier that creates an inhospitable environment for the mildew and its spores. When signs of mildew appear, spray neem on foliage until up to two weeks from harvest. Make sure to gently spray or wash the foliage off using pure, clean water a couple of times prior to harvest!

Hexagonal Water

■ Although controversial, this water filtration process has been said by some to eliminate powdery mildew and mold in gardens, and can also control spider mite infestations as well as some other pests.

■ By applying this water to the plant (but never the soil) botrytis and mold spores are exposed to water with a pH of 3.0 or less. A 2.5 pH water will kill any mold spore.

■ It can be mixed with neem oil to make an effective pesticide.

■ These units are very expensive, starting at $4000, but can save you that money by preventing the loss of a single crop.

■ The units are available from companies such as Kangen (www.enagic.com) as well as LIFE Ionizers (www.lifeionizer.ca).

Messenger

Messenger contains a naturally occurring protein called harpin, which stimulates a plant's immune system and promotes healthier plants and increased resistance to infection. It is used to prevent infection and reduce susceptibility to diseases.

Powdery Mildew

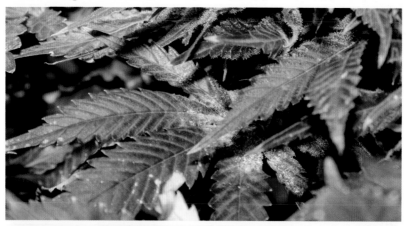

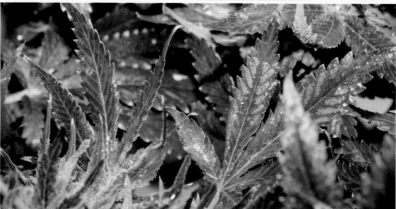

When signs of powdery mildew appear, it must be addressed immediately.

pH-up Liquid

pH-up is used for adjusting the pH of nutrient solutions. The active ingredients usually consist of either lye (KOH) or potash (K_2CO_3). Fungi thrive in an acidic environment and quickly die in an alkaline environment. Changing the pH of a leaf's surface from acidic to alkaline helps to kill the fungi. This is a very basic method of control and works well in advanced stages of infection. Place liquid pH-up onto a Q-Tip and swab off any mold / mildew present, or slightly spray on a plant surface by using a hand-mister.

Serenade and Sonata

Serenade and Sonata's active ingredients include different beneficial bacteria

Photos: Samson Daniels

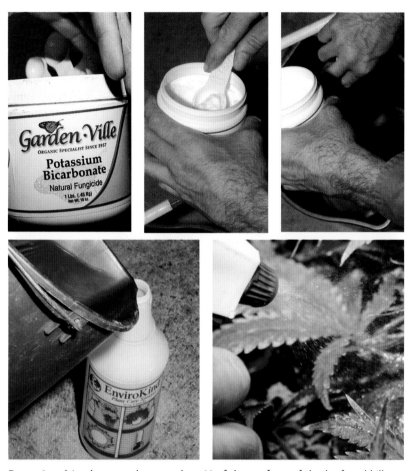

Potassium bicarbonate changes the pH of the surface of the leaf and kills the mildew and its spores.

that use various pathways to prevent and inhibit powdery mildew as well as botrytis. The living bacteria attack and kill fungi and mold organisms, creating a live protective barrier on the surface of the leaf. Both are safe and non-toxic to humans and animals; they are also easy to use as well as being effective. Apply as a foliar spray.

Potassium Bicarbonate

Potassium bicarbonate $(KHCO_3)$ comes in powder form and when mixed with water and sprayed on a leaf surface changes the pH of the surface toward alkaline. Another benefit is that the fungi's cell wall ruptures upon contact with potassium bicarbonate.

Be careful not to saturate your medium with it. Potassium bicarbonate should be used with neem oil (Azamax) and a spreader for optimum results. For application, mix 2 teaspoons of bicarbonate, 1 teaspoon of neem oil, 3 drops of surfactant, and one pint of distilled water. Spray the solution on all infected leaves and new vegetative growth, but not on the buds—trapped neem oil and bicarbonate are difficult to wash out of the inner core of developed buds.

Environmental Control

A good quality climate controller can help avoid fungus and mold problems associated with growrooms and green houses, which are often caused by nighttime dew point—the same phenomenon you see when the evening dew in spring and fall suddenly makes the leaves on trees wet. This is caused by the rapidly falling temperature that occurs in the transition from day to night.

The best way to reduce the chance of this dew point phenomenon is to control the temperature fall and potential condensation. Using large fans to intake and exhaust the air in the room can actually make the condition worse, if cool night air is brought in. Instead, you should use smaller fans that make slower, less drastic changes to the room's climate by lowering the humidity and temperature uniformly and together, so that the dew point does not occur. Climate controllers limit the temperature drop as well, monitoring environmental conditions to prevent dew-point formation and thus fungi proliferation.

Powdery Mildew and Hash

Mature buds that contain fungus or mold should only be used to make butane or water hash (explained in the chapter on Hash Making). The water captures mold, fungus, and their spores, separating them from desirable trichomes. You must thoroughly rinse the resin after collection to ensure that all the mold and fungi spores are washed away, rendering the hash safe to consume. If the resin does retain mold, you must not consume it! Throw it away. Consuming mold is harmful.

> **Caution:** Never consume mold or fungi-infected hashish or cannabis. It must be considered toxic and will make you ill. Do not consume, vaporize, or smoke. Trust me, it's not worth it.

Pest Prevention

The best piece of advice I can offer concerning pests and diseases is that you purchase and read *Hemp Diseases and Pests* by J. M. McPartland, R. C. Clarke, and D. P. Watson. This definitive masterpiece is the best book ever written on the subject.

Air Filtration

An important component to prevention. Try charcoal filters or Hepa filters (on all intake ventilation), which filter air pollutants, dust, insects, and some fungi with minimal restriction of airflow. They are available in many sizes and lengths, are very light, and are easy to install. When they become clogged, simply replace them.

The "Bug Net" is a prefilter for intake and exhaust ducts which is mildew and UV resistant and easily slips on and off for washing. It has a small weave screen that catches insects and traps dust, airborne particles, and some mildew spores. The Bug Net is available in custom sizes and restricts airflow less than 15%. It is like a very fine mesh hair net that is slipped over ducts before the charcoal filters. The prefilter extends the lives of the main filters and is an excellent choice for large-sized insect prevention.

Pyrethrum (Aerosol Bug Bombs)

This synthetic or botanical plant extract is derived from chrysanthemums. We find these bug bombs work for many pests. Use bug bombs for prevention: decontaminate growrooms with pyrethrum in between cycles; it kills and controls many pests. What follows is a schedule for the application of neem oil, baking soda, and pyrethrum. Add one to two teaspoons of potassium bicarbonate and neem oil (following manufacturer's instructions), plus three drops of a wetting agent, to one gallon of pure, adjusted water. Spray the mixture on the plant every other day for two or four applications, depending on the type of infestation or infection. Reapply as needed. Alternate between this and the pyrethrum application. Do not use neem oil on buds in mid to late flowering cycle and always wash off before harvest.

Turn off all lights, fans, ventilation, and ignition sources and leave pyrethrum bug bombs in the grow chambers / environment for one hour, then ventilate and allow new air into the space. Never use large foggers in a small chamber. Ventilate at the earliest opportunity, and foliar wash the

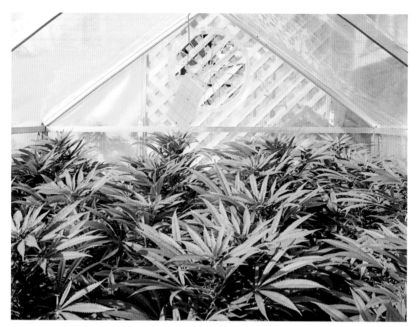

Yellow, pink, and blue sticky traps are excellent indicators for pest identification and rate of infection.

plants 24 hours later. Use foggers in the early morning period so the plants do not burn from being wet under too intense a light; this also allows them to dry completely before the night cycle.

Warning: Bug bombs contain petroleum-based products and are flammable, so use extreme caution and eliminate all ignition sources, i.e., pilot lights, propane burners for CO_2, water heaters, thermostats, fans, heaters, or dehumidifiers—all electrical appliances.

Aphid and Whitefly (Yellow) Sticky Traps

Use these traps to capture, monitor, and compliment your biological control program. Put them every seven feet or at the end of each row of plants, without letting them touch the plants. Note that these traps are highly visible and if you are a guerilla grower you may not wish to use them.

Thrip (Blue) Sticky Traps

The blue sticky trap attracts and catches thrips. Use in indoor, outdoor, and greenhouse environments as you would the yellow traps above.

Photo: K

BT: Bacillus Thuringiensis

BT is a bacteria that, when ingested, kills caterpillars, their larvae, and maggots. Bacillus Thuringiensis var. Kurstaki (BTK) is the most popular form of BT, and in addition to the insects listed it is toxic to moths. BT is non-toxic and completely safe for humans and animals, beneficial insects, and surrounding plants and vegetation. BT bacteria is short-lived and perishable. It becomes ineffective in one to three days and is very susceptible to UV light damage. Store and apply according to manufacturer's instructions. BT is also available in a microencapsulated form, which extends the life span of the bacteria to about a week, depending on environmental conditions.

> **Caution:** Some people have an allergic reaction to BT. Wear a filtration mask as you would when using chemicals.

Neem Oil

Neem oil is manufactured by cold pressing the seeds of a neem tree (Azadirachta indica). Neem oil does not clog the leaf's stomata. It can be purchased from most hydroponic supply stores. Trichome Technologies recommends Azamax by General Hydroponics.

Botrytis

Botrytis cinerea is a fungus that attacks many species of plants, including cannabis. It is typically called "gray mold" or "bud blight." There are different types of botrytis that can cause blight. Botrytis infections proliferate best in cool, humid, or rainy environments, such as summer / fall weather of around 60°F. It can be particularly damaging when these environmental conditions persist for several days. Note that botrytis is capable of becoming dormant in winter and reemerging the following spring.

Pruning to Reduce the Risk of Mold

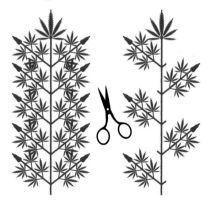

To reduce risk of mold in dense buds, eliminate every other bud site where larger / dense buds may form.

In such a humid environment, it is important to examine any brown, spotted brown, dead, or dying leaves or leaf material that appears on the plant. Botrytis blight is capable of infecting stalks, stems, leaves, and buds; every part of the plant except the roots. Inspect the inner core of the buds and look for masses of gray or silver spores on the dead or decaying tissue. The spores spread easily and can sometimes appear as dust falling off of a heavily infected bud; the dust is actually millions of spores, all looking for a host plant to infect.

Prevention and Control Tips

Molds such as botrytis that attack plants are endemic, meaning the spores are airborne and that there is no way to prevent them from proliferating and contaminating surrounding vegetation. The best tactic for prevention is to arrest spore germination by creating an undesirable environment for the spores. Botrytis germinates in cooler, humid, acidic environments, so to discourage it keep the humidity below 50% and the temperature between the high 60s to low 70°F range during both light and dark periods.

Another way to control botrytis is to maintain plant and leaf surface pH as alkaline rather than acidic. By using phosphorous (P) and potassium (K) foliar spray with a pH of between 8.5 and 9 on all plant surfaces, you will create this alkaline environment. The use of potassium bicarbonate as a foliar spray (1–2 teaspoons per gallon) also controls botrytis growth; it is available from beer brewing stores under many brand names. Organic compost tea, used as a foliar spray, will also work well as a mold preventative, as will beneficial bacteria and fungi.

One simple method of management is regular, thorough inspections and extreme cleanliness. While inspecting the plants, carry a sealable plastic bag and cut off any dead, infected, or unhealthy leaves and properly dispose of them. Do not cut while the plants are wet with dew, mist, rain, or water from foliar sprays, since this will spread the fungal spores that you are trying to eliminate. Prevention is easier and better than the cure.

Pests

Snails and Slugs

Snails and slugs can and will eat cannabis plants outdoors. Both are most active at night. When you see visible evidence of snails or slugs, as in the shiny trails) that we've all seen before, you must eliminate them immediately. We

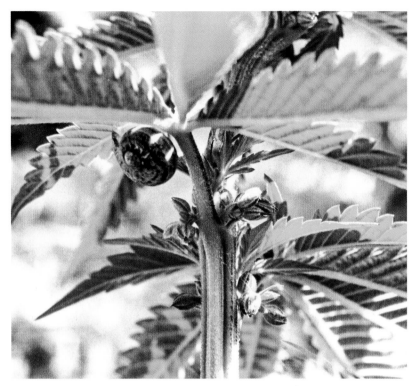

Snails can ruin your cannabis crop. Get rid of them immediately.

use Slug Magic, available from arbico-organics.com. This all-weather formula kills any snails and slugs and is biodegradable; it can be used up to the
day of harvest. The product lures snails and slugs from their hiding places;
they eat the Slug Magic and promptly die.

Animal Repellant

Deer, squirrels, and rabbits can also eat cannabis plants. We use Plants Kydd,
but there are many other products that work very well available from your
local nursery supply store. Deer-Off, available from arbico-organics.com also
works very well. Spray it on surrounding vegetation, not your cannabis
plants. It acts as an odor and taste barrier and protects against deer, squirrels,
and rabbits.

Rattle Snakes or Other Poisonous Snakes

Snakes love to curl up at the base of cannabis plants outdoors. If this is a

Identifying Budworms and Related Problems

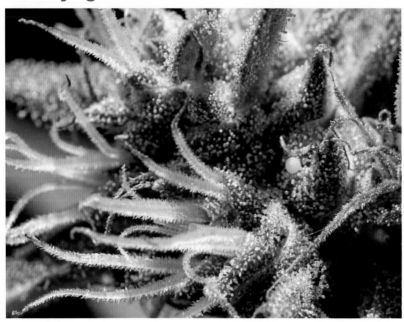

The tobacco budworm egg (yellow) is about 0.5mm wide.

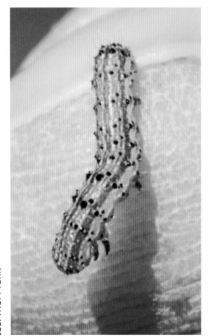

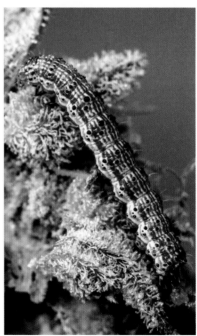

Photos: Mel Frank

Baby budworm.

Adult tobacco budworm.

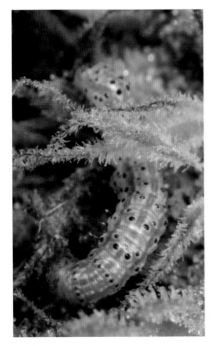

Budworm.

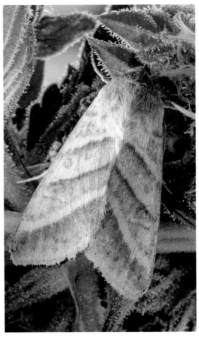

Tobacco budworm moth.

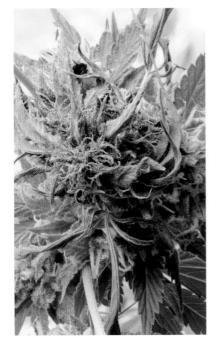

Bud rot due to budworms.

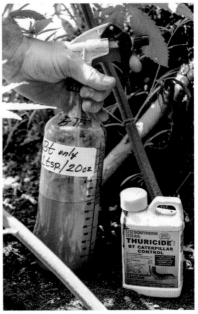

BT spray to get rid of bud worms and caterpillars.

problem for you use Snake Stopper, available from arbico-organics.com. It is a blend of all-natural and USDA recommended ingredients—clove oil, cedar oil, cinnamon oil, and sulfur. It effectively repels snakes from gardens without harming them. Treat the perimeter of the garden.

Caterpillars

Caterpillars are approximately ¹/₄-inch to four inches in size and usually only infect outdoor or greenhouse plants. They are usually light or dark green, sometimes with spots or white stripes running the length of their top or sides. Caterpillars are very detrimental to cannabis. They eat plant tissue and leave behind feces that looks like little black specks. This feces, combined with the dead tissue, promotes botrytis, which quickly spreads and infects whole buds. The infected buds quickly die and are useless for making anything but butane or water hash. If mature infected buds are hung to dry the caterpillars emerge and try to seek refuge in the closest living bud! You may find the caterpillars hanging off the drying buds by a long web, kind of like they are bungee jumping off your buds. Sometimes this will be the first indication you have that your plants have caterpillars.

BT (described above) is effective on young caterpillars, their larvae, and maggots. Apply as soon as a caterpillar infestation is noticed, remembering that caterpillars are most likely to show themselves at night. They seem to crawl out onto leaf tips at night and return to the confines of the inner bud during daylight hours. If possible, inspect plants in the dark with a flashlight (that has a green bulb). If you see any abnormalities in the bud such as yellowing or dying leaves, you must closely inspect the inner bud, deep inside, to make sure there are no caterpillars inside, nor feces or mold.

Spider Mites

There are many types of spider mites. They are the most common pest found in indoor growrooms. The two-spotted spider mite (Tetranychus urticae), also known as the glasshouse red spider mite, is the most prevalent mite. It has been estimated that a single two-spotted spider mite can produce thousands of progeny in one month. This illustrates the seriousness of even a low-level mite infestation.

Spider mites appear as small specks to the naked eye. They come in many colors, including brown, red, white, and yellow. Under magnification (10–50x)

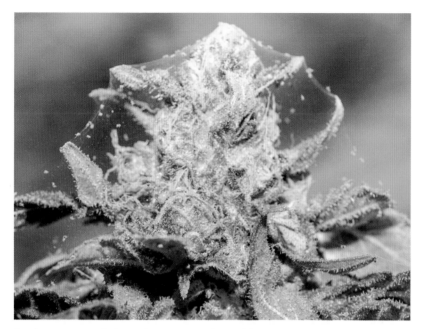

Spider mites in all their glory. Notice the webbing that will rapidly cover the entire bud.

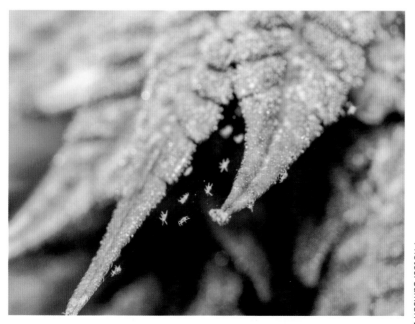

The mites have completely destroyed the natural vigor/health of this plant and must be eliminated immediately.

Photos: Samson Daniels

Identifying Spider Mites and Their Problems

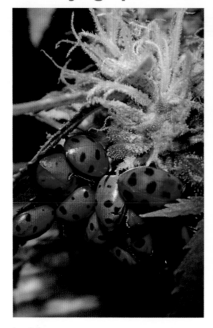

Ladybugs.

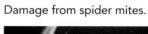

Damage from spider mites.

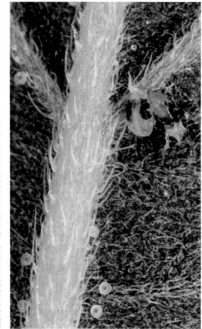

Two spotted spider mites with eggs.

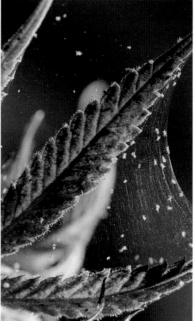

Spider mite webbing.

Top Left Photo: Krane Other Photos: Mel Frank

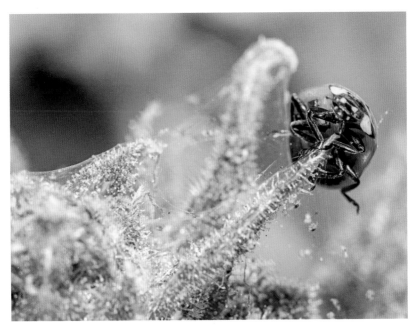

Ladybugs seek out, kill, and eat spider mites and are a valuable resource outdoors, but indoors they tend to fly directly toward the hot light and ultimately die.

you can see that they are indeed spiders, with eight legs. Spider mites appear in mass on the undersides of leaves in the beginning stages of infestation. This is also where they lay their eggs. Later, they proliferate through the plant. Adolescent and adult mites feed on the leaves' undersides and deplete its essential fluids, eventually killing it. While the mites can be difficult to see, the damage they cause becomes rapidly apparent. Yellow and white spots appear on the top side of older and younger leaves. As infestation continues, mites proliferate and can be found everywhere, including on buds. In advanced stages, mites will completely cover entire buds in thick spider webbing and form colonies—a spider mite orgy of plant death. Webbing is most visible after foliar feeding. When spider mite infestation is this advanced, it renders the buds and leaves useless for consumption.

Control

Cleanliness is paramount. Keep everything clean and disinfected. Regularly inspect the undersides of leaves and plants. Regularly spray with neem oil. When

Photo: Samson Daniels

mite infestation is rampant and neem oil and pyrethrums become ineffective, it is best to discontinue growth and eliminate all plants, disposing of all infected material and sterilizing the growroom.

The perfect climate for spider mite proliferation and reproduction is a drier one, with a temperature range of 70–80°F. Spider mites can reproduce every five days in temperatures above 80°F, when reproduction and populations expand exponentially. When your crop is infected you must create a hostile environment for the mites. Lower the growroom temperature to 60°F and foliar spray the underside and tops of all leaves with baking soda and neem oil (explained earlier in this chapter). This will disturb the mites and make the foliage slightly inedible for them; it also raises the humidity, which will slow their reproductive cycle. Reapply and alternate between a neem oil and baking soda mix, and pyrethrum. Isolate all infected plants and avoid cross contamination from one plant to another. Remove any tissue that is more than 50% damaged and dispose of it so that it doesn't infect the other plants.

Strict spraying schedules must be adhered to when treating spider mites with pyrethrum. You must use two or three applications minimum, at three to five day intervals. The infestation should be dramatically reduced or gone after three or four applications. Since spider mite eggs hatch in approximately five to 10 days, the first pyrethrum application kills all adolescents and adults, while the second kills the adolescents that have hatched from eggs and any remaining adults. The third application kills all remaining mites that may have hatched late or since the last pyrethrum application. Spider mites quickly develop a resistance to pyrethrum, so it is recommended that you rotate your application of pyrethrum and neem oil / baking soda. You can also use Spray Safe and Bugzyme, which work very well for controlling spider mites; use as directed by manufacturer.

Thrips

Thrips are tiny insects with four feather-like wings. They vary in color from pale yellowish-white to greenish to gray and dark brown, depending on the time of year. Greenhouse thrips are usually tiny black insects with translucent wings. Adult thrips lay eggs deep inside the folds of leaf tissue. Adolescents and adults cause damage by piercing and sucking out essential plant fluids from individual plant cells in newer leaf tissue. The prepupal and pupal stages (larval stage, prior to adulthood) are often found in the soil or chosen medium.

Whiteflies, Gnats, and Lacewings

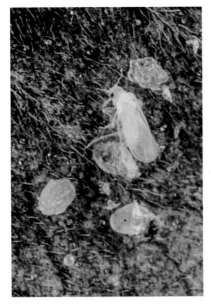

Silver leaf whitefly (*Bemisia argentifolii*) emerging from pupa.

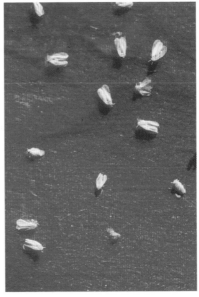

Whiteflies captured with Tanglefoot on red, yellow, or orange paper.

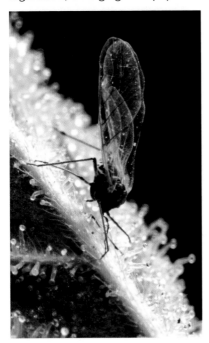

Gnat trapped by resin.

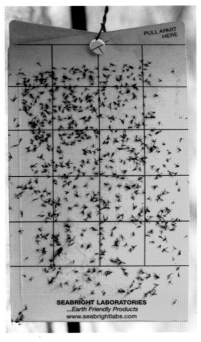

Yellow gnat trap.

Photos: Mel Frank

Typical damage can be seen on new, developing leaves and leaf tissue, which can cause leaf deformation and death and premature dropping. Another symptom is the dried black spots of thrip feces that develop near feeding sites.

Thrips can be difficult to completely eradicate but can be controlled by many biological means and with a variety of insecticides such as Azamax or Entrust, a bacterial byproduct that is effective against many foliage feeding pests but which does not harm beneficial insects. These are available from arbico-organics.com.

Damage

Thrips remove plant tissue and suck out essential fluids from individual plant cells. Small yellow-whitish holes appear on the top side of leaves and new tissue can become deformed. Damaged leaves discontinue photosynthesis and chlorophyll production, whereupon leaves dry out, become brittle, and drop off. Thrips prefer to feed on young, new tissue and inside buds. They often wrap up and distort leaves.

Physical and Cultural Control

Cleanliness is paramount, both for your grow environment and air intake. Use charcoal filters to filter incoming air and maintain a clean grow area. Regularly inspect and replace all clogged air-intake filters. Blue and pink sticky traps, available from nursery supply stores or online, act as a first indicator for thrip infestation. Thrips are very difficult to completely eradicate. Completely decontaminate all surfaces and rooms after completion of harvest and eliminate all infected plant material. Pyrethrum and neem oil are good for control and prevention.

Aphids

Aphids are commonly referred to as plant lice. They are very small and are easy to see with the naked eye, but a 10–50x magnification loupe is recommended for positive identification. Aphids are present in many climates and environments. Aphids range in color, including black, green, brown, rust, and even pink. The majority of aphids do not have wings, but a small percentage of them do, which aids in their proliferation. Aphids give live birth to predominantly female larvae and do not have to mate; these larvae begin to reproduce soon after birth.

Aphids and Aphid Damage to Plants

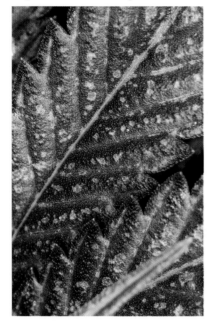

Damage caused by aphids.　　　　Aphids on an indoor plant.

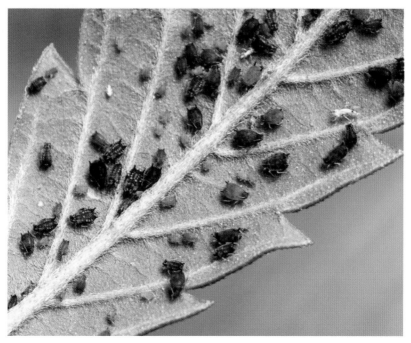

Aphid infestation.

Photos: Mel Frank

The number one source of aphids is poorly or unfiltered incoming ventilation air. As such, indoor gardens are most susceptible to aphids when populations increase outdoors, in spring and summer. We use sticky traps as a pest indicator, and these are placed at the base and canopy level.

Damage

Aphids are most commonly found under leaves, colonizing around stock and branch nodes and on newer tissue tips. Aphids suck internal fluids and sap out of the vegetation and foliage, causing leaf wilt, yellowing, and, finally, necrosis. Furthermore, they can spread destructive viruses and secrete a sticky fluid— a substance misleadingly called honeydew—along with their feces. This honeydew can form a sooty mold that can become a major problem, inhibiting productive growth and diminishing quality and yield. Aphids usually infest stressed, weakened plants first. Some species of aphids prefer to feed on new, succulent tissue and others prefer older vegetation, or even bud tissue.

Ants

Ants literally raise aphids like cattle! They feed on the aphids' so-called "honeydew" and will carry the aphids from plant to plant as they multiply. Therefore all ants must be rapidly eliminated from your growing environment. Aphids eat plants and produce honeydew as waste along with their feces, particularly in the fall, going into winter. Ants will try to infest greenhouses and indoor gardens and bring along a food source (aphids) so that they can have a warm winter with food. You must eliminate all ants and their access to the growing environment. Period.

Prevention

Seal any and all gaps or cracks in the walls and windows. Ensure excellent air intake filtration and placement of ant traps around the perimeter of the growroom; regularly apply neem oil.

Control

Remove any and all infested tissue and dispose of it so that it does not reinfest the growing environment. Destroy any plants that are completely infected right before harvest. Spraying pyrethrum or neem on buds before harvest only produces undesirable buds.

Nutrient Deficiencies

Re-familiarize Yourself With Nutrients

■ Primary Nutrients:

(N) Nitrogen

(P) Phosphorous

(K) Potassium

■ Secondary Nutrients:

(Mg) Magnesium

(S) Sulfur

■ Micronutrients:

(Ca) Calcium

(Fe) Iron

(Mn) Manganese

(Zn) Zinc

(Cu) Copper

(B) Boron

(Mo) Molybdenum

(Cl) Chloride / Chlorine

(Na) Sodium

(Ni) Nickel

(Co) Cobalt

(F) Fluoride

(Si) Silicon

■ Elements Absorbed from Air and Water

(C) Carbon

(H) Hydrogen

(O) Oxygen

Introduction

Dealing with the exact nutritional needs of a plant can be a balancing act. Not too little, not too much: it must be just right to achieve maximum results. Listed below are typical symptoms of deficiency and excess for the essential elements of plants. Also listed are the ways to correct these, where they apply. In most cases of nutrient excess, the only correction that can be made is to flush the medium with pure, 0 PPM, 6.2 pH-adjusted water at 72°F. Flush until runoff water is at an acceptable pH and PPM range, 5.8–6.8 pH, preferably 6.2, with the PPM progressively dropping in runoff water measurements as you flush. Of course, you should also lower the particular element in your nutrient mix or tank that your excess relates to.

In organic soilless mix you must be very careful not to include more organic fertilizers than the plant can use. Lower amounts of fertilizers are safer than higher amounts. It's easier to add nutrients than it is to take them away or eliminate them. However, nutrients in a hydroponic system are sometimes used up faster than they can be replaced. The quickest fix for most deficiencies is foliar feeding. However, this is a temporary fix, and does not solve the original problem; to do so, you must replace the nutrient solution every week instead of every two, as recommended. In some situations it may be necessary to switch to a different type of hydroponic fertilizer if the same deficiencies continue.

Salt Buildup

Fertilizer minerals and salt buildup is a problem most often experienced by growers using "hard water" in soilless situations (see the water purity section in the Water and Feeding chapter). Salt takes time to build up and it needs to be constantly monitored and flushed using pure, adjusted water.

The problem caused by buildup can be depletion, which is when the plants in a recirculating system do not utilize all available nutrients and minerals in the water, leaving some levels higher and others lower. The plant only takes what it wants when it needs it, and its needs are ever-changing. The fertilizers left in the solution will eventually build up, resulting in unhealthy plants and diminished yields. The same applies to aeroponic systems.

Using General Hydroponics' Flora Kleen Salt Clearing Solution can eliminate buildup. It removes fertilizer residue that can accumulate over time and can be used as a final flush to purge your system of excess salts and fertilizers. It is completely safe, will not harm plants in any way, and can be used to clean and maintain both hydroponic and soil-based environments.

Nutrient Deficiencies and Excesses
Antagonistic Effects
In order to fully appreciate the coming pages you will need to know what

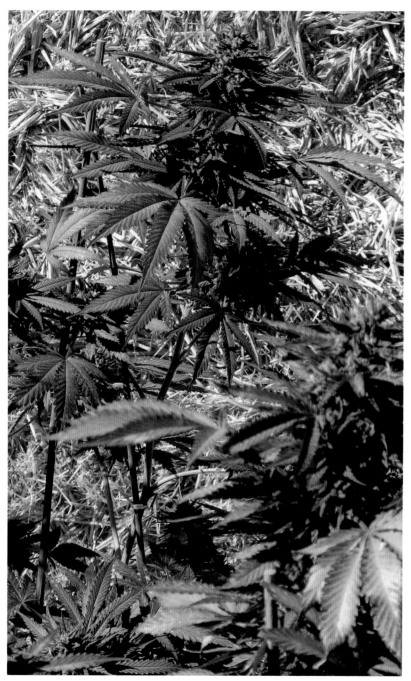

Purpling and yellowing in the final phases of flowering is not unusual, especially after all nutrients are utilized or flushed out.

Photo: K

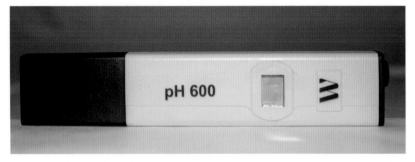

Check pH regularly with a calibrated pH tester.

"antagonistic effects" means. In this context, antagonistic effect means that chemicals (nutrients), when in excess or deficient, can bond together and cause symptoms of an altogether different nutrient deficiency or excess. Simply put, an excess or deficiency of one (or more) elements can cause an excess or deficiency in another.

Remedy
Periodically flush your medium and use properly balanced nutrient regimens and proportions. In recirculating hydroponic systems you must completely replace (drain and refill) water and nutrients every one to two weeks. You must always have a proper growing medium; an improper medium, one that's mineral rich or dominant in one characteristic or another, can cause an antagonistic effect.

Nitrogen
General Information
Cannabis prefers a high nitrogen level in the vegetative stage and lower nitrogen levels in the flowering stage. There are two basic forms of nitrogen—nitrate and ammonium—but for practical purposes they are commonly mixed together by some manufacturers, so you usually have little or no control of the level of either, unless you are using proper, custom-blended, specialized nutrients. Nitrogen's basic purpose is to aid in foliage and stem production, as well as the overall health and vigor of the plant.

Deficiency
A nitrogen deficiency causes general chlorosis or uniform yellowing of the leaf tissue, beginning with the older tissue. It also causes reduced leaf size

340

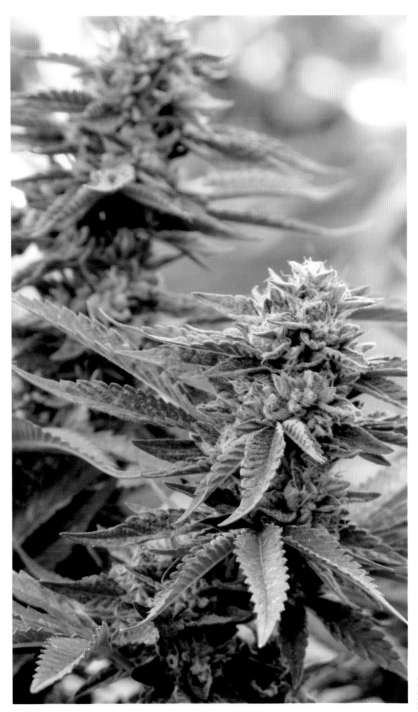

Sun-grown cannabis has the lowest cost of production.

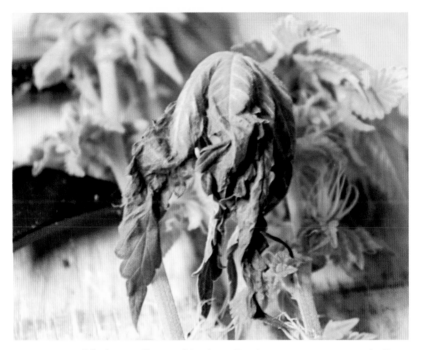

No amount of flushing will save this plant. Don't waste resources on it. Start over and try again.

and leaf dropping, beginning with tip burn on older leaves. When deficiency is severe the older tissue (fan leaves) will turn brown while the younger tissue (small leaves and vegetation) will be light green or yellow in appearance. Plants will look spindly, weak, and their growth will be stunted, if they do not stop growing altogether. Nitrogen deficient plants tend to mature early with reduced yields, and the finished product will be undesirable with a very harsh smoke.

Excess / Toxicity
Nitrogen excess will cause dark, thick green leaves with extremely lush foliage that will have delicate, weak stalks and stems. Bud development will be poor and airy and lack proper color. Overall the plant will have a high susceptibility to insect and fungal attacks and overall poor health. Leaves may wilt on high atmospheric demand days, caused by vascular tissue deterioration; leaves can turn a brown / copper color, dry up, and fall off. Again, the finished product will be undesirable and its smoke harsh.

Photo: Stoned Rosie

Excess Treatment

Excess amounts of nitrogen must be flushed out using pure, adjusted water. Readjust and replace nutrient solution at lower nitrogen (N) levels.

Deficiency Treatment

Nitrogen deficiencies call for a fertilizer with higher N levels on the N-P-K scale. Alternately, you can add calcium nitrate or potassium nitrate to your nutrient solution at 20 to 50 PPM increments, until symptoms disappear. And as explained previously, slight deficiencies may be corrected with foliar feeding.

Soil Treatment

In soil situations, organic soil amendments that are high in nitrogen are used to correct nitrogen deficiency, and can be used as a direct soil application—as a tea—or as a tea foliar feed. The high nitrogen amendments include but are not limited to fish emulsion, blood meal, and sea bird guano, just to name a few.

Phosphorous

General Information

Cannabis prefers a nutrient formula with a high phosphorous level in the germination, seedling, cloning, and flowering stages. Phosphorous is a vital component to the photosynthesis process and contributes to seed production, resin production, healthy root growth, and overall health and vigor in the early and late stages of growth. There are many root and bloom enhancers on the market and they all contain high levels of phosphorous.

Deficiency

A phosphorous deficiency causes the entire plant to develop a dark green or blue-green color, which may turn into a purple, reddish-bronze, or dull purple-green leaf coloration on older leaves, especially along the veins and stems. Symptoms occur in older leaves first. Plants will be stressed and susceptible to insect attack and diseases. When the deficiency is severe, older, lower leaves may be yellow, drying to a greenish brown or black, with eventual drop off. Eventually, plants will become stunted and stop growing, shoot growth will be short and thin, with very poor flower / bud production. The finished product will be undesirable and harsh.

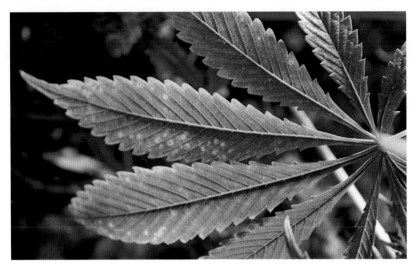

Chlorosis visible on a leaf indicates there is a nutrient problem of some sort.

Excess / Toxicity

Cannabis utilizes high levels of phosphorous in all stages and is capable of tolerating higher levels, but excess will result in variable symptoms that may induce iron, copper, zinc, calcium, and magnesium deficiency symptoms. These symptoms can take days, even weeks to appear. Plants can be slow growing but otherwise look normal. Excess phosphorous can cause cannabis to sparkle and burn poorly when smoked. A joint or bowl will not completely burn or turn to ash, but rather to charcoal-like clumps.

Excess Treatment

Excess amounts of phosphorous must be flushed out using pure, adjusted water. Readjust and replace nutrient solution at lower levels.

Deficiency Treatment

Phosphorous deficiencies call for a fertilizer with a higher phosphorous (P) level on the N-P-K scale. Increase the level of phosphorous you are using or switch to General Hydroponics hydroponic or organic fertilizer products. Alternately, you can add mono potassium phosphate (MPK) to your nutrient solution at 10 to 20 PPM increments until symptoms disappear—which should take approximately one week. Phosphoric acid (H_3PO_4) added at 10 to 20 PPM increments is also a good source.

Soil Treatment

In soil situations, high phosphorous organic soil amendments are used to correct phosphorous deficiencies, and can be used as a direct soil application—as a tea— or as a tea foliar feed. The high phosphorous amendments include but are not limited to bone meal, various animal manures, and bat guano, just to name a few.

Potassium

General Information

Cannabis requires potassium throughout its entire growth cycle. It increases natural resistance to infections, bacteria, molds, and mildew. It is also an important component in essential oil production, which is responsible for flavor and odor. Potassium is required for vigorous root growth.

Deficiency

In the early stages of potassium deficiency, plants will appear to be healthy and normal but will then turn dark bluish-green in color—similar to phosphorous deficiency—and then dead or dying spots will appear on the leaf margins, particularly older leaves, giving them a scorched appearance. Stems can become weak and brittle. Plants will become susceptible to pests and disease and will become stunted when the deficiency is severe, ultimately resulting in poor yields. Finished product buds will be undesirable and harsh with diminished flavor and smells.

Excess / Toxicity

Potassium excess can be difficult to diagnose because potassium buildup can cause symptoms that also appear with iron, calcium, magnesium, manganese, and zinc deficiencies, magnesium being the most likely one. Potassium buildup is rare in closely monitored situations, but must be addressed immediately when it occurs.

Excess Treatment

Excess amounts of potassium must be flushed out using pure, adjusted water. Readjust and replace nutrient solution at lower levels.

Deficiency Treatment

Potassium deficiencies call for a fertilizer with a higher potassium (K) level on the N-P-K scale. Increase the level of potassium you are using or switch to General Hydroponics fertilizer products. Alternately, you can add potassium nitrate to your nutrient solution at 50 PPM, in increments, until symptoms disappear, after approximately one week. Make sure to adjust the pH.

Soil Treatment

In soil situations, soluble potash (wood ash), an organic soil amendment that is high in potassium, should be applied directly to the soil after being mixed with water and pH adjusted to 6.2. Potash has a very high pH that must be lowered. Check the PPM of the solution prior to feeding and add at 20 to 50 PPM increments. Never use potash solution as a foliar feed.

Calcium

General Information

Cannabis requires calcium (Ca) throughout its life cycle in a balanced nutrient solution mix accompanying other micronutrients. Calcium increases natural resistance to bacteria and fungi, and is an essential component of cell manufacture and growth. It is essential to the preservation and development of membrane permeability, which increases the plant cells' resistance to environmental attacks, and cellular integrity, which is the composition of plant cells. Calcium is also necessary for healthy root growth.

Deficiency

If you are using a good quality, over-the-counter fertilizer or have properly mixed your organic medium, calcium deficiency is fairly rare and sometimes difficult to detect. However, it can present itself in high humidity situations of 80% and above. Calcium deficiency will cause younger leaves to stop growing and eventually die. The margins of the leaves may become chlorotic (yellow), a situation that is followed by necrosis, distorted leaves, and leaf drop. New growth / buds will develop "blossom-end-rot" and root growth will be severely reduced and readily susceptible to infection by bacteria and fungi, resulting in stunted plants with poor bud development and yield: ultimately, an undesirable finished product.

Excess / Toxicity

Calcium excess can cause either potassium, magnesium, manganese, or iron

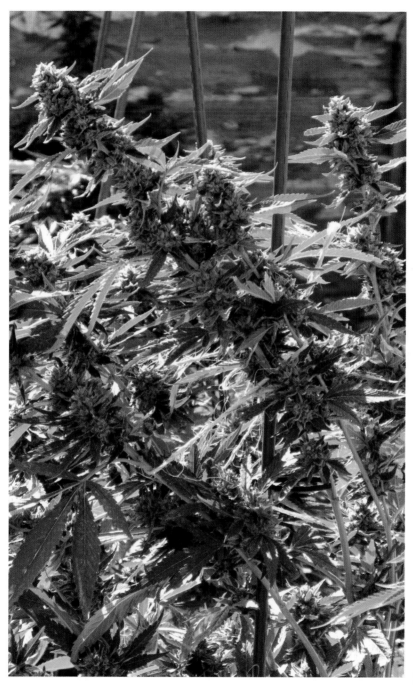

Photo: K

When nearing harvest, buds can become so heavy that they break the branch that they are on, so you must tie them up or secure them.

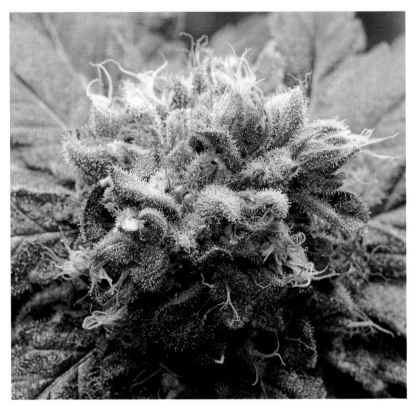

Stigmata are turning brown, and this plant is beginning to ripen.

Photo: Samson Daniels

deficiency symptoms due to antagonistic effects: imbalance of fertilizer micro- and macro- nutrients. It can affect the proper balance that is necessary for maintaining good, healthy growth. Early warning signs include leaf wilt, and excess will stunt early development. Cannabis can typically process more calcium than is available; it is usually washed out of leaves during the foliar feed process.

Excess Treatment

Excess amounts of calcium are rare, but if they occur must be flushed out using pure, adjusted water. Spray off the plants using pure, adjusted water as well. Readjust and replace nutrient solution at lower levels.

Deficiency Treatment

Potassium deficiencies call for a fertilizer with higher calcium (Ca) levels. Increase the level of calcium you are using or switch to General Hydroponics fertilizer products. Alternately, you can add calcium nitrate to your nutrient solution at 50 PPM in increments, until symptoms disappear, usually after one week. Conversely, you can add ¹/₂ teaspoon of hydrated lime to one gallon of purified water and adjust the pH to 6.2. Add this to your reservoir or media at 10 to 20 PPM in increments until symptoms disappear, usually after about one week. This solution can also be used as a mild foliar feed when plants are calcium deficient.

Soil Treatment
In soil grows, a high-calcium organic soil amendment in the form of fine dolomite lime can be mixed and applied as recommended in the organic soils section.

Magnesium
General Information
Cannabis utilizes and requires high levels of magnesium (Mg), so growers find that magnesium deficiency is a common occurrence, especially in non-balanced nutrient reservoirs and acidic pH media. Magnesium is required throughout the plant's life cycle and is essential to a plant's ability to absorb and use light energy; it also helps plants facilitate nutrient utilization and neutralizes soil acids as well as increasing the plant's natural resistance to fungus and disease.

Deficiency
Magnesium deficiency is common. Symptoms will first appear on the older plant tissue, especially the lower leaves and vegetation, as a marginal chlorosis and wilting between the veins of the leaves. Severe deficiency causes the death of older leaves and eventually the chlorosis of the entire plant. A magnesium deficiency will also increase a plant's susceptibility to fungus and disease, cause stunting of growth, resulting in poor bud development and, ultimately, undesirable product.

Excess / Toxicity
If you are using a properly balanced nutrient formulation, magnesium excess is extremely rare, almost non-existent, and is difficult to detect. Toxic levels of magnesium may induce a potassium or calcium ion conflict, particularly in hydroponic solutions. Visual symptoms may not appear, although the plant may be growing poorly.

Excess Treatment

Excess amounts of magnesium must be flushed out using pure, adjusted water. Readjust and replace nutrient solution.

Deficiency Treatment

Magnesium deficiencies call for a fertilizer with a higher magnesium level. Increase the level of magnesium you are using or switch to General Hydroponics fertilizer products. Alternately, you can add two teaspoons of the finest Epsom salts available for plants to one gallon of water. Add this to your nutrient mix in 20 to 30 PPM increments until symptoms disappear, after about one week. You can also foliar spray with this solution after it is pH adjusted.

Soil Treatment

In soil situations, high magnesium organic soil amendments are available in the form of dolomite lime, as recommended in the organics section. Also, the Epsom salt remedy noted above works in soil.

Sulfur

General Information

Cannabis uses sulfur to produce essential oils that are responsible for the odor and flavor of the final product. It is also an essential element in the production of plant cells and seed formation, for aiding respiration and photosynthesis, and for the breakdown of fatty acids. All quality fertilizer products contain some level of sulfur and therefore deficiency rarely becomes a problem. Sulfur is required throughout the plant's life cycle.

Deficiency

Symptoms of sulfur deficiency are not too dissimilar from nitrogen deficiency, with plants appearing light lime green to pale yellow in color, depending on the severity of the deficiency. Symptoms appear in older fan leaves first, but normally they are generalized over the whole plant. As the deficiency progresses, the plant will become spindly and stunted and lack vigor. Older yellowed leaves turn brown and die. Younger leaves yellow but veins remain green with progressive purpling of the petiole and smaller stems. Leaf tips can burn, turn brown and crispy, and curve downwards. Sulfur deficiency causes elongated stems that become woody at the base, with more

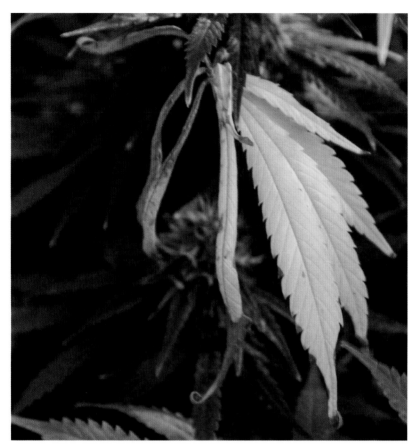

This leaf is completely yellow and dead. Remove it and keep an eye on your plant for other signs of problems.

and longer roots than usual. In hydroponic situations, sulfur deficiency can occur when the pH is too high (6.8 and above) or when calcium levels are too high. Always use properly balanced hydroponic nutrient formulas.

Excess / Toxicity

Sulfur excess seldom occurs, but when it does, as in a hydroponic situation, it causes a lockout of other essential elements and nutrients. When the excess is severe, leaf tips and margins will develop chlorosis and become discolored (brown) and burnt. Visual symptoms include leaves that are stunted, small, and dark green, as well as premature leaf death and poor growth and yields.

Photo: Stoned Rosie

Excess Treatment

Excess amounts of sulfur are rare, but if they occur, must be flushed using pure, adjusted water. Readjust and replace nutrient solution.

Deficiency Treatment

Sulfur deficiencies call for a fertilizer with a higher sulfur (S) level. Alternately, you can add two teaspoons of the finest Epsom salts available for plants to one gallon of water. Add this to your nutrient mix in 20 to 30 PPM increments until symptoms disappear, after about one week. Lower reservoir pH to 5.5–6.0.

Soil Treatment

Natural forms of sulfur include many animal manures (use sterilized manure, preferably; never use raw manure as it will burn tender roots), mushroom compost, and Epsom salt solution. Symptoms should disappear after about one week.

Iron

General Information

Cannabis uses iron (Fe) through its entire life cycle, therefore it must be present in all professional-quality fertilizers. Iron aids in allowing plants to use sugar, which is a catalyst for chlorophyll production. It is also an essential element in the process of photosynthesis and respiration. Acidic soil situations are usually perfect in terms of iron content.

Deficiency

Iron deficiency symptoms include a general chlorosis of the new leaf tissue while the veins remain green, though they will turn brown and if left untreated will drop off. Symptoms will eventually spread to the whole plant. An iron deficiency can often be directly attributed to an excessive amount of available copper. When severe, plants become stressed, growth is slowed, and the plants become stunted, producing poor yields and undesirable product. Iron deficiency situations can present themselves when the pH is above approximately 6.8.

Excess / Toxicity

Under reasonable conditions, iron excess or toxicity is rare and will not occur. Excess levels will not damage plants but may cause magnesium and phosphorous deficiency symptoms due to antagonistic effects.

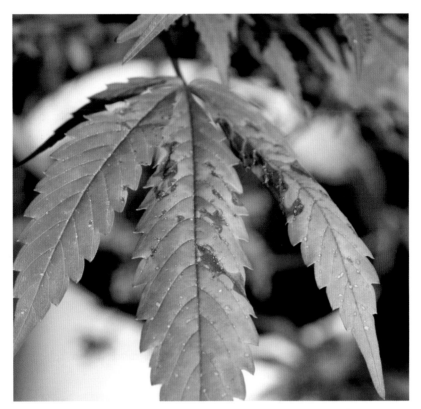

Signs of necrosis on this leaf. Over or under fertilization could cause this. Unhealthy leaves can be caused by a myriad of things. You must always monitor environmental conditions and nutrient supply.

Excess Treatment

Excess amounts of iron are rare but if it occurs must be flushed out using pure, adjusted water. Readjust and replace nutrient solution.

Deficiency Treatment

Iron deficiencies call for a fertilizer with a higher iron (Fe) level or a switch to General Hydroponics fertilizer products. Lower the pH of the soil and fertilizer mix to 6.5 or less, which will allow plants to uptake more iron. Discontinue fertilizers that contain high levels of copper, manganese, phosphorous, and zinc, all of which inhibit iron uptake. Foliar feeding is a perfect remedy for iron deficiency; use a mild fertilizer mix containing iron and the deficiency will quickly disappear, after about one week.

Photo: David Strange

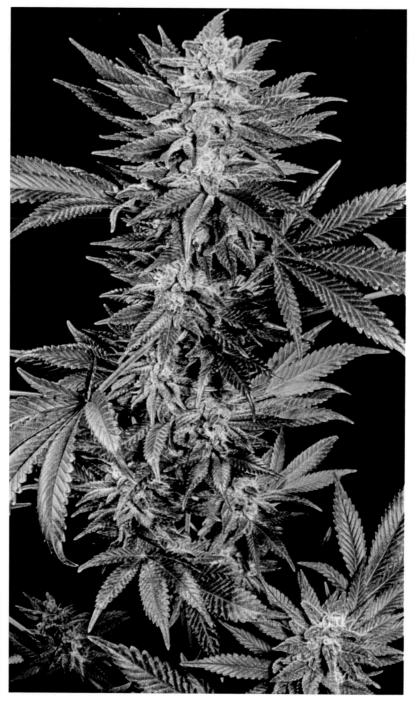

This plant is in perfect health

Soil Treatment

Have a pH of 6.8 or below and a quality fertilizer in proper proportions with a matching pH. Iron excess or toxicity is rare when using a tea fertilizer or by foliar feeding.

Manganese

General Information

Cannabis uses manganese (Mn) throughout its life cycle and it must be present in all stages of growth. Manganese is present in all professional-quality fertilizers. When combined with other elements, manganese contributes to plant photosynthesis and in the facilitation and utilization of nitrogen. Manganese and iron are both essential elements for chlorophyll production.

Deficiency

Manganese deficiency is quite prevalent in indoor and hydroponic situations. Younger tissue leaves express symptoms first, becoming yellow between veins, a condition known as interveinal chlorosis, while the veins themselves remain green. When severe deficiency occurs, symptoms rapidly migrate from younger tissue to old, and necrotic spots will appear on the leaves, which will eventually die and drop off. Plants will be stunted and new leaves can be misshapen. Manganese deficiency can also extend the ripening of buds, and severe deficiency can mimic a magnesium deficiency.

Excess / Toxicity

Excess manganese symptoms may not be very different from deficiency symptoms at first. Manganese toxicity may include iron, magnesium, molybdenum, and zinc deficiency symptoms as antagonistic effects. Necrotic rust and brown spots appear on young leaves before spreading to older foliage. Plants can become stunted or stop growth entirely. Note that manganese excess can result from poor soil aeration, and that conditions may be made worse in low humidity and low pH conditions.

Excess Treatment

Excess amounts of iron are rare but if they occur they must be flushed out using pure, adjusted water. Readjust and replace nutrient solution and keep the pH above 5.8.

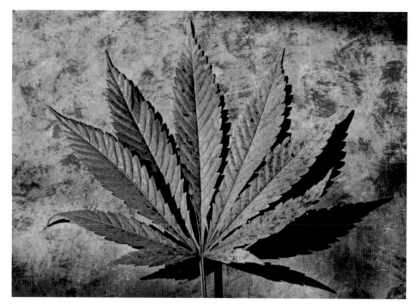

This leaf is not healthy. Note the brown spots and yellowing of the leaf on the right side.

Deficiency Treatment

Manganese deficiencies call for a fertilizer with a higher manganese (Mn) level. Lower the pH to approximately 6.2 for soil and in a foliar mix. Foliar feeding is a perfect remedy for a manganese deficiency: use a mild fertilizer containing manganese and the deficiency will disappear in about one week.

Soil Treatment

In soil situations, most complete hydroponic and organic fertilizers and soils with amendments usually contain ample amounts of available manganese. Using tea is perfect for fixing any manganese deficiencies.

Zinc

General Information

Cannabis uses zinc (Zn) throughout its life cycle and it must be present in all stages of growth. Zinc is an essential element in the production of sugar proteins and is required for the formation and manufacture of chlorophyll. It is also an important element for stem growth and formation. Zinc is present in all professional-quality fertilizers.

Deficiency

Zinc (Zn) deficiency is prevalent in low humidity environments and soil, as well as soilless situations with a pH above 7. It is fairly common in cannabis cultivation. Young tissue will develop interveinal chlorosis, with leaf tissue between the veins becoming lighter in color. It will also develop small, narrow, and distorted blades and leaf tips and margins, which eventually become brown and discolored. A deficiency will spread to the entire plant, causing necrotic spots to become larger; leaves will slowly dry out and drop off. Plant growth will be stunted and give poor yields as well as an undesirable finished product. Zinc deficiency symptoms can be mistaken for manganese or iron deficiencies, the difference being that zinc deficiencies cause new tissue, vegetation, and buds to deform, become misshapen, dry out, and die.

Excess / Toxicity

Zinc excess may produce copper and iron deficiency symptoms due to antagonistic effects. Furthermore, zinc excesses are toxic and will cause plant death.

Excess Treatment

Excess amounts of zinc must be flushed out using pure, adjusted water. Readjust and replace nutrient solution, keeping the pH above 5.8 and below 6.8, preferably 6.2.

Deficiency Treatment

Zinc deficiencies call for a fertilizer with a higher zinc level or a switch to General Hydroponics fertilizer products. Keep the pH at about 6.2 in the soil and the fertilizer mix. Foliar feeding is a perfect remedy for zinc deficiency; use a mild fertilizer mix and it will disappear after about one week.

Soil Treatment

Most complete hydroponic and organic fertilizers with amendments usually contain ample amounts of available zinc. Using tea is perfect for fixing any zinc deficiencies in soil situations.

Copper

General Information

Cannabis uses copper (Cu) throughout its life cycle and it must be present in all stages of growth. Copper is an essential element in part necessary for nitrogen fixation, oxygen production, carbohydrate metabolism, and the plant's production of a multitude of beneficial proteins and sugars.

Deficiency

Copper deficiencies can be fairly common. Young tissue may wilt, leaves will turn yellow, deep bluish green, or slight copper color with edges curled up; young leaves may permanently wilt or have a reduced size; young shoots often die back and fruiting stops or is dramatically reduced. A copper deficiency can cause the entire plant to wilt and droop even when it is properly hydrated. In short, plants with a copper deficiency may become poorly stunted and the finished product will be of poor quality at best.

Excess / Toxicity

A copper excess may produce molybdenum, iron, or zinc deficiencies—or even a copper deficiency—due to antagonistic effects. Even a minor copper excess is toxic, and will severely effect plant growth, causing slow growth and stunting. When severe, symptoms include the yellowing of leaves and less branching, and the roots become affected, turning brown and thick, ultimately resulting in plant death. Toxic situations can be exacerbated rapidly in acidic soil situations.

Excess Treatment

Excess amounts of copper must be flushed out using pure, adjusted water. Readjust and replace nutrient solution and keep the pH between 5.8 and 6.8, preferably 6.2. Regularly change nutrients in a reservoir to avoid buildup.

Deficiency Treatment

Copper deficiencies, which are rare, call for a fertilizer with a higher copper level or a switch to General Hydroponics fertilizer products. Keep the pH at 6.2 in soil and fertilizer mix. Foliar feeding is a perfect remedy for copper deficiency, and a mild spray containing copper will resolve problems in about one week.

Soil Treatment

Most complete hydroponic and organic fertilizers contain ample amounts of available copper. Using tea is a perfect solution for fixing any copper deficiencies in soil.

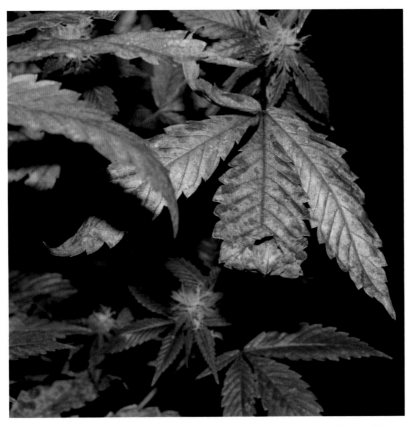

This leaf is extremely unhealthy. The plant has a problem. Check pH of the soil or hydro medium right away. Remove all unhealthy leaves.

Boron

General Information

Cannabis uses micro-amounts of boron (B) throughout its life cycle and it must be present in all stages of growth. Boron is an essential element that rarely becomes a problem either in excess or deficiency and is available in trace amounts in most professional-quality fertilizers. Experts state that boron aids the plant in calcium uptake, cellular division, and many other basic functions of the plant, including but not limited to bud maturation, differentiation, respiration, and pollen germination.

Deficiency

A boron deficiency may distort or thicken new growth; roots may swell,

Photo: MoD

darken in color, stop growing, or become readily susceptible to bacteria and fungus. Leaves may become brittle; young leaves may be scorched at the tips and margins, as well as contorting and turning black. This is followed by symptoms on lower foliage. When severe, leaves wilt and necrotic spots develop on foliage, especially along margins; interveinally, shoot tips discolor or die. Roots eventually become completely infected and die, flowering is affected and the finished product will be unacceptable at best.

Excess / Toxicity

Boron toxicity will severely affect growth by stunting plants. Leaf tips become yellow, then the margins become necrotic and scorched and eventually the leaves fall off. On older leaves, chlorosis is followed by necrosis in irregular patches along leaf margins or in the serrations of the leaves. Foliage usually drops off soon after. If the toxicity is severe, the plant will quickly die.

Excess Treatment

Excess amounts of boron must be flushed out using pure, adjusted water. Readjust and replace nutrient solution and keep the pH between 5.8 and 6.8, preferably 6.2. Regularly change nutrients in a reservoir to avoid buildup.

Deficiency Treatment

Boron deficiencies call for a fertilizer with a higher boron level or a switch to General Hydroponics fertilizer products. Keep the pH at 6.2 in soil and fertilizer mix. Foliar feeding is a perfect remedy for boron deficiency, and a mild foliar spray containing boron will resolve problems in about one week.

Soil Treatment

Most complete hydroponic and organic fertilizers contain ample amounts of available boron. Using tea is a perfect solution for fixing any boron deficiencies in soil.

Molybdenum

General Information

Cannabis uses molybdenum (Mo) throughout its life cycle and it must be present in all stages of growth. Molybdenum is an essential element that rarely becomes a problem and is available in trace amounts in most profes-

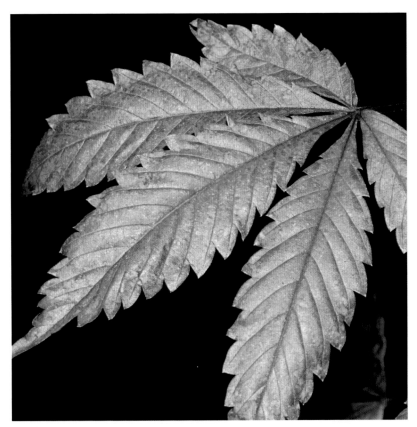

This fan leaf is exhibiting signs of a problem along its outer edges. Nutrient burn could be to blame.

sional-quality fertilizers. It is important in the conversion of nitrate to ammonium and is essential for root and seed formation and production.

Deficiency

Molybdenum deficiency rarely develops in cannabis. When it does, it can cause nitrogen shortage; therefore molybdenum deficiency symptoms will be very similar to nitrogen deficiency symptoms. Older fan leaves and vegetation will yellow and become stunted and malformed, with interveinal chlorosis and necrotic spots. Leaf tip burn is common, too. When severe, yellowed leaves develop rolled up edges and as symptoms progress will become severely malformed and twisted, become dried up and brown, and eventually die and drop off. Overall plant growth and development is stunted, resulting

Photo: MoD

in a final product of unacceptable quality and quantity. Molybdenum deficiencies often present themselves in acidic soil situations.

Excess / Toxicity

Molybdenum toxicity is rare in cannabis, but when it does occur can induce iron and copper deficiencies (see those symptoms above).

Excess Treatment

Excess amounts of molybdenum must be flushed out using pure, adjusted water. Readjust and replace nutrient solution and keep the pH between 5.8 and 6.8, preferably 6.2. Regularly change nutrients in a reservoir to avoid buildup.

Deficiency Treatment

Molybdenum deficiencies call for a fertilizer with a higher molybdenum level or a switch to General Hydroponics fertilizer products. Keep the pH at 6.2 in soil and fertilizer mix. Foliar feeding is a perfect remedy for molybdenum deficiency, and a mild spray containing molybdenum will resolve problems in about one week.

Soil Treatment

Most complete hydroponic and organic fertilizers contain ample amounts of available molybdenum. Using tea is a perfect solution for fixing any molybdenum deficiencies in soil.

Chlorine (Chloride)

General Information

Cannabis uses chlorine (Cl) in micro-amounts throughout its life cycle and it must be present in all stages of growth. Chlorates are an essential element that rarely become a deficiency problem, yet is usually not a component of fertilizers. Chlorine is present in most municipal water supplies. Cannabis will tolerate low levels of chlorine, but chlorine does kill any beneficial bacteria, nematodes, or other positive life forms in soil situations, and thus too much must be avoided (see the section on water purity). Chloride availability is mandatory and is partly responsible for the cellular division of foliage and roots, as well as for photosynthesis and the regulation of internal moisture. Excessive amounts can be toxic.

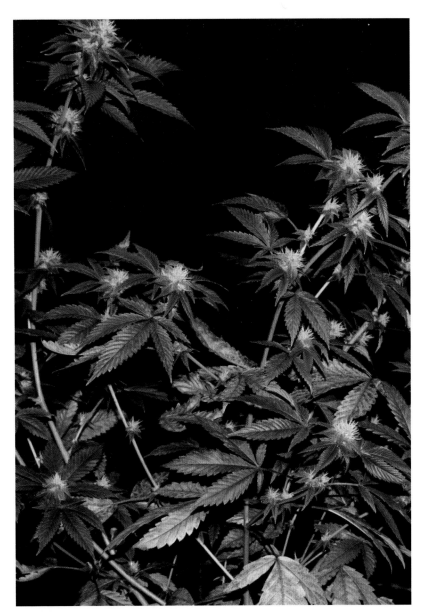

This plant is just beginning to flower, but its fan leaves are exhibiting signs of a problem. Check your nutrient mix and pH right away.

Photo: MoD

Deficiency

Chlorine deficiency rarely develops in cannabis. Only in the most unusual circumstances is a deficiency likely to occur. Deficiency symptoms would include a yellowing / pale green color in all leaves at the onset of deficiency, progressing to a bronzing of the leaves, which would be followed in turn by chlorosis and necrosis and leaf death and dropping. Roots may become thick and stunted. Deficiency and excess in this case produce similar bronze-colored leaf symptoms.

Excess / Toxicity

Chlorine excesses are fairly difficult to produce, but if they occur will result in a wilting of young tissue, with burned tips and edges; marginal and leaftip necrosis on older leaves; and, as the excess progresses, leaf wilt (on high atmospheric demand days), overall stunting, the bronzing of yellow leaves, and the eventual death and dropping of leaves. Clones and seedlings are the most vulnerable to chlorine excess. Note that a chlorine excess can also interfere with the uptake of nitrogen.

Excess Treatment

Excess amounts of chlorine must be flushed out using pure, adjusted water. Readjust and replace nutrient solution and keep the pH between 5.8 and 6.8, preferably 6.2. Regularly change nutrients in a reservoir to avoid buildup.

Deficiency Treatment

Add chlorinated water to your purified water. Mix 2 gallons of chlorinated water (normal unaerated city tap water) with 8 gallons of purified water. Keep the pH at 6.2 in soil and fertilizer mix. Foliar feeding is a perfect remedy for chlorine deficiency, and a mild spray containing non-filtered city water adjusted to pH 6.2 will resolve problems.

Soil Treatment

Chlorine excesses and deficiencies rarely occur, but as mentioned before, when they do arise chlorine will kill all beneficial living organisms in a medium. If deficiency symptoms appear, you can follow the advice above; otherwise, never give chlorinated water to your plants unless you absolutely have to.

Fluoride

General Information

Many municipal water suppliers fluorinate tap water. Deficiency and excesses never or rarely occur, and will probably never cause you problems. However, toxic levels of fluoride (F) could cause leaf wilting, marginal necrosis, and tip burn. To remedy you must purify and filter your water before use (see water filtration section).

Nickel

General Information

Cannabis uses nickel (Ni) throughout its life cycle and it must be present in all stages of growth. Nickel is an essential element; it is crucial to iron absorption and nitrogen utilization. That said, nickel deficiencies or excesses rarely develop in cannabis, and most quality fertilizers contain ample amounts of available nickel. If nickel levels did become toxic, symptoms would mimic other nutrient deficiency symptoms—too many to list, but they usually take the form of nitrogen deficiency symptoms.

Cobalt

General Information

Cannabis uses cobalt (Co) throughout its life cycle and it must be present in all stages of growth. It is in part responsible for the proliferation and health of beneficial bacteria, nematodes, and other beneficial life forms in a medium. Cobalt is also necessary for nitrogen absorption and the production of volatile aromatic compounds. A deficiency may cause antagonistic effects and interfere with nitrogen uptake. Cobalt is an essential element that is not typically included on a fertilizer's list of ingredients but is usually present in the mix. Trace amounts of cobalt are available in most hydroponic fertilizers. Cobalt deficiencies and excesses rarely develop in cannabis.

Sodium

General Information

Cannabis uses sodium (Na) in micro-amounts throughout its life cycle and it must be present in all stages of growth. Although sodium is an essential element, water containing more than 50 PPM of sodium is considered toxic and will cause antagonistic effects and severe deficiencies of many other essential elements. Always purify water that is above 50 PPM in sodium. Although trace amounts of sodium are utilized by the plant's root system, the less sodium you have in your water, the healthier your plant will be.

Deficiency

Sodium deficiencies rarely develop in cannabis. In the unusual event that they did occur, symptoms would mimic many other nutrient deficiency symptoms—too many to list.

Excess / Toxicity

A sodium excess will induce calcium, magnesium, or potassium deficiencies due to competitive effects, i.e. excessive amounts of sodium can lock out other essential elements, causing nutritional deficiency symptoms.

Excess Treatment

Excess amounts of sodium must be flushed out using pure, adjusted water. Readjust and replace nutrient solution and keep the pH between 5.8 and 6.8, preferably 6.2. Regularly change nutrients in a reservoir to avoid buildup.

Deficiency Treatment

Sodium deficiencies rarely develop in cannabis, as discussed above. Most quality fertilizers contain ample amounts; if yours does not, switch to General Hydroponics fertilizer products.

Soil Treatment

Most complete hydroponic and organic fertilizers contain ample amounts of available sodium. Using tea is a perfect solution for fixing any sodium deficiencies in soil.

Silicon

General Information

Cannabis uses silicon in trace amounts throughout its life cycle and it must be present and available in all stages of growth. Toxicity and excess rarely develop in cannabis under normal conditions. Silicon is found in soil and water and is utilized in maintaining a balance of iron and manganese levels. It is also a component of cell walls, and promotes stronger cell walls that are more resistant to mold, fungus, disease, and pest attacks, as well as increasing a plant's tolerance to heat and drought. A deficiency of silicon may cause deformation of new tissue and a decrease in yields and the overall health of the plant, as well as increased susceptibility to mold, fungus, pests, and disease.

Acceptable Limits and Average PPM Information

These are the recommended fertilizer levels for cannabis, measured in PPM.

Element	Limits	Average
Nitrogen	150–1,000	250
Phosphorous	50–100	80
Potassium	100–400	300
Magnesium	50–100	75
Sulfur	200–1,000	400
Calcium	100–150	200
Iron	2.0–10	5.0
Manganese	0.5–5.0	2.0
Zinc	0.5–1.0	0.5
Copper	0.1–0.5	0.5
Boron	0.5–5.0	1.0
Molybdenum	0.01–0.05	0.02

A Final Note on Nutrient Excesses and Deficiencies

The aforementioned elements, frequently referred to as heavy metals, can be extremely toxic to plants at elevated levels in nutrient solution, especially when cultivating in a solution without a root-supporting media, such as soil, to act as a buffer. These heavy metals may cause antagonistic effects and create imbalances of other nutrients, as you have read above. Extreme care should be given to prevent excessive or deficient levels from occurring in the mixing of the nutrient solution, or as a result of buildup in the growing media. Correct pH levels are paramount at all times. Excesses must be flushed out immediately. Good luck and pay attention.

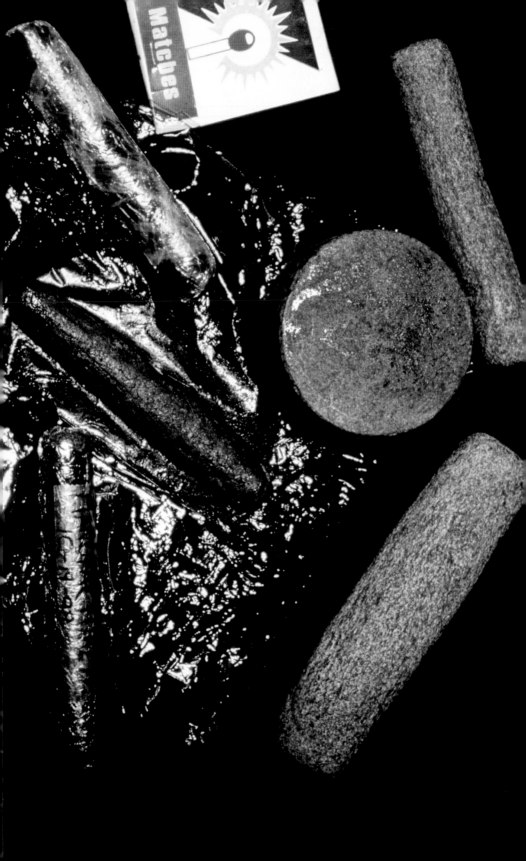

CHAPTER 17

Hash Making

If you have access to any sizable amount of quality cannabis buds or resin-covered leaves, you already have the most important component for producing excellent hashish. Good quality hashish is a concentration of isolated resin heads from mature capitate-stalked glandular trichomes containing Delta 9 THC; in plain English, hashish is made up of the resin gland heads containing THC, the psychoactive element of the cannabis plant. Together with these glands are naturally occurring contaminates such as immature glands, gland stalks, broken stigmata, and leaf matter, as well as a whole host of other cannabinoids and terpenoids—the effects of which have yet to be fully explored. Look up the International Cannabinoid Research Society for more information.

It is important to use only leaves that have an abundance of resin glands on them. The large fan leaves, for instance, will produce no hashish, whereas the smaller leaves, the leaf trimmings from the floral clusters, and the (normally useless) small, airy flowers will produce a considerable amount. When in doubt, check the leaf surface using a 10–20x magnifying glass.

There are several low-tech, basic methods of making hashish, all of which can produce an extremely potent and satisfying product. Several factors will govern the

◀ There is nothing like perfectly cured and aged hashish.

Photo: Andre Grossman

Cross Section of a Female Bract

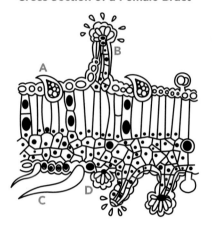

Close up of a Trichome

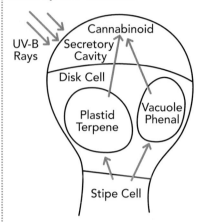

A) Cystolith Hair

B) Large Glandular Hair (with several heads)

C) Thick Walled Conical Trichome

D) Large Developing Glandular Hair

Note the interaction between UV-B rays and the trichome.

Depiction and Explanation of Types of Trichomes

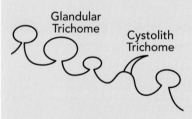

Cystolith Trichome: a plant hair, and not technically a gland at all.

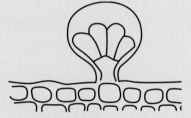

Bulbous Trichome

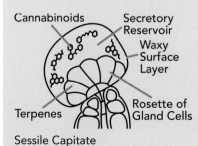

Sessile Capitate

Capitate Stalked Glandular Trichome

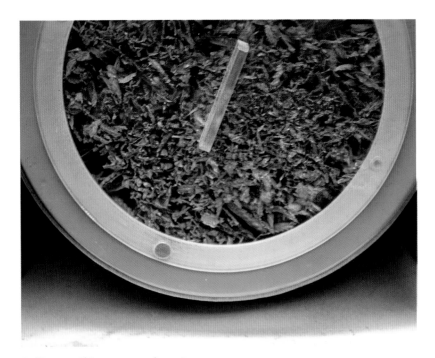

Pollinator sifting top-grade resin.

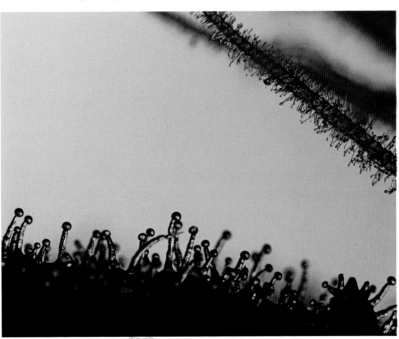

Examine the heads of the resin glands closely to determine peak ripeness.

Top Photo: Samson Daniels Bottom Photo: Andre Grossman

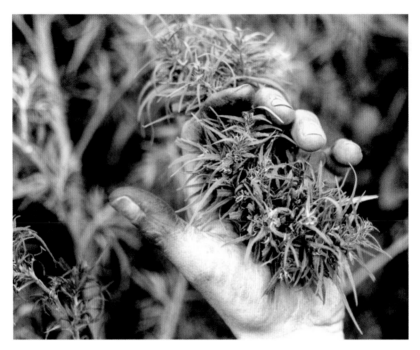

Finger hashish in 1979.

quality and quantity of your final product, in addition to the quality of your original plant product. These include:

Temperature and Humidity: Quite simply, THC glands become brittle and separate more easily from the leaf matter when cold. Either your working environment or the product you're working with must be at a temperature of 25°F or lower, with a relative humidity of 35%. Although this sounds complicated, it is easily achieve by putting your product in the freezer for about 45 minutes prior to sieving, or, in the case of the water extraction method, by using very cold ice water.

Debris (plant particulate): This is determined by the screen size used for filtering the separated resin glands. This will be explained further in the section on sieving.

Scissor and Finger Hash

Finger hash is commonly produced in Nepal, Tibet, India, and other climates that are too humid to sieve in. To make your own, always use natural or synthetic surgical gloves when manicuring and handling buds. Resin will

Photo: Mel Frank

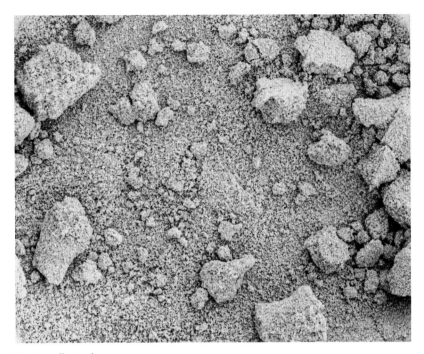

Resin collected on a screen.

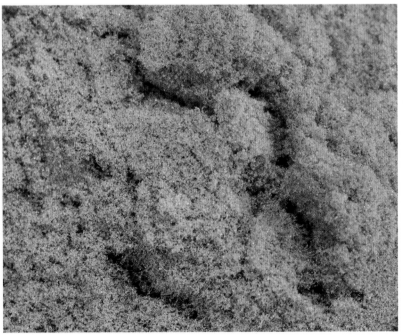

Resin glands.

Top Photo: Mel Frank   Bottom Photo: Samson Daniels

Making Sieved Hash using the BubbleBox

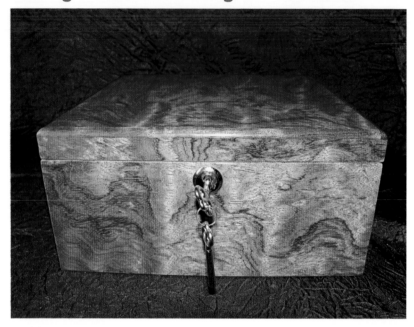

BubbleBox is closed.

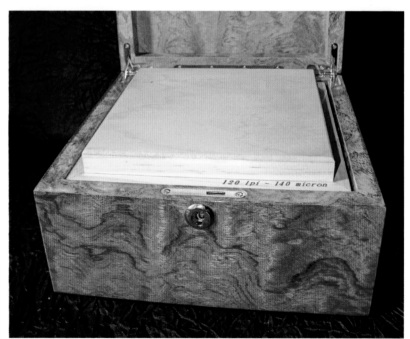

Open BubbleBox to reveal the screens and extraction system.

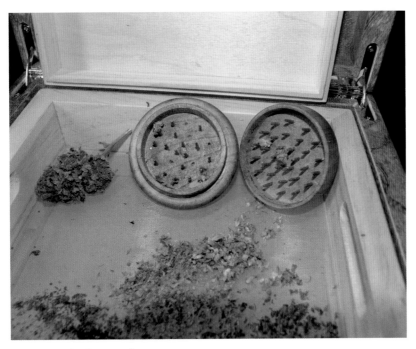

Grind your buds onto the top screen.

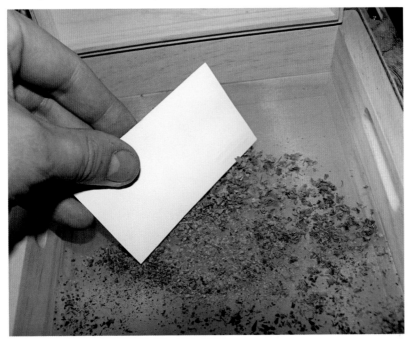

Use a card to spread the ground cannabis over the top screen.

Making Sieved Hash using the BubbleBox

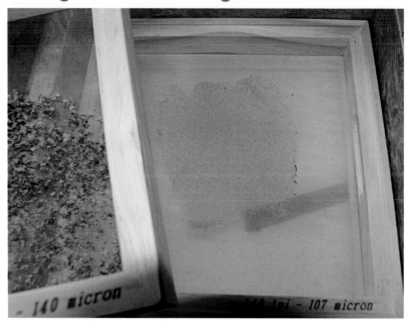

The trichomes fall through to the lower micron-size screen. The top screen has a larger size sieve screen than the screen below it, so the trichomes fall through.

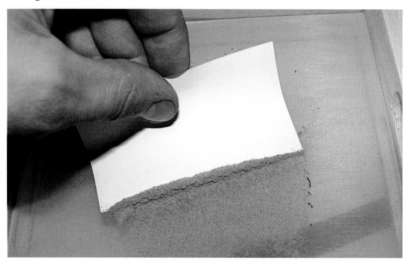

Use the card to agitate the matter over the smaller size screen. The finer material that can fit through the 107 micron screen will then collect on the 70 micron screen.

Photos: BubbleMan

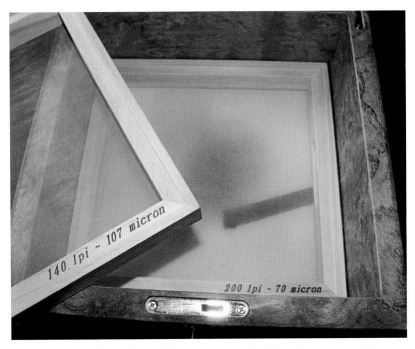

Here we see the hash that's fallen through to the 70 micron screen. You collect each layer and label it individually as each layer has its own unique properties.

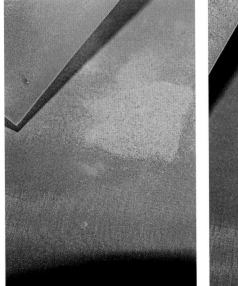
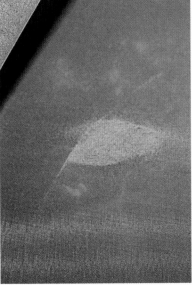

Collect the powdered hash and either press it, or enjoy it as is.

Making Sieved Hash using the BubbleBox

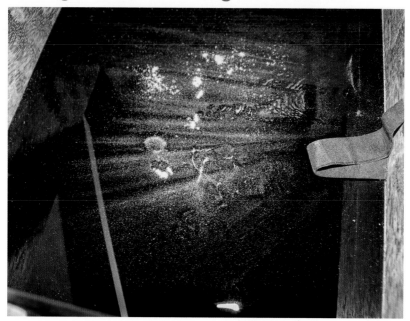

Here the sieved hash is spread on a clean glass surface area.

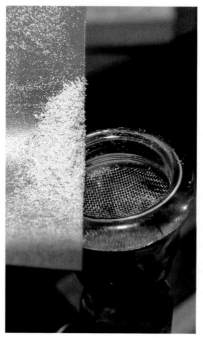
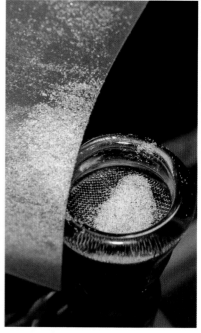

Feel free to put the hash directly into your pipe or bong and enjoy!

collect on gloves and scissors. Periodically scrape clean scissors and change gloves when resin builds up. Place collected resin on open-air, dust-free surfaces to dry for 24 hours. Fresh resin collected from a wet bud still contains moisture, which can cause mold. To collect the resin from the gloves, after two hours in the freezer turn them inside out and partially inflate the glove; slightly stretch the fingers. Resin will collect in the tips of fingers. Transfer all resin to one finger, and then cut it off. Pour resin onto an open-air, dust-free surface and allow to sit for 24 hours. This form of hashish is strong yet crude, in that it contains large amounts of vegetative material and stigmata fragments; yet it has a magnificent aroma and taste, though unless you have very large amounts it is not worth a large effort to press.

Sieving

(Refer to the screen size measurement chart in appendix one, as needed.)

Dry sieved hash is more flavorful and aromatic than water-extracted hash because dry sieving does not wash away any water soluble flavonoids or terpenoids. The sieving process is the most commonly used process in the world, probably because it is very straightforward and can be easily set up at home. First, make a wooden frame and stretch tightly over it a silkscreen with a pore size of between 25 and 220 microns. These silkscreens are available from art supply shops or you can purchase a product called the Resin Reaper from AquaLab Technologies. The micron chart in Appendix 1 is useful for determining what screens or hash making products to purchase. Quality, pre-made screens for hash making, are available from your local art supply store. (See micron chart). Place a sheet of glass or mirror on the table underneath the screen. Gather the leaf trimmings left over from manicuring your buds, and, after having chilled them in the freezer for at least 45 minutes, place them on the screen and thresh them around for between 5 to 15 minutes. You will start to see dislodged resin gland heads appear on the glass surface under the screen.

Once you see particulate (non-resin, vegetable matter) start to appear under the screen, stop! Anything you collect after this point will be low grade. The remaining resin on the leaf can be collected later using the water extraction method. Don't crush the leaves or try to push them through the screen. To do so would only serve to increase the undesirable particulate content.

Large mechanized sifters, available from AquaLab Technologies, such as Tumble Now and APE pollen extractors, as well as the Pollinator, are perfect for dry resin separation. They come in an assortment of sizes, depending on your needs, and are available in any desired micron size. These separators work like a non-heated tumble dryer in which the drum is typically a 150-micron screen. As the drum turns, the resin glands dislodge and fall through the screen onto the bottom of the sifter where they can be collected. Allow the leaf to tumble for between 5 to 15 minutes. As with the home- made set up, it is best to keep an eye on the collected resin glands and stop the process the minute that you see any vegetable matter appearing or resin color darkening from gold / blond to greenish.

An archeology separator will not only rapidly process large amounts of material, but, unlike the other dry sifters, it will separate the various sized resin glands all in one process as well. It works by stacking eight circular screens that are 4 inches tall and 12 to 24 inches in diameter, and clamping them together. Unseparated resin or vegetative material is placed onto the top screen. All 8 screens vibrate at once and separate resin glands by size as they fall through the screen. After just a few minutes, separation is complete. The clamps are released, and resin is poured into separate containers one at a time. The screens are restacked, clamped, and the apparatus is ready to refill. This equipment is very efficient and simple to use. They are available in many sizes from globalgilson.com, and they vary in price. With an unlimited variety of screens, they will have the exact size you need.

If indeed you wished to continue either of these processes beyond the point at which you see particulate appearing, it can be done, but the resulting

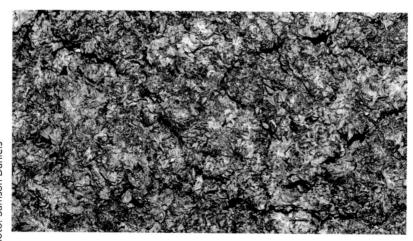

Photo: Samson Daniels

These buds are destined for hash production.

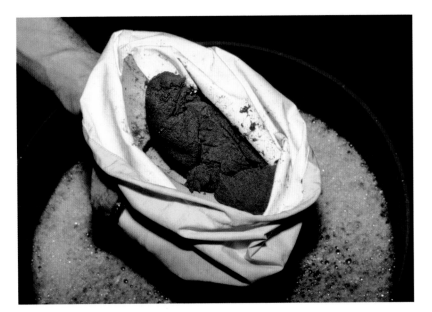

Water hash in a filter bag.

product would be slightly contaminated and would need to be cleaned out later using the water extraction method. Hashish that is produced purely using the sieving method is likely to have a slightly different taste when smoked than that which is made using water extraction, due to the fact that the water will wash away some of the terpenes and other water-soluble substances which are responsible for aroma and flavor.

Once you have collected your resin glands, take them and gently shake them on a 25-micron screen, or indeed envelop them loosely in a 25-micron screen and gently shake it for about 30 minutes over a piece of glass or mirror. The small, immature, sessile trichomes, debris, mold spores, dirt, and small plant material will fall through the screen, leaving only the purest resin glands of very uniform size and consistency. You may still find particles of foreign matter such as human or pet hair, carpet fluff, etc., in this resin. The way to remove these contaminates is by gently sifting the product through a fine metal mesh strainer over a clean piece of glass or mirror, which is best done after refreezing for a period of time, and picking out the foreign matter with a pair of tweezers. At this point, you should have pure white to golden (not green or dark) powder. This resin should stick together easily between your thumb and forefinger at body temperature.

Photo: Mel Frank

Ice Water Hash Extraction with BubbleBags

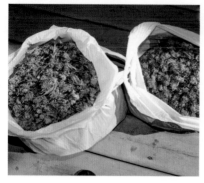

Cannabis buds or shake can be used for BubbleBag extraction.

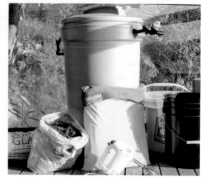

Garbage can, bubble bags, and a bunch of bud, then you just add ice and water.

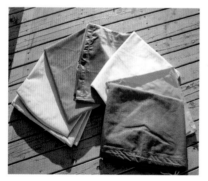

Each filter bag has a different micron size to allow you to get different grades of bubble hash.

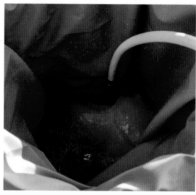

The water goes into the bag.

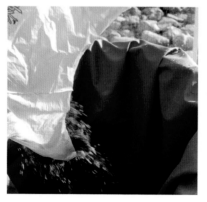

Add your cannabis to the top bag (largest filter size).

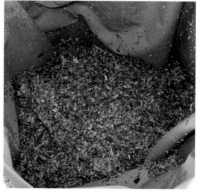

Cannabis sits in the filter bag and waits for ice and water.

Photos: BubbleMan

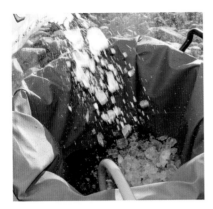

Add ice with the water. Bagged ice is fine. Just pour it in.

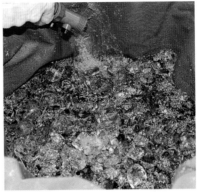

Some more water to ensure the buds are all covered.

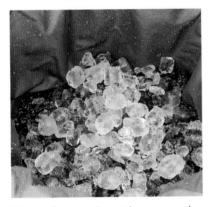

The ice freezes the trichomes on the cannabis and they fall off.

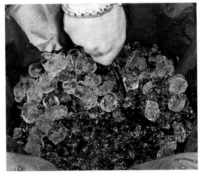

Agitate the buds and ice water to encourage trichomes to break off and fall through the filter.

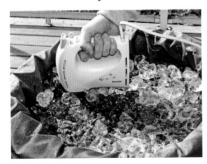

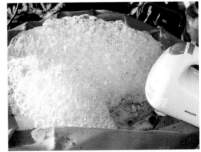

You can use a kitchen blender to agitate the buds and ice. Mix it up really well to get all the trichomes off the cannabis. It is a tradeoff between quantity and quality. Do not agitate too much or too long unless you want an increase in quantity.

Large Micron Sieves to Small

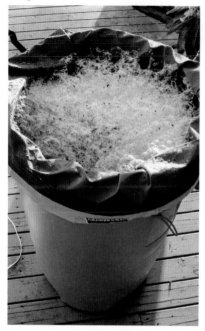
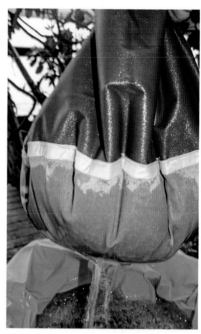

Let ice melt then remove top bag and let drain into bag below.

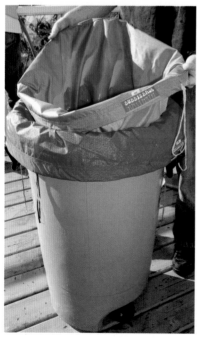
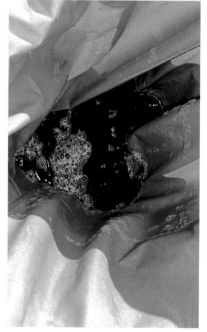

Photos: BubbleMan

Remove the next bag which has a slightly smaller filter size. Let drain.

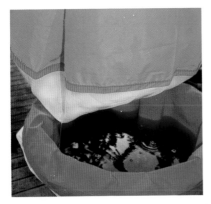
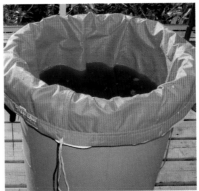

As you remove each successive filter bag the hash accumulates in the bottom. Let the bag drain into the bag below and allow the smaller sized resin glands to filter through.

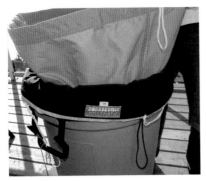
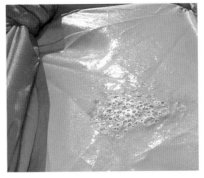

Here we see the next smallest size being removed and the bubble hash is visible collected at the bottom of the filter bag.

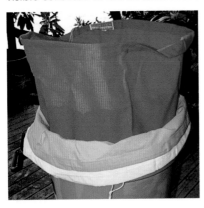
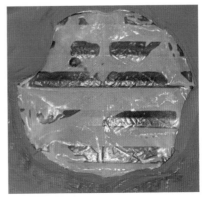

Each bag collects a different grade of hash. Just let the water drain through and collect it all.

Large Micron Sieves to Small

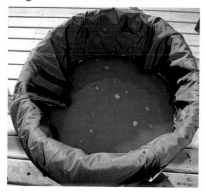 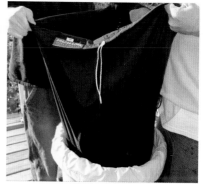

The water is drained down to the smallest micron sieves here and the hash is of a very fine grade.

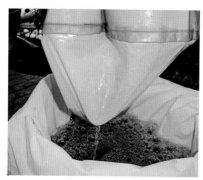 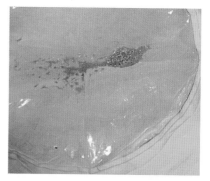

Smaller micron sieves at the very bottom of the BubbleBag system. Which screen the best quality is captured in is dictated by the resin gland size of the starting product.

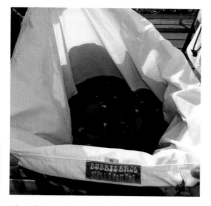 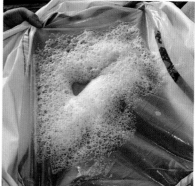

The final bag has the least amount of hash collected, but it is still enough to be useful. This system is very efficient, effective, and safe.

Photos: BubbleMan

Dry the Sieved Product

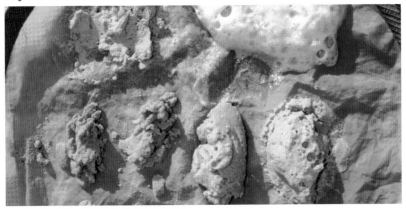

Each sieve size is represented here as the product dries.

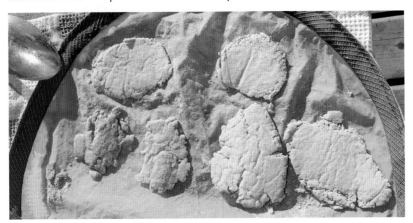

This resin has been pressed to get the majority of water out.

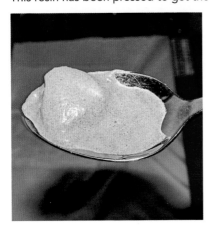

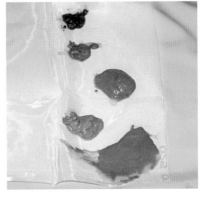

A spoon full of wet resin glands.

Different grades of resin collected off different sized screens.

Properly Drying Water Hash

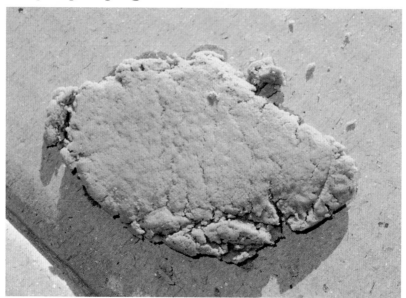

This resin has had the majority of water pressed out of it, but needs further drying.

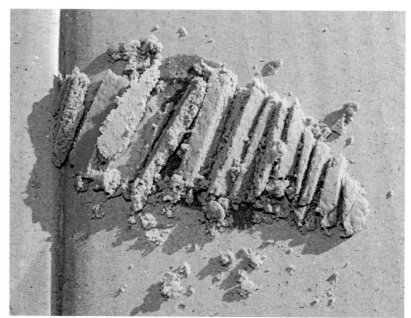

Slightly dried resin requires further drying by breaking the material into smaller pieces.

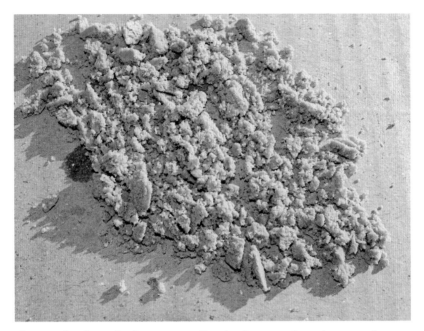

The resin has been broken into smaller chunks, exposing a larger surface area to facilitate complete drying.

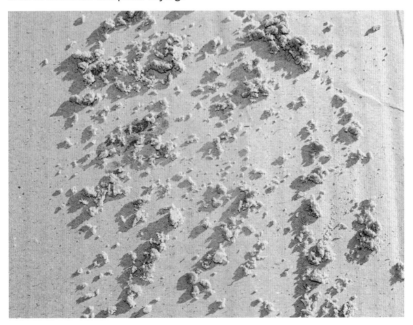

The resin has been allowed to sit out and completely dry and is now ready for storage or pressing.

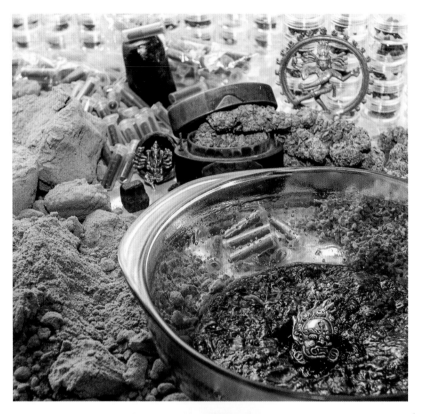

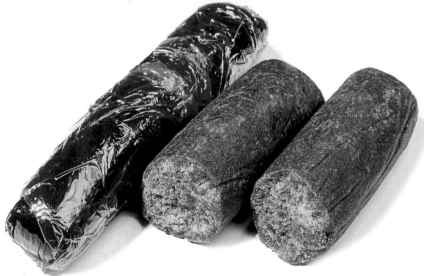

Top Photo: Samson Daniels Bottom Photo: Andre Grossman

A plethora of hashish and other goodies.

If you want to press this hash immediately, simply pour it into a piece of natural cellophane, double wrap it in a thick plastic bag, and, after warming your hands on a hot cup of tea, work it and mold it with your hands. Otherwise, you can wrap it in a very thick plastic (like that used to line water beds) and repeatedly pound it with a small mallet or bat. This heats the hash to 80°F and thoroughly homogenizes it, releasing the volatile oils and terpenes which make for a perfect smoke. Never apply excessive external heat such as a flame or oven temperatures to hashish and never use a microwave.

For creating the finest hashish, the Afghans used to wrap their resin in a very tight weave linen or cotton bag and store it in an airy, cool, dark, and dry place for up to two years. This allows time for further 'curing,' converting other cannabinoids into Delta 9 THC and releasing any remaining water molecules.

Cold Water Hashish Extraction

The water extraction method of hash-making has many advantages. If you have used a crude sieving method and have a lot of contaminate mixed with your resin, the water method will purify it; it will also separate resin from mold spores in the case of botrytis / bud rot and powdery mildew caused by excessively damp conditions during the drying phase. This method may be performed in hot, humid climates like those of Jamaica and Thailand; even fresh, undried leaves and flowers may be used; and large quantities are easily handled.

The taste and smell is different (not necessarily better or worse, just not as intense) than that of dry sieving due the fact that the water-soluble terpenoids can been washed away by water. But, at Trichome Technologies, we had the end product of this method tested and the result was hashish with 68% THC purity. Yet much higher levels are easily achievable.

Basic Water Extraction Method

The general overriding principle for this method is easy: leaves float, and resin is heavier than water. Taking this concept one step further, the more potent, mature resin gland heads are heavier than less mature glands, which in turn are heavier than sessile resin glands. Therefore, the hash maker has two choices. After agitation, they can let the water stand for a short period of time to extract the purest high quality resin glands, or let it stand for a longer period of time and be happy with a greater quantity of a slightly less potent product.

For the small hobby grower, an easy, inexpensive method of water extraction

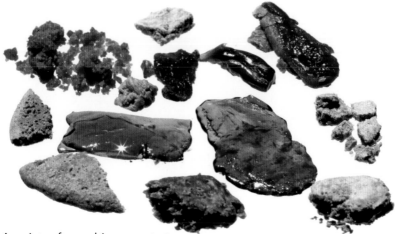

A variety of cannabis concentrates.

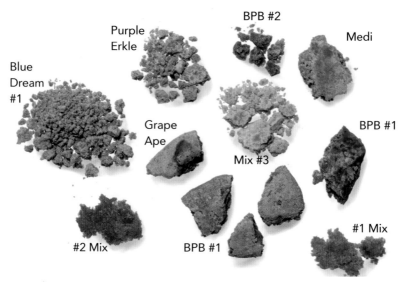

Blue Dream #1

Purple Erkle

BPB #2

Medi

Grape Ape

Mix #3

BPB #1

#2 Mix

BPB #1

#1 Mix

Cannabis concentrates come in many colors and consistencies.

is very much attainable. Take a one-gallon (5 liter) clear jar and fill to about 20% full with frozen, resinated wet or dry leaves and / or bud, or previously contaminated resin from sieving. Fill the jar up with very cold water, preferably containing ice; the colder the better. Let the mixture stand for 15 to 20 minutes to freeze the resin glands. Use a spoon to stir or shake the mixture vigorously for five minutes; let it stand for five to 10 minutes for the purest quality, or 30–50 minutes for the maximum quantity. The resin will separate and drop to form a layer at the bottom of the jar, and the leaf will float at the top. Using a tea

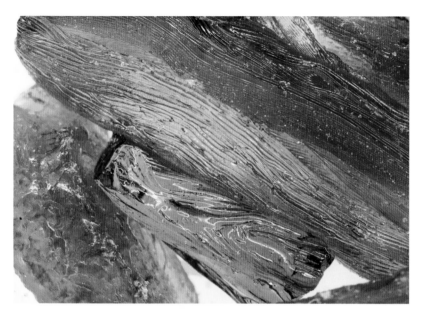

A closeup of super refined cannabis concentrate.

strainer or spoon, scoop off the leaf that is floating at the top without disturbing the resin on the bottom. Once this is done, pour off the water without pouring out any resin. If left to stand for only fifteen minutes, this water will appear colored and cloudy, but will be relatively clear after 50 minutes of standing. Refill the jar with water and shake and let the water absorb any residual contaminants. Now, pour the leftover, water-soaked resin into a coffee filter. To further purify, pour through a 50-micron screen and rinse through with more cold water. Squeeze out the water and remove the wet lump of resin. Sieve the lump into powder, and after the resin completely dries, press and work it in the palm of your hand using your thumb. When it is homogenized, sticky and black, it's done.

Water extracted hashish can be made by using many different sized micron bags. There are many water hash-making kits available, some good and some not so good. The better kits use superior materials for construction, thus extending the life of the collection bags and screens. A good bag kit should offer many different micron-sized collector bags. The cultivar and resin gland size will dictate which bag sizes are best suited to your needs. Many different manufacturers offer different sizes. Test run a small portion to determine which size bags best suit your purposes. A wide size variation of bags will yield higher

Photo: Mel Frank

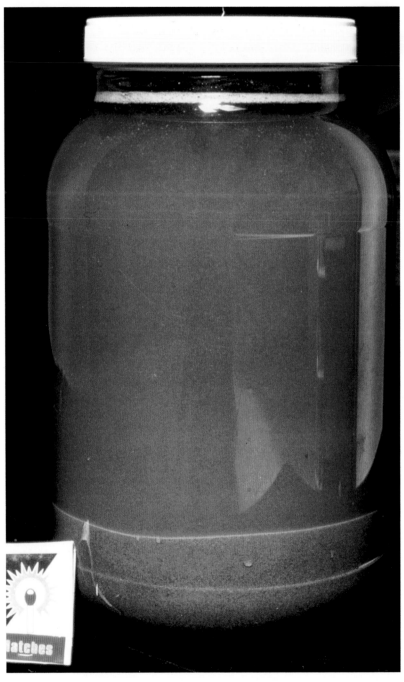

Photo: K

Resin glands at the bottom of a one-gallon jar. The leaf was on top of the jar and has been eliminated. The resin will now be filtered using a coffee filter.

separation of resin, i.e., different grades. Theoretically, 10 different micron-sized cleaner bags will yield 10 different grades / sizes of resin glands, separated immature glands, trichome stalks, and other material. One or two of the cleaner bags will yield superior quality resin. Thereafter, the quality will decrease, which in turn is determined by the quality of the starting material. The idea is to find the perfect screen / resin gland size match, resulting in every gland being separated by size. You must experiment and discover which screen size yields the best resin. We also recommend BubbleBag.com.

Note: wet leaves and buds produce better quality end product than dry leaves because they reduce the level of leaf-matter and stigmata as contaminate, and produce a terpene-rich hash. Immediately freeze the wet leaves and place them in cold water and ice in the extractor or collector bags.

Because the water washes away some of the terpenes, it is advisable to add some dry-sieved hash powder to the water hashish to replace lost aroma and flavor. Add the dry-sieved resin after the water hash is completely dry. It will impart the original flavors and aroma.

Resinizer (from Aqualab Technologies)

The Resinizer uses a quick and gentle agitation system to separate trichome glands into water in fifteen to twenty minutes. It's the quickest, cleanest, easiest, and most effective small sized resin extraction method there is. This cold water extraction appliance is also available in five-and twenty-gallon sizes. It is basically a miniature washing machine, but it works very well. All you need to do is turn it on and switch loads. They advance the technology of nylon bag gravity extraction.

The machines can hold up to a pound per load, depending on the model, but reducing the amount to about 300 grams can increase yield by a small margin. Getting a 5% increase may not sound like much, but it quickly adds up. The 185-micron bag produces the best and cleanest quality product and the 220 produces the greatest quantity, but anything above 185 is more like commercial-grade hash.

The Resinizer and similar machines work by placing cannabis into a zippered mesh bag containing ice; this bag is then placed in an ice and water mix in the agitation chamber, which gently knocks off the resin heads from the vegetable matter and releases them into the water. After washing off the resin heads and turning off the machine, the resin heads are collected and drained into multiple cleaner bags for further separation. They are available in three- and five-bag systems.

Collected resin is further separated by using multiple cleaner bags in a 5-gallon bucket; the resin is drained directly into the screens in the bucket, the bucket is topped with water, and then the resin is separated by size to isolate the best grade.

Note: When making water hash, always use the purest, cleanest water possible (for small quantities, use distilled water). The purer the water, the better.

Clear Jar Resin Cleaning Method

This method is originally from "Sadhu Sam" and uses water separation to separate lower quality leaf and vegetable matter (broken stigmata parts) and adulterated resin. Place impure or adulterated frozen trichomes in a one-gallon clear plastic jar with a screw top. Fill the jar $^2/_3$-full with distilled water and ice, screw on the cap, and shake up the contents. Completely mix it up. After the contents settle, open the jar: the trichome heads have sunk to the bottom of the container while the unwanted contaminate is at the surface, where it can easily be skimmed off. This process can be repeated as many times as it takes to completely purify the resin glands.

Slowly pour out the water without losing any resin. Pour the last remaining water and resin through a coffee filter that sits in its holder on top of a coffee can with holes in the bottom for water to escape. Do this over the sink. When all water has drained from the coffee filter, use a spoon to scoop out the resin and place it on a drying screen. Fold the screen and put it between a folded towel. Squeeze the towel where the lump of hash is and squeeze out the remaining water. Sift and repowder the hash using a kitchen colander and allow to dry on a clean surface for one to three days. After this time, the resin glands can be pressed or stored in a sealed glass jar as you would with other hash; make sure the resin is completely dry or it will mold and become unsmokable.

Hash Oil

Warning: it is important to note that the solvents used here are highly flammable and therefore great care must be taken to avoid an accident. Careful attention must be paid to temperature and ventilation, or you will face an explosion! It's best to work outdoors when using solvents. Low heat (the heat of the sun is sufficient during the hot summer months) and plenty of ventilation are a *must*. Also, be forewarned that in most countries throughout Europe, as well as in most of America, cannabis oil or hash oil is regarded as a Class A, Schedule 1 drug, as it involves a refinement process using flammable chemical solvents, and thus harsher legal penalties come with its manufacture.

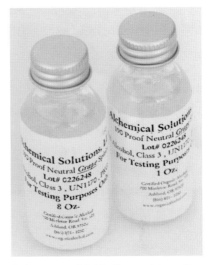

Solvents are highly flammable so it is best to work outdoors with them.

Equipment

■ 5-gallon standard plastic bucket with a lid for soaking

■ 5-gallon plastic tub with a large surface area for evaporation

■ Large metal sieve or strainer

■ Large plastic glass funnel

■ Paint scraper or a couple of razor blades

■ Rice cooker with multiple heat settings

■ Large plastic spoons

■ Several large pieces of silkscreen, or, alternatively, a couple large pieces of cheesecloth

■ Coffee filter

■ Large Pyrex dish for the final evaporation refinement process

■ Solvent. Pure, 99% food grade ethanol alcohol. Ethanol alcohol is available at Alchemical Solutions: www.organicalco-hol.com and Kleen Extract Ethanol is available at www.kleenxtract.com.

Note: Ethanol alcohol extracts more chlorophyll from the plant material than other solvents; oil made with ethanol alcohol is much darker in color but is still very potent. Butane and many other solvents produce oils that range from amber to translucent because butane extracts less chlorophyll.

Optional Extras

A heat source. If using heat, it's important that you use Pyrex glass utensils rather than plastic tubs. Do not use an open flame heat source or a heating apparatus that causes sparks.

If planning to do an evaporation collection on your solvent, you will need a "condenser." This is a glass chemistry apparatus that is used for condensing gasses into liquid for collection, using cold water to condense the hot vapors.

Starting Materials

You can use a wide variety of starting materials to make oil. I use my bud trimmings covered in resin glands, but you can use the buds / flowers, hash, or loose trichomes from a Resinizer machine, a Pollinator, BubbleBags, or commercial grade hash itself.

For the purpose of this exercise, I will use what I normally use when I make oil: bud trimmings and any small wispy flowers from my plants. These are basically the same materials that I use to make water hash with.

Preparation

To make the small amount of oil, empty the starting cannabis into a 5-liter container. Now, pour in the solvent at about a ratio of 60% solvent to 40% starting material. Then cover this and place it outside to soak, stirring it from time to time for 24 to 48 hours. Commercial hash with any form of contaminant or impurities would require a longer soaking period than leaf trimmings or bud, which need about 24–48 hours. You will need approximately two gallons of solvent to strip the resin glands off of one pound of dry leaf / buds, and about 500 ml is enough to strip the resin glands from an ounce.

After this period, take a fresh, clean glass dish with a large surface area. This will be used for evaporation. Take a large funnel and line it with a coffee filter, silkscreen, or cheesecloth, ensuring that there is a fair bit of overlap hanging down the outside of the funnel.

Pour the entire contents of the soaking container through the silkscreen or cheesecloth-lined funnel and into the evaporation container. When the soaking container is completely empty, fold the top of the silkscreen over and squeeze out the last of the liquid through it before throwing it away. By running this through the silkscreen or cheesecloth, all the valueless particulate matter is removed, and all the THC (now infused in the solvent) is sitting in the evaporation container and ready for the next step.

Cover the evaporation dish or rice cooker (explained later in this chapter) with a clean piece of silkscreen or cheesecloth, and put outside in a warm shaded area to evaporate at its own speed. To boil off the solvent with a rice

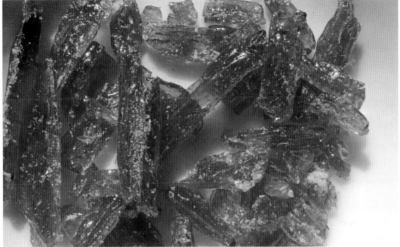

Extracts in their purest form, such as this amber glass, are one of the purest forms of cannabinoids and terpenoids available today.

cooker, the rice cooker should have at least two settings (high and low) and hold over half a gallon of solvent. It is important to come back to it from time to time and stir it, in order to release possible pockets of solvent that can be trapped in the oil. You should at this point add a few drops of water (depending on the amount of oil / solvent); 10 to 20 drops per container. The remaining solvent gets infused in the water, making the trace amounts of solvent easier to evaporate. This is the easiest and safest way to evaporate the excess solvent, leaving you a thick, dark, tarry, viscous-looking material as an end product. It is important to keep in mind that light and heat can degrade the THC content. A temperature between 93°F and 100°F is fine for the evaporation process. Never exceed 100°F! Too much higher and you reach the boiling point for most solvents, and you risk degrading the THC and lessening the potency of the oil as well as causing an explosion!

To test that the oil is solvent free, take a spoon, extract a small amount of oil and go far away from the main evaporation area and oil. Pass a flame over the oil in the spoon without touching the flame to the oil. If the oil ignites—blow it out—you now know that the oil still contains solvent and you must continue to stir and evaporate the oil and solvent. If the oil does not ignite, then it is probably solvent-free. Double check: smear some of the oil on a piece of glass and apply a flame. If the oil ignites rapidly, it still has solvent present and

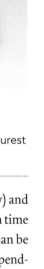

Photo: MedicinalAlchemy.com

you must continue to evaporate the solvent. When you feel that the oil is solvent free, it's time to take it through its last and final stage of purification.

Using the large sheet of glass, spread the oil thinly over the surface and leave in a completely dust-free, well-ventilated environment for another 24 hours, so that the last residues of solvent can evaporate. With the paint scraper or razor blade, scrape the oil off the glass sheet and into whatever container you have chosen for storage. Head shops sell small glass vials with screw tops that are ideal for this purpose. They normally come in one, five, ten, and 30 gram sizes.

Using a Heat Source

In certain countries, where warm sunshine is not abundant, a heat source may have to be used in order to extract oil from your starting material. This has to be done outdoors. It is important to pay close attention to ventilation and temperature. Whenever you are using a head source, use Pyrex containers for the evaporation stage.

There are several heat sources that can be used for oil extraction. A stove is *not* one of them. *Do not use open flame heat sources*, either.

Keeping in mind that you don't want your temperatures to exceed 100°F, the following methods of warming your evaporation container are readily available:

■ A rice cooker with at least two settings that will hold at least a half-gallon of oil / solvent mixture.

■ A heat mat, ordinarily used for warming the roots of seedlings in a grow-room. Use these only if you are sure of which setting will warm your container to the right temperature. You can use a Pyrex dish filled with water and a thermometer to establish this beforehand.

■ A metal cylinder (such as a coffee can) made by chopping the top and bottom off a large tin, with a low wattage heat lamp inside. Again, test before using!

■ Hot oil. Heat the oil to the appropriate temperature, then warm the Pyrex container in the warm oil. This method can be a little labor intensive, but it is basically just a double boiler setup, common in many kitchens.

These are just a few methods suitable for oil production. Whatever heat source you use, be sure that the temperature never exceeds 100°F; 90°F to 95°F is even safer. Whatever you use, it is important to keep it out of the house at all costs. But never evaporate in a garage by a hot water heater either. Fires and explosions are no fun.

The four most common ignition sources responsible for explosions are

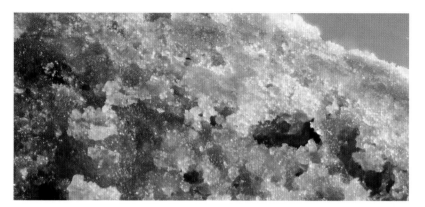

Layered macro photo of a cannabis concentrate.

static electricity, electronics from refrigerators, the spark from electrical switches, pilot lights on furnaces, or stoves, and the careless fool who sparks up some form of smoking material without thinking.

Using Condensers

Condensers that are designed to cool vapor and turn it back into a liquid are available through chemical supply companies. A condenser is only necessary if you feel the need to reclaim your solvent. This would make sense:

■ if you are safeguarding the environment;

■ if you are using huge amounts of solvent and wish to save money;

Pressing Hashish

There are many techniques for pressing hashish. Small amounts are best when pressed by hand. Another nice method is to place the resin into a natural cellophane envelope sealed with a small piece of scotch tape. Place pinholes in 3 or 4 evenly spaced areas to allow air to escape. Lightly wet a sheet of newspaper and completely wrap the resin envelope in the moist newspaper. Preheat a cast iron skillet. Place the moist newspaper-covered resin in the pan and place a brick on the newspaper packet, essentially steam heating the resin. This melts it without vaporizing or destroying the potency or essential oils or terpenoids and flavonoids. When the outside of the newspaper becomes slightly dry, remove it and place the packet on a clean hard surface. Fill a resealable glass bottle with extremely hot water. Put on oven mitts so you do not burn your hands. Using the bottle as a rolling pin, gently flatten out the resin completely until

Photo: Todd McCormick

How to Hand Press Hash

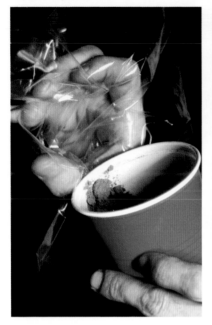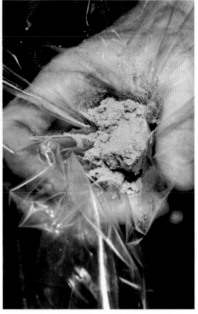

Collect the loose resin glands in a container.

Place collected resin into one area of the cellophane.

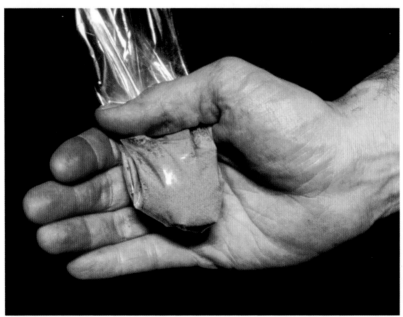

Photos: Mel Frank

The resin is then tightly wrapped into a ball.

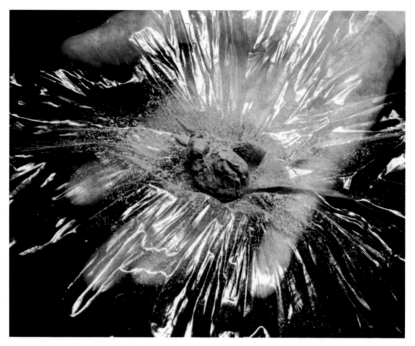

After a slight bit of pressing the resin will begin to stick together.

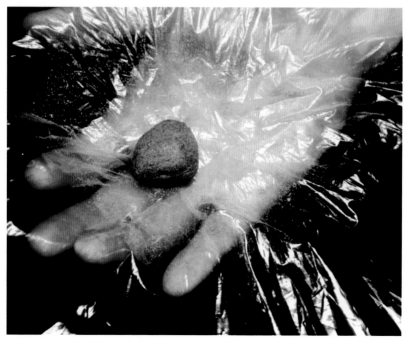

After applying more pressure, the resin will begin to form a ball of hash.

Pressing Hash Photo Guide

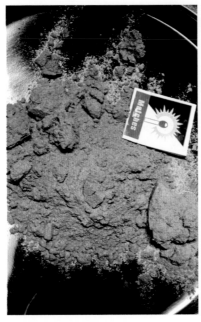

Sieved cannabis resin.

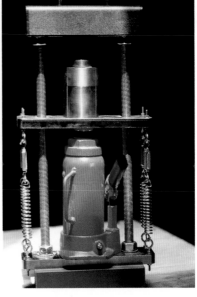

This press and hash mold can be utilized to expedite hash pressing.

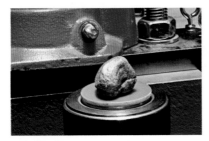

A ball of hash placed into the forming mold.

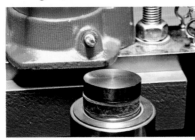

Finished product being extracted from the forming mold.

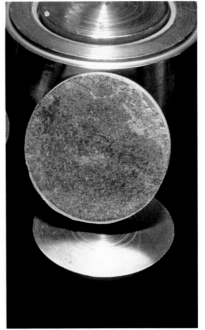

Finished pressed hash.

it becomes a homogenized solid form. After pressing, place into the freezer for 1 hour. The hashish is then ready for consumption or may be stored in the freezer almost indefinitely. Remove cellophane before consumption.

Recently, I was introduced to a gentleman who had taken large quantities of the purest, best quality resin and processed it through an industrial strength, small-sized meat grinder and had the photos and samples to prove it. It ground up and extruded the resin glands, releasing, exposing, and homogenizing all essential oils, flavonoids, and terpenoids. After grinding, the resin is hyper-compressed, extruded, and forced through small holes as if making hamburger meat. The resulting final product was incredible. At room temperature and above it resembled an oily black liquid, but when frozen it was a solid. The smell and flavor were magnificent. Because all resin glands have been pulverized, this hashish will oxidize and degrade rapidly. Large quantities should be stored in the freezer.

Pressing—Pros and Cons

To press or not to press? That is a question only you can answer.

When trichomes and resin glands are pressed, many become ruptured. This starts the process of degradation and loss of potency through oxidation, especially on the outside surfaces. This is why amber and gold colored resin and trichomes turn black when heated, pressed, or ruptured. Outside surfaces turn black while the inner core maintains a much lighter color because it is not exposed to the heat, air, light, or the environment. After curing, it is still best to press large quantities of resin, as it will slowly degrade and lose potency. Aside from the outside surfaces, the inside resin is protected from the environment, and will retain potency for a very long time if stored properly in a freezer or cool, dark, dry area. When working with smaller amounts, there is really no reason to press, as you will probably consume it before it starts to lose potency. Store loose unpressed resin and trichomes in airtight glass containers and place them into the freezer or a cool, dark, dry area. Simply remove the amount you desire and place the bulk back into storage. This ensures that all of your precious resin and trichomes are unbroken / unruptured, and that all essential oils are available for your full benefit and pleasure.

A Note on Powdering and Pressing

You must always re-powder the pressed hashish before consumption, except for pure sticky or water extracted hash. Be it in a pipe or joint, breaking up the chunk of hash into fine bits of powder will make all the aroma, flavor, and THC available. Some use a coffee grinder for this purpose. If you just place a single chunk into a pipe and apply a flame, it simply burns the outside surface area and turns the hashish into a charcoal-type lump that will never express the wonderful flavor and aroma contained inside.

Advanced Methods

The methods described above are basic. Much more advanced methods are possible, including large-scale production and hi-tech methods of manufacturing honey oil. These methods require large volumes of cannabis starting material.

Hash Tips

1. Always use the purest, cleanest, coldest water possible. Water chillers work very well.

2. Save all shake and leaves that contain resin as well as any wispy buds or trichome heads for hash.

3. Immediately wash and dry all water hash manufacturing screens with clean water or they will become clogged and begin to smell bad.

4. Separate resin heads by cultivar or create a mixture of resins from different cultivars to produce incredibly unique, strong, aromatic, and flavorful hashish.

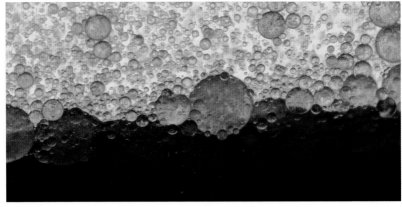

Photos: Todd McCormick

Cannabinoids being super-refined utilizing H_2O and sodium sulphate.

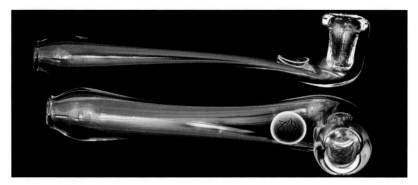

A heavy-walled clear pipe from iyqglass.com.

5. Do not carry hashish or unpressed trichomes (or buds) in ziploc bags. Resin glands bind to and stick to plastic and cannot be recovered. Use glass containers for storage whenever possible.

6. Please note that hashish of this purity should never be touched with an open flame. Using a clean glass pipe with a titanium or stainless steel mesh screen, vaporize the hash by adjusting the distance between the pipe and the flame so that you are watching the hash bubble as you inhale. This way you can enjoy the true flavor of this fine product.

7. Warning, proper storage of hashish is very important. If it is not completely dry, it will mold, destroying the hashish and making it unhealthy to smoke. At the first sign of a white mold appearing, remove the affected area and either consume what's left immediately, or freeze it. Again, when storing hash, always store it in a cool, dry place.

8. If you do manage to properly store and age it for two years or more, you will have one of the finest products in the world today.

Useful Products

■ Grasshopper Extractor (www.grasshopperextractor.com)
■ Zenport EC-101 Plant Oil Essence Extractor (www.zenportindustries.com)
■ Extraction Contraption Pro System (www.friendlyfarms.com)
■ SuperC from OCO Labs, Desktop CO_2 Extractor (OCO LABS INC www.ocolabs.com)

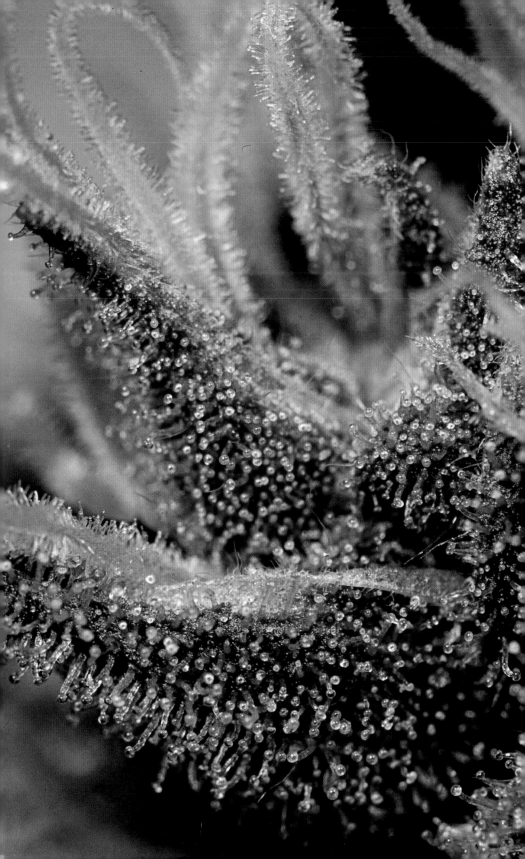

Screen Sizes

Screens are sized by the amount of space between the threads, and are measured in microns. Most water-extraction screens / bags are available in a variety of sizes, from 25 to 220M. With most bag kits you will only use three bags (or as many as eight), and ultimately the decision is yours, but these bags must be used in the proper order. Basically, the first two top nylon bags (the bags placed on top of all of the others) are used to remove plant material and other contaminants while allowing resin and trichome heads to dislodge and fall through and be collected by the succeeding bags and screens. Contaminants can include insects, dust, mold, nutrient buildup, and useless parts of the cannabis plant (such as capitate stalks).

The 220M bag is sturdiest and can't get wrapped up in hand-held mixers, so it should be your top one. 190M should be next as it will trap everything unwanted that passes through the 220M. The remaining bags will contain the desirable trichome heads. Different cultivars of cannabis have larger and smaller trichome heads, so it is impossible to predict which bag will produce the best quality or yield. However, the best trichome heads are usually found in the 73 or 90M range. The more bags you use, the easier it will be to find the exact grade of trichomes you desire. With cannabis, practice and experimentation are the keys to success.

◀ All of these resin glands will be captured, cured, and later pressed into amazing blocks of hash.

Photo: Andre Grossman

Screen Size Measurement

A micron is one millionth of a meter (1/1,000,000m) or one-thousandth of a millimeter (1/1,000mm). This length is also referred to as a micrometer. The symbol used to denote a micron is "M."

Microns (M)	Thousandths of an inch
220M	8.66
190M	7.48
160M	6.30
150M	5.91
120M	4.72
104M	2.87
73M	2.87
66M	2.60
45M	1.77
43M	1.69
25M	0.98

APPENDIX 2

Terpene Extraction: The Future of Cannabis Extracts

At this moment, extract artists worldwide are producing, or trying to produce, an absolute – a hard piece of see-through shatter / glass. A stable piece of concentrate that is not sticky and can be held in one's hand, without sticking to it.

To achieve this goal they utilize various methods and equipment, such as: winterization and vacuum drying ovens. THC levels in concentrate trends are getting higher. Some exceed 80% THC (either in THCA form or as activated delta nine form).

But pursuit of elevated THC levels has come at the cost of terpenoids.

Terpenes / terpenoids are oil and alcohol-based, thus the more of them present in a concentrate, the softer and more fluid it will be. Terpenes and terpenoids are responsible for the aroma and flavor of the plant / bud / concentrate. The more flavor and smell it has, the more terpenoids are present. That being said, the harder the glass / shatter is, the less terpenoids that are present.

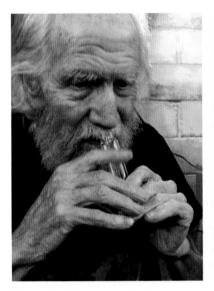

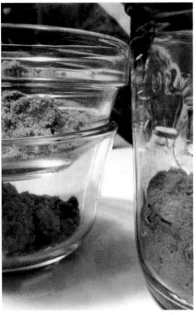

Alexander Shulgin smelling terpene compounds isolated by Trichome Technologies.

Dry sieve resin

The act of winterization removes fats and wax, but also traps terpenes, and then the act of utilizing a vacuum oven / drying oven removes even more terpenes. The reason it is referred to as a drying oven is because it dries the product, whether the product is a computer chip or a cannabis concentrate, the act of 'drying out' removes both solvents and terpenes. When combined with heat, the solvent as well as the terpenes evaporate rapidly.

This results in a concentrate that is devoid of solvent, but also a concentrate that is devoid of many terpenes. It doesn't get rid of all the terpenes, just the lighter oils that are predominately responsible for smell and flavor. And all this does not even take into account the synergistic effects of combined levels of cannabinoids and terpenoids that majorly contribute to both the medicinal effects and the desired effects of the cannabinoids that are responsible for the high.

Pure THC does not taste pleasant, but the addition of terpenoids can make it taste pleasant. In addition, the terpenoids contribute to and accentuate the medical benefits and effects of the THC / CBD / cannabinoids. So the problem becomes evident as reflected in the academic article "Cannabis Oil: Chemical Evaluation of an Upcoming Cannabis-based Medicine" by Luigi L. Romano

Photos: K

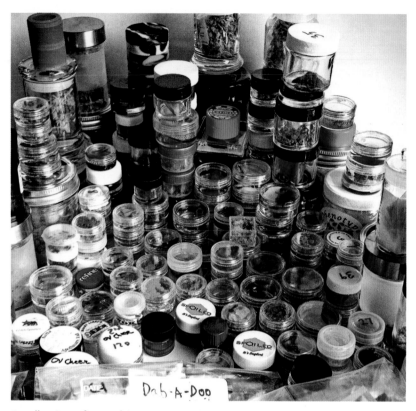

A collection of cannabis concentrates.

Photos: K

& Arno Hazekamp in conjunction with the Department of Pharmacy at the University of Siena, Italy, Plant Metabolomics Group, and the Institute of Biology, Leiden, Leiden University, Netherlands and the International Association for Cannabinoid Medicines.

This paper essentially concluded that the scientists could not figure out how to decarboxylate the concentrate without evaporating all the terpenoids. They also could not manage to rid the concentrate of solvent without (again) evaporating the terpenoids, which produces a cannabinoid-rich concentrate that has lower than desired levels of terpenoids.

It has been proven time and time again that the THC requires terpenoids to have the maximum benefit to the consumer (first proven by David Watson of HortiPharm). Therefore the logical answer is to first remove and concentrate all essential oils / terpenoids.

By first removing the terpenoids, they remain whole in their composition

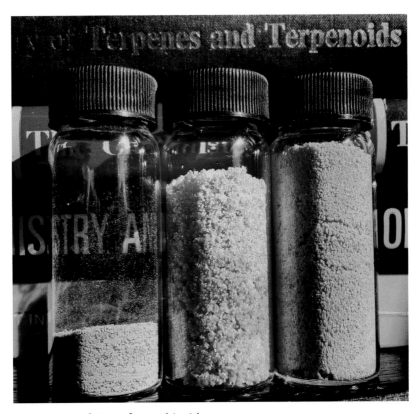

Micro encapsulation of cannabinoids.

and the closest aroma that is true to the original varietal / plant. They contain as many of the lightest and heaviest oils as possible. Once the terpenoids are separated and safe in airtight sealed containers, they are placed in a dark refrigerator to prevent degradation from heat, light, or oxygen.

From there the cannabinoids can be extracted without losing or destroying any terpenoids. The final composition of the extract will be determined by the extraction method and the solvents utilized.

For infused goods / edibles etc, ethanol extraction may be preferred, while extract artists will utilize both ethanol and butane to produce extracts. The revolutionary change will be caused by the advent of the patented whole-terpenoid isolator from Trichome Technologies' Kenneth Morrow.

This apparatus took 3 years to design and develop. It is the single most important cannabis development since the THC molecule was first isolated by Dr. Mechoulam in 1964.

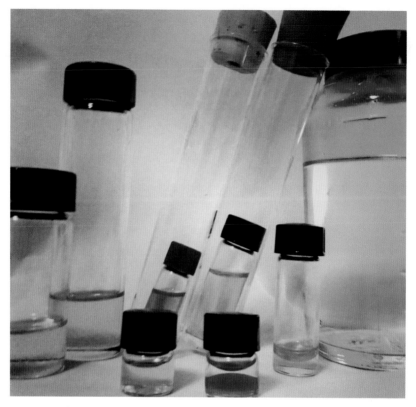

Pure cannabis terpenes extracted using Trichome Technologies' patented technology.

Dr. Alexander Shulgin authored and published a paper entitled "Recent Developments in Cannabis Chemistry" that was printed in the Journal of Psychedelic Drugs, Volume II. From 1972 when this article was published until David Watson independently with Robert Connell Clarke performed synergistic effect studies by smoking 25 mg of 100% pure THC.

Then they blended 50% THC with 50% dry sifted resin, and then combined various cannabinoids and terpenoids to perform double blind studies with many cannabis experts and scholars who wish to remain nameless. The whole process took more than a year to accomplish and included a dozen subject volunteers who all kept notes and discussed their findings.

This study only recently came to light and for that I thank David and Robert, as this work validated what is now called by Dr. Lester Grinspoon, the 'entourage effect / synergistic effect.' From then until now there have been

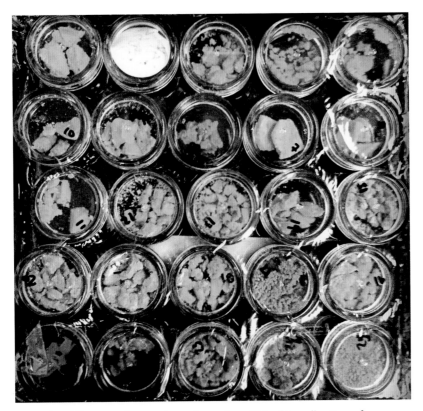

Note the different colors and consistencies within this collection of cannabis concentrates.

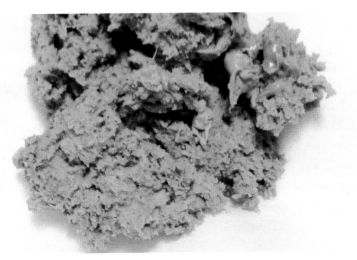

A closeup of a cannabis concentrate classified as a budder.

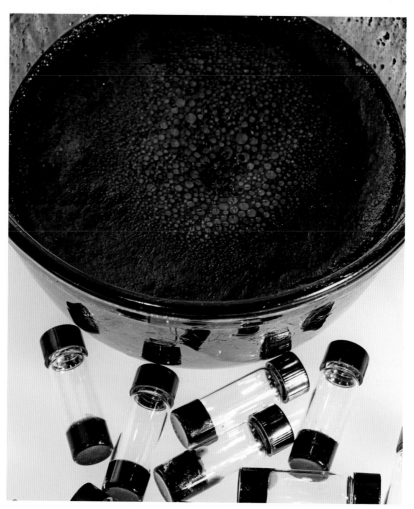

Unrefined raw whole plant cannabis extract.

few studies or scientific research projects into cannabis-derived terpenoids.

Why is this so? Because until now it has not been feasible to extract whole-composition cannabis derived terpenoids. Plant terpenoids are available en masse: ie limonene, pinene, etc. However, they are derived from citrus fruit and pine trees.

It is possible to extract terpenoids utilizing a GCMS, but only minute quantities that were subjected to heat, or by distillation and other means. This essential oil is only considered the artifact of the original composition, as the lighter volatile oils were destroyed by heat or carried off with the water vapor / steam.

Photo: K

The resulting product pales in comparison to the whole-terpene composition. Before this invention it has not been possible to capture cannabis-derived terpenoids in whole-composition form. This new technology will change the history of cannabis as medicine. From here, it will now be possible to research the true benefits of every aspect of the plant as it has never been before.

This one single advancement will change the future of cannabis and cannabis concentrates. Because the extract artist now knows that excessive vacuum purging and heating eliminates or vaporizes valuable terpenoids. With this new invention, they can capture the terpenoids during the vacuum drying process and then re-apply them to the original concentrate. However, this will also change the composition of the product / concentrate.

The second the terpenoids are applied back to the cannabinoids in the extract, the two will mix and combine to make an oleoresin: a sap that is oily in nature, which is the complete opposite of what is popular with consumers today.

So quit struggling to make the extract hard. You are breaking it. Remember, the goal is to eliminate the solvent but NOT the terps! Leave in or re-apply the terps and you have sap. Sorry shatter lovers... I'm just telling the truth. Take the shatter and re-apply terps and the shatter melts. Simple.

Not to worry though, the sappy / syrupy concentrates of the future will taste amazing and that in itself is worth the hassle of dealing with sticky stuff once again. But the true advancements will come from the pharmaceutical industries. For 20 years all of these companies have had representatives in the ICRS (International Cannabinoid Research Society).

They have all been waiting for three events to happen: 1) The rescheduling of cannabis; 2) legalization; and 3) the ability to extract, identify, separate, patent, and profit off of all cannabinoids and terpenoids. Once they have the ability to isolate, research, and patent cannabinoid and terpenoid derivatives, they will produce their own synthetic versions.

The patent application office will be very busy for quite some time, I suspect. So now having the ability to isolate pure cannabis-derived terpenoids is truly groundbreaking. The compound is literally the holy grail of cannabis.

We now have the ability to eliminate the green vegetative matter / fiber, the fats, the wax, and end up with cannabinoids and terpenoids which possess the original flavor / aroma components which can remain intact throughout the process. Allowing one to reconstruct the compounds into any desired percentage of THC, CBD, terps etc of any desired flavor – ie Tangerine, Blueberry, Bubble Gum.

With this advancement, the future of cannabis extracts for both recreational and medicinal use seems bright. Hopefully it benefits mankind in some way.

Daily Logs for Cultivation Facilities

Date	STG	GAL	PH	PPM	Brand	Additive	Details

Daily Nutrient Log: Log every nutrient / amendment / adjustment etc made to water every day, changes to pH, everything. The daily nutrient log helps for recording all nutrients and amendments that go into your soil or media.

Date	STG	GAL	PH	PPM	Brand	Additive	Details

Nutrient Runoff Log: This log is to record all the run off water exiting the soil / media.

Date	Estimate (outside air)	Room 1	Room 2	Room 3	CL Room

Daily Temperature Readings Log

Date	Estimate (ouside air)	Room 1	Room 2	Room 3	CL Room
		hi / low	hi / low	hi / low	

Daily Humidity Readings Log

Date	Name	Actual Hours	Total Hours	Location	Job Description	Date Paid	Amount Paid

Time Card: keeping track of who does what and when is useful for larger grows that involve multiple workers.

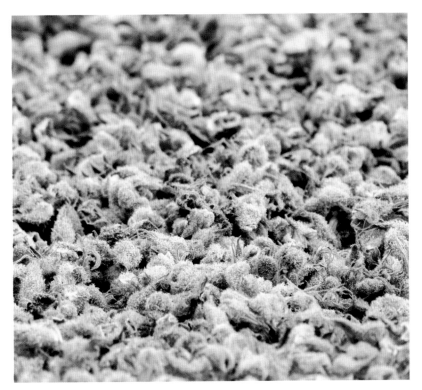

Thousands of collected bracts.

Photo: Samson Daniels

APPENDIX 3

Commonly Asked Questions

Q: What do my seeds need in order to germinate?

A: Seeds don't actually require light to germinate, but all seeds require proper medium temperature. The temperatures advised by seed companies refer to the medium, not the ambient temperature. When the medium temperature is too high or low, the seeds will germinate slowly or not at all.

Q: How much space is required for an indoor growroom?

A: Almost any space can be converted into a growroom. Visit your local growing supply store to find a specific system or method that works in your chosen space and fits your requirements. If this is your first indoor garden, you may want to experiment with a couple of differently sized plants in the first cycle. This will help you determine exactly when to induce flowering so

419

that the plants mature at the desired height, without getting to close to the lights, in a smaller space.

Q: How do I know if my indoor plants are getting enough light?
A: Plants get "leggy" when they don't receive enough light. A light meter can help insure proper light levels, as can proper placement of your plant in the grow space.

Q: How much will an HID light cost to run?
A: You can calculate the approximate cost by using the following equation: Kw/h (kilowatts per hour rate) x Kw (bulb wattage) x H (hours used in a day) x D (days used in a month) = monthly cost.

Q: Why do plants need such intense lighting to grow?
A: Natural outdoor sunlight is up to 100 times brighter than indoor / artificial lights. Therefore, you must try to replicate outdoor sunlight conditions. Plants convert nutrients and sunlight into the food they need for growth.

Q: How much light do my clones / seedlings require?
A: For optimum results, clones / seedlings must have 14 to 18 hours of light each and every day. Cool white fluorescents, compact fluorescents, LEDs, or induction lights are used for this purpose; the light should be kept 18 to 24 inches from clones or seedlings, raised or lowered as needed.

Q: What is the difference between metal halide (HID) lights and high pressure sodium (HPS) lights?
A: A metal halide light produces a white light that promotes vegetative growth (similar to sunlight). A high pressure sodium light produces a light spectrum that is more in the orange / red range. HPS lights encourage the plants to produce buds, so we prefer a 60% HPS and 40% HID mix, i.e., one of each bulb or a 400-watt HID bulb and a 600-watt HPS bulb.

Q: What wattage high intensity discharge bulb should I use?
A: Many factors determine what wattage you will need! They include the size of the area to be lighted, ceiling height and clearance, and the size of ventilation. All of these factors dictate what size of light you need.

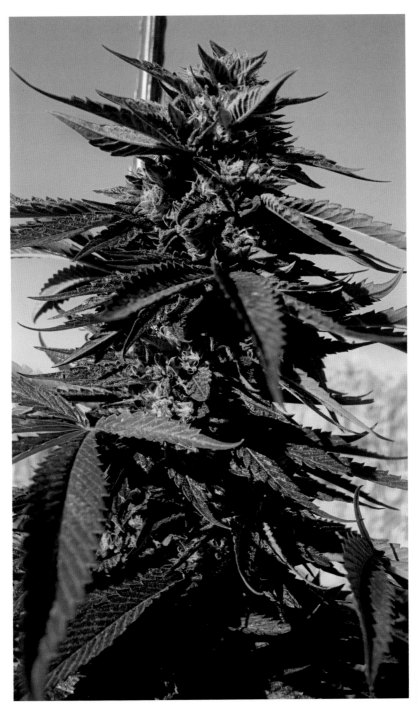

Sun-grown outdoor plant.

Photo: K

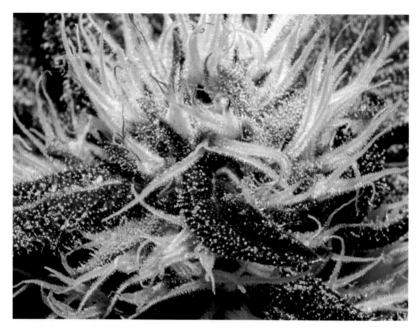

This bud is just beginning to ripen.

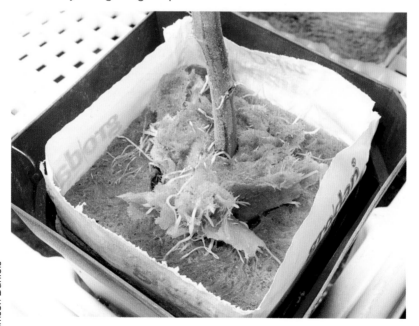

Photos: Samson Daniels

The wrapper around the rockwool has been slid up approximately two inches to encourage water to drain through the rockwool cube instead of run off the top/sides.

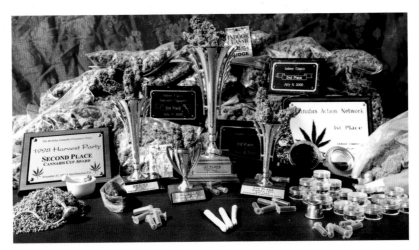

K from Trichome Technologies' many awards from California cannabis competitions.

APPENDIX 4

Six Simple Preventative Tips

These simple tips will help prevent many basic problems you may encounter; they cover many types of growth methods and systems.

1. Keep good records: keep a journal or chart that lists the PPM, pH, temperature, CO_2, light levels, and runoff for each day. By doing this you can learn from your experience and correct any anomalies.

2. If you have a large reservoir and many plants, it is best to replace reservoir solutions. It is recommended that you completely change the nutrient solution once a week, every week. During the week you can top up the tank and adjust the PPM and pH, but if you don't change the solution it will rapidly become depleted of vital nutrients and micronutrients or infected with disease, causing root rot.

3. Keep everything clean: always cut off dead leaves and remove them from the growroom. Decaying organic matter encourages fungus, gnats, mold, and disease. You should remove infected or diseased plants so that the problem does not spread. Clean the system and non-plant surfaces with a 10% bleach and water solution or hydrogen peroxide and rinse before using it again.

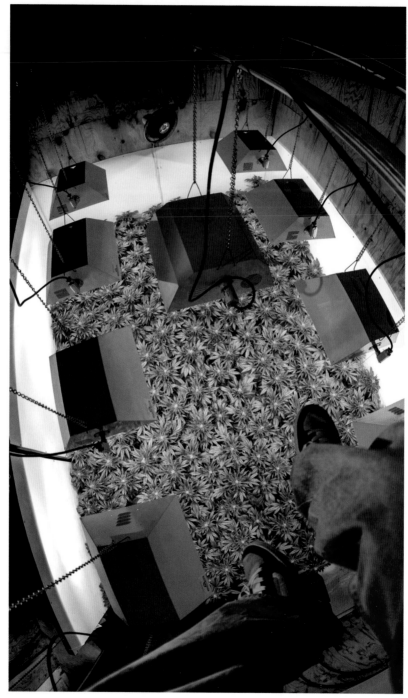

The photographer at work.

4. Use less fertilizer for soil than for rockwool. In properly amended soil, most of the nutrients are available to the plant in its early stages of development.

5. If you use a drip, spray, or mist system, purchase a few extra drippers, sprayers, or misters so that you can change them if any become clogged. Keep a bucket of vinegar and drop the clogged unit into it so that they will be unclogged and ready to use the next time you have to change them over.

6. For ebb and flow systems, get a quality, heavy-duty timer that you can set to 5-minute intervals so that a full cycle will only soak the rockwool for ten minutes.

Dedication

This book is dedicated to all cannabis prisoners—past, present, and future—and all victims of the senseless, criminal "war on drugs." Together we battle as true, righteous outlaws and patriots. Our forefathers would be proud. Fight on.

Jeff Goldberg, June 13, 1970 – March 17, 2015

Within this book there are many photos by Jeff "Freebie" Goldberg. Jeff was one of the most prolific cannabis photographers I have had the pleasure of working with. As a High Times Magazine photographer, he had an impressive number of cover and centerfold credits, as well as an incredible amount of photos (from many magazines) that went with amazing stories, some of which I had the honor of being the subject of.

Sadly, Jeff passed away on March 17, 2015, at the age of 44.

Jeff and I worked very well together and we had a lot of fun. Together, we produced many cover and centerfold shots. We both recognized the artistic side of cannabis photography. We produced a great body of work over a 15 year period.

Besides being an artist and photographer, Jeff was a friend, and I will always miss him and his infectious smile. I have no doubt Jeff touched many people and will be missed by all of them.

Much love, Jeff.

– Kenneth Morrow

Index